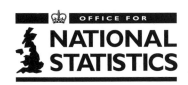

TI
A
18

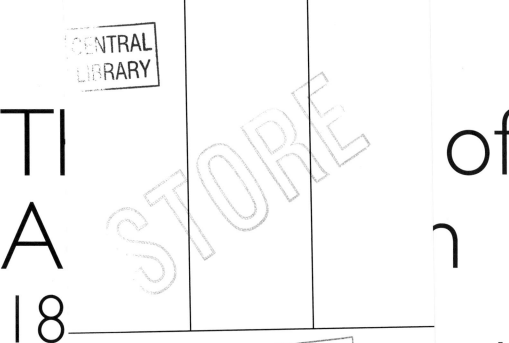

of

Volume 1

Chapters 1-14

Editors: John Charlton
               Mike Murphy

Decennial Supplement No. 12

London:

X400 000020 1866

ISBN 0 11 691695 8

Front cover photographs: details of photographs reproduced with permission of
Sally and Richard Greenhill and the Sidery Collection.

Other reports in this series

Occupational Health - decennial supplement
ISBN 0 11 691618 4 price £29

The Health of our Children
ISBN 0 11 691643 5 price £21

The views expressed in this report are not necessarily those of the Office for National Statistics

Contents

Tables and figures

7 Trends in diet 1841-1993

8 Trends in alcohol and illicit drug-related diseases

9   Trends in mortality from smoking-related diseases

10   Housing-related disorders

14   Medical advances and iatrogenesis

Foreword

These two volumes bring together a wide range of information about the health of adults, covering a period of over 150 years. More than forty expert authors have generously donated their time to this comprehensive review, and our thanks are due to them for the result. The first volume presents general material on morbidity, mortality, and trends in behavioural and environmental factors known to be associated with health. The second considers specific major categories of diseases, the elderly, and changes in health generally in the most recent ten years.

The *Health of Adult Britain* is the third in a new series of decennial supplements, the previous two supplements being *Occupational Health* and *The Health of our Children*. A further volume, on socio-economic differences in health, is planned for publication in late 1997.

KAREN DUNNELL
Director of Health and Demographic Statistics

Acknowledgements

The editors are extremely grateful to the many colleagues in the ONS who have helped in one way or the other in producing these volumes, especially Anita Brock and John Waterman who laboured over proofs and graphs. They would also like to thank those people who kindly acted as referees and whose names are given in Appendix C.

About the authors in Volume 1

Ross Anderson is Professor of Epidemiology and Public Health at the Department of Public Health Sciences, St George's Hospital Medical School.

Dr Mel Bartley is Principal Research Fellow in the Department of Epidemiology and Public Health at University College London and has published widely on the social influences on health and illness.

Dr David Blane is Senior Lecturer in Sociology Applied to Medicine at Charing Cross and Westminster Medical School and has published on various aspects of medical sociology.

John Charlton is an epidemiologist and principal methodologist at the Office for National Statistics. His research interests include health outcomes, suicides and demographic trends.

Michael Curwen is a retired Statistician who formerly worked for the Office of Population Censuses and Surveys (now the Office for National Statistics).

Sarah Darby is a statistical epidemiologist working at the Imperial Cancer Research Fund Cancer Epidemiology Unit in Oxford.

Richard Doll is an epidemiologist, emeritus professor of medicine at Oxford University and an honorary consultant to the Imperial Cancer Research Fund in the Nuffield Department of Clinical Medicine in Oxford.

Douglas Fleming is the Director of the Royal College of general Practitioners Research Unit in Birmingham and has published widely on epidemiology in primary care.

Patricia Fraser is an epidemiologist who was holding a consultancy contract with the Office of Population Censuses and Surveys during the preparation of this volume.

Leicester Gill is the Chief Computer Scientist responsible for 30 years of pioneering work into record linkage techniques and technology.

Michael Goldacre is a reader in Public Health at the University of Oxford and consultant in Public Health to the Anglia and Oxford Regional Offices of the National Health Service Executive, and honorary director of Oxford Record Linkage Study.

Stephanie Goubet is a statistician at the Department of Primary Health Care and Population Sciences, Royal Free Hospital School of Medicine and University College London Medical School.

Andy Haines is Professor of Primary Health Care at the Department of Primary Health Care and Population Sciences, Royal Free Hospital School of Medicine and University College London Medical School.

Sonja Hunt is an epidemiological consultant with specific interests in housing-related health issues.

Elizabeth Limb is statistician at the Department of Public Health Sciences, St George's Hospital Medical School.

Alison Macfarlane is a medical statistician at the National Perinatal Epidemiology Unit, Oxford and Honorary Senior Lecturer in the Department of Epidemiology and Public Health, University College London School of Medicine.

Mike Murphy is a medical epidemiologist who worked for the Office for National Statistics. He now works for the Imperial Cancer Research Fund at the University of Oxford in General Practitioner Research. His main interests are in cancer and health care epidemiology.

Martin Plant is Professor/Director of the Alcohol and Health Research Group, Department of Psychiatry, in the University of Edinburgh. A sociologist, he has been engaged in research into alcohol and illicit drugs since 1970. His books include *Drugtakers in an English Town*, *Drugs in Perspective*, *Drinking Careers* and *Risk Takers*.

Antonio Ponce de Leon has returned to Brazil but continues to be an Honorary Research Fellow at the Department of Public Health Sciences, St George's Hospital Medical School.

Karen Quaife was a research officer for the Office for National Statistics.

Elise Whitley is a statistician working at the Imperial Cancer Research Fund Cancer Epidemiology Unit in Oxford.

Chapter 1

Introduction

By
John Charlton and Mike Murphy

The Health of Adult Britain draws together in two volumes data and commentary concerning health over the past 150 years. In planning the volumes we chose to use the broad World Health Organisation definition of health, i.e. 'Health is a state of complete physical, social and mental well being, and not merely the absence of disease and infirmity'. A wide variety of sources were tapped in order to cover the many dimensions of health. The only measure available for the earliest time period is mortality, although there were early census health questions. The earliest date from which consistent and relatively reliable data can be assembled is 1841, and this was chosen for the start date of our review. 'Adults' were defined for our purposes as those aged 15 and over. Where Scottish data were readily available these are presented alongside those for England and Wales, but this was not always practical. It was not possible for all chapters to relate to such a long time period, and some chapters cover only the most recent past.

The project was ambitious, with 43 authors and over 100 referees all contributing, to say nothing of the efforts of the ONS team. In the event these volumes have taken longer to produce than originally anticipated. While general chapters cover the period up to 1994, it is more usual for chapters to cover the period up to 1991, since with different chapters arriving at different times it was not practical to update them all. Changes in health occur relatively slowly, with the result that this is of little importance.

The review is presented in two volumes. The first is largely general, covering methods, data sources, trends in overall mortality and life expectancy, and trends by broad category of diseases (ICD chapter). The advantages and disadvantages of using data collected from health service utilisation are also described. Factors that may influence health are discussed in terms of their trends: wealth; public health legislation; diet; alcohol and illicit drug use; smoking; housing; family and household structure; air pollution and climate; medical advances and iatrogenesis. The second volume describes in depth the trends for specific diseases: infectious diseases, including sexually transmitted diseases and AIDS; cancers; cardiovascular, neurological, respiratory, renal, digestive and musculoskeletal diseases; and accidents. The final three chapters discuss the health and prospects for older adults, including centenarians, and health trends in the most recent past.

We wanted to include a chapter on trends in mental health but this was not possible. Data which describe national trends in mental health consistently over time are not available, although the ONS Surveys of Psychiatric Morbidity provide valuable information about current mental health in Britain. Wherever trend data exist that relate to mental health they have been included, for example in Chapters 4, 5, 19, 25 and 26.

Each chapter was typically refereed by three referees and also commented on by the Department of Health. We are grateful for everyone's hard work, and the many useful comments received from referees. The content of each chapter was ultimately decided by individual authors, and thus the views expressed are not necessarily those of the Office for National Statistics or the Department of Health. The data presented in these volumes will become available on CD ROM shortly after publication.

Chapter 2

Monitoring health – data sources and methods

By

John Charlton and Mike Murphy

Summary

- This chapter reviews the data sources used by the authors of the two volumes, including their special features and limitations. Statistical approaches that are widely used in the volumes are also described.

- Although some data on mortality were available from 1532, comprehensive data have been available only since 1841. This followed the implementation of the Births and Deaths Registration Act in 1837, which established the General Register Office (GRO).

- Since 1841 many changes have occurred which affect the completeness and accuracy of mortality data, and the categories into which a particular cause of death might be classified. These are summarised for the reader.

- The first population census undertaken by the Registrar General was in 1841, when more comprehensive information was obtained than hitherto. Selected health questions were asked between 1851 and 1911, and again in 1991.

- Intercensal population estimates have been prepared for the country as a whole and for large towns since the nineteenth century, and for local authority districts since 1911. A variety of data sources are employed to arrive at these estimates.

- Notification of infectious diseases began in 1889 (2 years earlier in Scotland) to combat 'dangerous infectious diseases', and weekly provisional returns were made by local authority Medical Officers of Public Health from 1922. The list of notifiable diseases has grown over time.

- In 1947, the GRO took over, from the Radium Commission, analysis of cancer incidence data supplied by local and regional registries. A comprehensive national cancer registration scheme became operational from 1962.

- Data linkage such as those achieved by the ONS Longitudinal Study, the Scottish Record Linkage System and the Oxford Record Linkage Study enhance the original data and enable analyses that would be impossible without linkage.

- In addition to data gathered from routine records there are a number of surveys, ongoing and *ad-hoc*, which address questions that the routine data cannot answer. These surveys include the General Household Survey, the Health Survey for England, the ONS Disability Surveys, the ONS Psychiatric Morbidity Surveys, Dental Health Surveys, National Food Surveys and the Labour Force Survey.

2.1 Introduction

This chapter reviews the routine data available for monitoring the health of the British population, namely the sources used by the authors of this book as appropriate. The first part of the chapter describes data sources, their special features and limitations. The final part describes a number of statistical approaches used widely by the authors.

2.2 What is health, and how can it be measured?

2.2.1 What is health?

The absence of health has always been easier to define than its presence. The biomedical model of health defines disease as deviations of measurable biological variables from the norm, or the presence of defined and categorised forms of pathology. These deviations are caused by: a) specific causes such as micro-organisms, nutrient deficiencies, toxins, other causative agents; b) multiple and interactive causation (such as susceptibility, genetic dispositions and influence of psychosocial factors). The World Health Organisation (WHO, 1979) proposed a wider definition of health: health is a state of complete physical, social and mental well-being, and not merely the absence of disease and infirmity. Blaxter (1990) surveyed British people's attitudes to health. They described health as a relative state, influenced largely by the normal ageing process. Although they generally saw health as the absence of disease, most people's concept of health approximated the WHO definition more closely than the biomedical model.

2.2.2 Measuring health

Jette (1980) suggested four criteria which determine the choice of health status indicator: (1) the purpose, for example whether we wish to measure the health of population groups or evaluate specific interventions; (2) the conceptual focus, e.g. whether symptoms, performance or pathology is to be measured; (3) properties of the measuring instrument such as reliability, sensitivity and validity; and (4) the source of data, for example routine data, record audits, or postal or interview surveys. The focus of this book is to describe trends in the health of the British population, and this aim to a large extent determines the measures that we can use, since they need to be consistently interpretable over reasonably long periods of time.

The most absolute measure of ill health is death. Mortality data have been collected nationally for the entire period covered by this volume. Death rates have traditionally been used as crude, but often effective, surrogates for more comprehensive measures of disease. This is often justified by the fact that death is unambiguous and the data collection are complete. However, sole use of mortality data could provide misleading impressions concerning the burdens of disease in society. For example, musculoskeletal disorders (including rheumatism and arthritis) are the most important causes of limiting long-standing illness (Breeze et al., 1991) but one of the least prevalent causes of death.

As one moves away from death towards more minor complaints, measurement becomes more difficult. Health service records for example provide a plentiful source of health related data, but they are strongly influenced by variations in access to health care and patient help-seeking behaviour. Also, doctors, when treating sick and dying people, are only aware of the disease presented to them. Apart from this there is a large 'iceberg of disease' (Last, 1963) that is not brought to the medical profession's attention. This includes diseases such as hypertension that have not yet caused symptoms, and problems that patients have chosen not to present to their general practitioner for one reason or another. General practitioners may not be aware of disabilities encountered by their patients. Although hospital and GP data only provide information on recognised demand they nevertheless complement mortality statistics.

In order to learn about health problems independently of service utilisation factors, a variety of studies are required. These include screening studies using standardised procedures to detect unidentified, as well as identified, disease levels in the population. Community surveys are required to elicit information on disability levels, self-rating of health and subjective experiences of health or its absence. 'Lifestyle', which describes choices about food, smoking, drinking, how leisure time is spent and social behaviour, can only be measured via surveys. Sometimes health-related behaviours which are likely to lead to ill-health, such as smoking, drinking and illicit drug use, are monitored as proxy health measures.

It is also important to collect and analyse trend data on environmental aspects that are suspected of influencing health status, or known to do so. Factors that may affect health and which are not always a matter of choice for the individual concerned include: poverty; diet; employment conditions; education; housing; water supply; sanitation; extreme temperatures; access to appropriate medical care; social isolation; genetic inheritance; violence in society/the home; transport; childhood neglect; environmental pollution; and so on.

2.3 The data available for studying trends in the population's health

It has been our intention in this volume to provide trend data from all the above sources over as much of the time period as possible, in order to provide as comprehensive a review as possible. Ideal measures of health would provide information on incidence, prevalence and severity of illnesses by age-group, sex, socioeconomic and geographical characteristics of the population. There are no ideal measures, and various sources are used in combination to gain a better understanding.

The varied sources of population health information provide different pieces of the overall health jigsaw. These include mortality data, censuses, inter-censal population estimates, notifications of infectious diseases, registry data, congenital malformation notifications, abortions, community and institutional surveys (including those undertaken by clinical professionals), health care records and proxy measures of health such as lifestyle. These are discussed below.

2.3.1 Mortality data

Availability of mortality data

Although some data on numbers of deaths and their causes first became available from the weekly London Bills of Mortality which began in 1532, they, like the parish records from which they were compiled, were not complete, and the terms used were often inexact. They excluded burials of dissenters, and many clerks of parishes made irregular returns or none (Ransome, 1893). The Births and Deaths Registration Act of 1836 came into operation on 1 July 1837. It provided for the registration of every death which occurred in England and Wales, with a space in the prescribed register for the cause of death. The General Register Office (now ONS) was established in order to carry out the requirements of the Act. Data collected as a consequence of this Act have been published from 1837 onwards. Registration of deaths in Scotland began with the Registration of Births, Deaths and Marriages (Scotland) Act of 1854. In 1839 the first classification of causes of death was introduced by William Farr, and this was published in the Registrar General's first report.

Mortality data for England and Wales became comprehensive from 1841 onwards, and are available in a computer readable form from 1901 onwards, classified by age, sex and detailed cause (the historic deaths database included on the CD-rom accompanying this volume). It is largely these data that are used in this volume to show trends. In 1841 the Registrar General conducted the national population census for the first time, which formed a sounder basis for population estimates than previous censuses. Censuses have been undertaken at 10-year intervals since (except in 1941), and provide reliable denominators from which mortality rates can be calculated.

When the death is registered, the registrar fills in a draft entry form (Form 310) which includes additional information such as occupation and marital status, and this information, used only for statistical purposes, is the basis of statistical data collected by ONS and GRO (Scotland).

Factors likely to affect interpretation

Accuracy and completeness of data

Care needs to be taken in using mortality data to examine health trends. The way that diseases have been described and classified has varied over time, affecting the interpretation (see Table 2.1). Mortality trends by cause could reflect variations in disease incidence, case fatality rates or statistical artefacts (Charlton, 1986). In the earlier years of death

registration the accuracy of certification was well below the standards we would find acceptable today, and it is also likely that some deaths were not registered (Wrigley and Schofield, 1989). There was no penalty for failure to register – the onus of registration was placed on the registrar rather than the informant, who could only be prosecuted if he/she refused to give information after being asked to do so by the registrar. Incomplete death registration was less of a problem than birth registration because bodies could only legally be buried after registration.

Cause of death data were also likely to be inaccurate because the 1836 Act did not require that the cause be obtained from a medical practitioner, and medical services were expensive. It is also worth noting when interpreting trends by cause for early years that many doctors certifying deaths would have been trained in the late eighteenth century, when medical knowledge was limited. Some of the causes of death described in the early tables published by the Registrar General seem somewhat unusual today; one of the oddest was a small 'epidemic' of 22 deaths from 'tight boots' between 1894 and 1900 – a cause of death that has not been described at any other time.

In 1874 a new law, the Births and Deaths Registration Act, led to an improvement in the accuracy of death certification. It placed a duty on the medical practitioners who were attendant during the person's last illness to provide a cause of death, unless an inquest was being held, in which case the coroner's verdict was recorded. A penalty was introduced if the death was not registered. It also improved the quality of certification for infants and stillborn children. However, even then not all deaths were in fact certified by qualified medical practitioners – in 1878, 5 per cent of deaths were still not so certified; by 1928 this proportion had fallen to 1 per cent (Ashley and Devis, 1992). In 1926 an Act made it unlawful to dispose of the body of a dead person before a registrar's certificate or coroner's order had been issued, and also required the registration of stillbirths.

Nowadays, few, if any, deaths escape registration, and the cause of almost every registered death has been certified by a medical practitioner or coroner. All deaths must be registered with a registrar of Births and Deaths, usually within 5 days in England and Wales, or 8 days in Scotland. In order to do this a medical certificate of cause of death is required, usually signed by the medical practitioner who attended the deceased during his/her last illness. In the case of sudden death, or where there is the possibility of an unnatural death, or when an industrial disease is suspected, the case will be referred to a coroner in England and Wales, or to the Procurator Fiscal in Scotland, who will certify the death, possibly after holding a post mortem and/or inquest. Coding of the underlying cause (see later) follows rules laid down by the World Health Organisation (WHO, 1977).

The way in which the descriptions on death certificates have been coded has varied. Farr's 1839 classification of cause of death was changed in 1881 and again in 1901. The second

International Classification of Diseases (ICD) was adopted by the Registrar General in 1911. The international classification has subsequently been revised approximately every 10 years, to keep pace with advances in medical knowledge, and incidence of 'new' diseases. The version in current use in Britain is the ninth revision (ICD9). The years for which ONS has used the various versions are given in Table 2.1. Since the 2nd/3rd revision change there have been 'bridge coding' exercises every time that the classification has been changed. These have involved coding a sample of death certificates according to both classifications so that the effect of the classification change can be measured, enabling appropriate adjustments to be made to trends (OPCS, 1983b) – for example, the user can group together causes in order to get a more consistent series over time.

Problems in identifying the underlying cause

Published mortality statistics are usually based on a single, underlying cause of death, selected by ONS from the several causes that may be mentioned on the death certificate. Methods for selecting the underlying cause have varied (see Table 2.1), and also the number of items on the death certificate has tended to increase, increasing the difficulty in arriving at a single underlying cause (Ashley and Devis, 1992). In 1927 the format of death certification changed – the new certificates were in two parts, the first for the disease or condition leading directly to the cause of death, and causes antecedent to it, and the second for 'other significant conditions contributing to the death, but not related to the disease or condition causing it'. Figure 2.1 shows the death certificate in current use, much the same as the 1927

Table 2.1

Factors which may have affected recorded mortality by cause

1532	London Bills of Mortality, some towns, parish records – incomplete picture of mortality.
1837	The Births and Deaths Registration Act of 1836, operationalised 1 July 1837, comprehensive registration data for deaths in England and Wales from 1841 onwards. But no penalty for failure to register, and doctors need not provide cause details.
1874	The Births and Deaths Registration Act of 1874 required the medical practioners who were attendant during the person's last illness to provide a cause of death unless an inquest was being held. A penalty was introduced if the death was not registered. Also improved the quality of certification for infants and stillborn children.
1881	Changes to classification of causes of death.
1901	Changes to classification of causes of death. ONS used a variant of the first International Classification of Diseases (IDC1*).
1911	Adoption of 2nd ICD revision (ICD2†).
1921	Adoption of the 3rd ICD revision (ICD3†).
1926	1926 Act made it unlawful to dispose of the body of a dead person before a registrar's certificate or coroner's order had been issued. Also required the registration of stillbirths.
1927	Format of certification changed – new certificates in two parts, the first for the disease or condition leading directly to the cause of death, and causes antecedent to it, and the second for 'other significant conditions contributing to the death, but not related to the disease or condition causing it'.
1931	Adoption of the 4th ICD revision (ICD4†).
1940	Adoption of the 5th revision of the ICD (ICD5†). Major changes made to method of selecting the underlying cause of death when more than one cause was mentioned on the certificate. Now the underlying cause would be selected in accordance with the certifier's preference, as expressed in the order on the certificate (Campbell, 1965).
1950	Adoption of the 6th revision of the ICD.
1958	Adoption of the 7th revision of the ICD.
1968	Adoption of the 8th revision of the ICD.
1978	Criminal Law Act of 1977 – amendments to Rules and Regulations affecting compilation of mortality data for Injury and Poisoning (see DH2 no 11).
1979	Adoption of the 9th ICD revision.
1981	Registrars work-to-rule (1981–82) significantly affected Injury and Poisoning data for 1981 and to a lesser extent for 1982, especially cause of injury (no coroners' data).
1984	ONS made a change in their method of applying the WHO's coding rule 3. For effects see DH2 no 11.
1986	New neonatal death certificate introduced which abandoned the concept of a single underlying cause of death and instead requested separately details of maternal and of foetal contributions to mortality - affects neonatal and all-ages cause-specific mortality data.
1993	Redevelopment of computer systems for processing mortality data, resulting in: 1) reversal of ONS policy on rule 3 that was introduced in 1984, due to the introduction of automatic cause coding which follows internationally agreed rules; 2) medical enquiries suspended until 1998.

*Notes: *ONS used an un-numbered list instead of the International Classification during 1901–10.*
†As amended for use in England and Wales.
A listing of codes and explanations for ICD1–5 used in the ONS Historic Deaths Database is available on disk in 'Paradox' or text format.
Other factors affecting certification are: improvements in medical diagnosis; improvements in access to care; changes in diagnostic fashion and certification practice.

Source: ONS

Figure 2.1

Death certificate in current use

SPECIMEN   MED A 751753
21

BIRTHS AND DEATHS REGISTRATION ACT 1953
(Form prescribed by the Registration of Births and Deaths Regulations 1987)

MEDICAL CERTIFICATE OF CAUSE OF DEATH

For use only by a Registered Medical Practitioner WHO HAS BEEN IN ATTENDANCE during the deceased's last illness,
and to be delivered by him forthwith to the Registrar of Births and Deaths.

Registrar to enter
No. of Death Entry

Name of deceased

Date of death as stated to me .... day of .... Age as stated to me

Place of death

Last seen alive by me .... day of

1 The certified cause of death takes account of information
   obtained from post-mortem.
2 Information from post-mortem may be available later.
3 Post-mortem not being held.
4 I have reported this death to the Coroner for further action.
   [See overleaf]

Please ring appropriate digit(s) and letter

a Seen after death by me.
b Seen after death by another medical practitioner
   but not by me.
c Not seen after death by a medical practitioner.

CAUSE OF DEATH

*The condition thought to be the 'Underlying Cause of Death' should
appear in the lowest completed line of Part I.*

I(a) Disease or condition directly
      leading to death†
(b) Other disease or condition, if any,
     leading to I(a)
(c) Other disease or condition, if any,
     leading to I(b)

II Other significant conditions
    CONTRIBUTING TO THE DEATH but
    not related to the disease or condition
    causing it.

*These particulars not to be
entered in death register*

Approximate interval
between onset and death

The death might have been due to or contributed to by the employment followed at some time by the deceased.

Please tick
where applicable

†*This does not mean the mode of dying, such as heart failure, asphyxia, asthenia, etc: it means the disease, injury, or complication which caused death.*

**I hereby certify that I was in medical attendance during
the above named deceased's last illness, and that the
particulars and cause of death above written are true
to the best of my knowledge and belief.**

Signature

Residence

Qualifications as registered
by General Medical Council

Date

For deaths in hospital: Please give the name of the consultant responsible for the above-named as a patient.

Source: ONS

certificate. As defined by the 9th revision of the International Classification of Diseases (WHO, 1977), the underlying cause of death is:

(1) the disease or injury that initiated the train of events leading to death, or
(2) the circumstances of the accident or violence (e.g. suicide) that produced the fatal injury.

Prior to 1940 the selection of this cause had been determined on the basis of certain rules whereby conditions of various types – violence, infectious diseases, malignant tumours and so on – were given an arbitrary order of precedence, no notice being taken of the order in which the certifying practitioner wrote down the various causes of death (Logan, 1950).

In 1940 the 5th revision of the ICD was adopted, and ONS made major changes to the method of selecting the underlying cause of death when more than one cause was mentioned on the certificate. Now the underlying cause was to be selected in accordance with the certifier's preference, as expressed in the order on the certificate (Campbell, 1965).

In 1984 ONS made a further change in their method of selecting the underlying cause, using a broader interpretation of the WHO's coding rule 3 (OPCS, 1985). This rule states that where the condition in Part I is clearly a direct sequel to a condition in Part II, the latter is to be preferred as the underlying cause. The cause entered in Part II was thus selected more frequently, resulting in a fall in deaths from less specific causes such as bronchopneumonia (ICD-485) and pulmonary embolism (ICD-415.1). The changes resulted in increases in more specific categories, particularly chapters III (Endocrine, nutritional and metabolic and immunity disorders), IV (Blood and blood forming organs), V (Mental disorders), VI (Diseases of the nervous system and sense organs), XII (Diseases of the skin and subcutaneous tissue) and XIII (Diseases of the musculoskeletal system and connective tissue). These changes are discussed in detail elsewhere (OPCS, 1985), and in Chapter 4 of this volume. In 1993 when automatic cause coding was adopted (Birch, 1993) the decision taken in 1984 was reversed, moving back to the internationally accepted interpretation operating before 1984. The changes and their effects are described in an ONS publication (OPCS, 1995a).

Because it can be difficult to select the underlying cause from a multiplicity of recorded causes, ONS has from time to time produced tables based on more than one cause. The first were in the Registrar General's Annual Reports from 1911 to 1914, the next in the 1931 decennial supplement. The first modern analysis covered a sample of deaths in 1951. Subsequent analyses were published for 1966–67, 1976, and most recently in 1985–86 (OPCS, 1988). Here tables include causes with which people died as well as those from which they died. Some conditions, such as cancers and cerebrovascular disease, frequently appear alone on a death certificate, while causes such as diabetes appear many times more often as 'mentions' than as the underlying cause.

Other considerations affecting interpretation

Problems arise when death certificates do not include sufficient information for accurate cause classification. Since 1964 ONS has sent a 'medical enquiry' form to certifying doctors where this occurs, requesting further information. In recent years about 3 per cent of all deaths have been subject to this procedure, with an 80 per cent response rate (Ashley and Devis, 1992). Most changes resulting from these are small, and a substantial proportion of these enquiries relate to redefinition of the site involved for cancer deaths (ONS, 1996). Medical enquiries have been suspended from 1993 to 1998 to enable new computer systems to be adopted.

In 1978 the Criminal Law Act of 1977, the Coroners (Amendment) Rules 1977 and the Registration of Births, Deaths and Marriages (Amendment) Regulations altered rules and regulations affecting compilation of mortality data for Injury and Poisoning – see DH2 no 11 (OPCS, 1985). The coroner's jury was no longer required to name a person it finds guilty of causing a death, and the coroner no longer need commit that person for trial. Furthermore, where an inquest is adjourned because a person has been charged with an offence in connection with the death, provisions were made for the death to be registered at the time of adjournment rather than having to wait for the outcome of criminal proceedings. Such deaths were assigned to ICD-9 code E988.8, or in the case of motor vehicle accidents, to the appropriate traffic accident code. The result of this change was that reported homicide deaths were reduced, and open verdicts correspondingly increased – this is discussed in more detail elsewhere by Noble and Charlton (1994).

In 1986 new neonatal and foetal death certificates were introduced for stillbirths and deaths occurring in the first 28 days of life. These certificates abandoned the concept of a single underlying cause of death and instead requested separate details of maternal and of foetal contributions to mortality. This affects cause-specific mortality data under age 1, since tables by cause now omit deaths in the first 28 days of life. Recently an algorithm has been introduced to derive an underlying cause grouping from the information provided (Alberman *et al.*, 1994). Scotland has not adopted a new stillbirth and neonatal certificate so this problem in interpreting trends has not arisen there.

Post mortem examinations can be a means to a more precise diagnosis (see Figure 2.2). A substantial proportion of death certificates, 74 per cent, are currently signed without one. This figure was 91 per cent in 1928, when statistics on post mortem examinations first became available. Post mortem rates vary according to cause of death, with nearly all coroners' cases (cases of death by injury, poisoning or sudden unexplained death, about a quarter of all deaths) involving post mortems. Only 3 per cent of doctor-certified deaths not referred to the coroner involve post mortems (Ashley and Devis, 1992). Deaths from neoplasms, a major cause of death (see Chapter 4), rarely require post mortems because diagnoses are usually confirmed by surgery, histology, blood tests and other investigations. Improvements in the accuracy of medical diagnosis and improvement in access to care may lead to an increase in specific causes (including hard to diagnose conditions such as multiple myeloma), and falls in less specific causes such as symptoms and signs. A large study comparing clinical and autopsy diagnoses of underlying cause of death (Heasman and Lipworth, 1966) examined 9,501 patients in 75 hospitals in England and Wales and found considerable differences, with agreement in only 45 per cent of cases. However, the overall numbers in most disease groups, regardless of method of diagnosis, were similar, since the errors tended to cancel each other out. For example, 183 patients were coded as dying from malignant diseases on the basis of clinical diagnosis, and 182 by pathologists. A later study of 1,126 patients from the Birmingham area comparing autopsy and death certificate diagnoses found 48 per cent complete agreement, 26 per cent partial agreement and 22 per cent total disagreement (Waldron and Vickerstaff, 1977). Alderson has reviewed a number of validation studies to determine the accuracy of cause of death certification for specific diseases, and discusses how these have been affected by changes in diagnosis and coding (Alderson, 1981). There is greater certainty regarding diagnoses in individuals aged under age 65, and for men rather than women. In an analysis of data from Bristol, making use of hospital and death certificate data together, he found that in 70 per cent of cases

Figure 2.2

Autopsy for IHD: 1959–91

England and Wales

Rate per 1,000 deaths

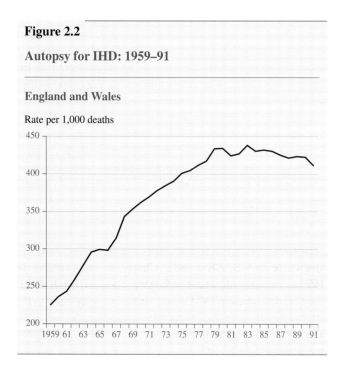

the initial coding was correct, in 20 per cent a minor alteration was required and in 10 per cent a major alteration, but this varied according to whether the certificates were signed by hospital doctors, those recently qualified, those in non-teaching hospitals and whether the patients were elderly or had respiratory diseases (Alderson, 1965). It was suggested that greater accuracy would result from linking together different data sources such as hospital and mortality data. The Oxford Record Linkage Study (Acheson, 1967) is one such linkage exercise.

Another cause of apparent change in mortality rates, especially crude all-ages rates, is changes that occur in the make-up of the population, for example, when the age distribution changes. If the average age of the population increases then a higher crude mortality is to be expected even if death rates at each single year of age remain constant. This statistical artefact is overcome by 'age standardisation methods' (see Section 2.4). The effect of this is shown in Figure 3.12 of Chapter 3.

Up to 1992, deaths recorded in mortality statistics for England and Wales have been those registered in England and Wales in calendar periods. From 1993 onwards ONS has published data by year of occurrence. The effect of this change is small (OPCS, 1995a; ONS, 1996).

No distinction is usually made between deaths of civilians and non-civilians. The deaths of persons whose usual residence is outside England and Wales are included in the total figures for England and Wales if they died in England or Wales. Similar procedures apply to Scotland – deaths of English residents in Scotland will appear in Scottish statistics but not English statistics. An assessment of the impact of registration of non-residents on the comparability of mortality statistics, with particular reference to Scotland, has been made (Carstairs, 1991). The problems are greater for some causes of deaths (such as heart diseases and injury and poisoning) than others (such as malignant neoplasms). Deaths of non-residents appear to be more common in Scotland (0.9 per cent of all deaths) than in England and Wales (0.3 per cent). About half of non-resident deaths occur under age 65. Somewhat fewer deaths are referred to the Procurator Fiscal in Scotland than to the coroner in England and Wales, and fewer postmortems are therefore conducted. This may affect the comparability of the data since 'sudden death' is more common in Scotland (Ashley and Devis, 1992).

2.3.2 Censuses availability and reliability of census data

It is difficult to interpret counts of medical events without adequate population denominators against which rates can be calculated. The first national census of population was conducted in 1801, with further censuses at 10-year intervals apart from 1941. There was, however, population registration in 1939. The 1841 Census was the first to be conducted by the Registrar General, when the method of enumeration changed from a count of houses and persons by local Overseers of the Poor to self-enumeration by household,

directed by the registration service. Apart from counts of the population by age and sex, the census has provided a wealth of information about the socioeconomic characteristics of the population, such as household composition, marital status, education, employment, accommodation and lack of amenities, enabling trends to be studied. Some health questions have been asked from time to time: from 1851 to 1911 the number of 'idiots', blind, deaf and dumb were enumerated, and in 1991 a question was included on limiting long-term illness (LLTI). The availability and validity of past census data have been reviewed (Ashley et al., 1991). Since 1961 it has been standard practice for ONS to carry out a census evaluation programme, to check the coverage and quality of replies entered on the census form. The method used is to repeat the enumeration for a sample of the households shortly after census day, using a team of skilled interviewers. In 1981 the net under-enumeration was 0.5 per cent – in 1991 there was an estimated 1 per cent shortfall, which was concentrated in men and to a lesser extent women aged from 19 to 31 (OPCS, 1993a). The discrepancy was as high as 6 per cent at age 27, and it is thought that avoidance of the recently introduced council tax was a factor.

2.3.3 Intercensal population estimates

The main source of detailed data comes from censuses, but based on these and estimates of census population under-counts, annual mid-year estimates are produced which take account of births, deaths, and migration into and out of the country, local and health authorities. These have been prepared since the nineteenth century for the country and large towns, and for local authorities since 1911 (Whitehead, 1985). The current methodology has been published (OPCS, 1993b), and includes using data from the International Passenger Survey for international migration, the National Health Service Central Register (NHSCR) for movements between Family Health Services Authorities, electoral roll statistics and comparison of censuses for the Republic of Ireland and Great Britain. Population projections for future years are also made (Daykin, 1986; Armitage, 1986). The validity of annual population estimates depends heavily on the quality of the data sources and methodology. Of the elements discussed above, migration is the most difficult to estimate. ONS continually monitors the accuracy of its estimates (see for example OPCS, 1982a).

The population covered by population estimates has varied over time. From 1915 to 1920 and from 3 September 1939 to 31 December 1949 for men and 1 June 1941 to 31 December 1949 for women the civilian population was used, i.e. the home population excluding all members of HM Forces and Forces of other countries stationed in England and Wales. Between 1950 and 1970 the population estimates related to the home population – those living in England and Wales, including overseas visitors to the country and the Forces of other countries temporarily in England and Wales, but excluding residents and members of HM Forces who were outside the country on census night. From 1971 onwards the estimates relate to the resident population – those resident in

England and Wales including members of HM and non-United Kingdom Forces stationed in England and Wales, and residents who were outside the country on census night, but excluding overseas visitors and HM and non-United Kingdom Forces stationed outside the country.

2.3.4 Notifications of infectious diseases

National notification of infectious diseases was introduced with the Infectious Diseases Notification Act of 1889, which aimed to combat 'dangerous infectious disorders'. In Scotland notification was introduced 2 years earlier. The first figures to appear in the Registrar General's weekly return were published in 1895, giving the numbers of five diseases which had been admitted to certain London hospitals. From 1922 onwards weekly provisional returns made by each Medical Officer of Public Health were published. The list of notifiable diseases has been enlarged over time, as shown in Table 2.2. In England and Wales notification by medical practitioners is made to the 'proper officer' of the local authority in which the disease is identified or suspected, usually the consultant for communicable disease control (see McCormick, 1993). In Scotland notification is to the Chief Administrative Medical Officer in the area where the case was diagnosed.

Table 2.2

Notifiable diseases in England and Wales

Date made notifiable	Infection
Under the Public Health (Control of Disease) Act 1984	
1889	Cholera; relapsing fever; smallpox; typhus
1900	Plague
1949	Food poisoning
Under the Public Health (Infectious Diseases) Regulations 1988	
1889	Diptheria; scarlet fever; paratyphoid fever; typhoid fever
1912	Acute poliomyelitis; tuberculosis
1914	Opthalmia neonatorum
1918	Acute encephalitis
1919	Dysentery (amoebic or bacillary); malaria
1940	Measles; whooping cough
1951	Leprosy
1960	Anthrax
1968	Leptospirosis; meningitis; viral hepatitis; yellow fever; tetanus
1976	Rabies; viral haemorrhagic fever
1988	Meningococcal septicaemia (without meningitis); mumps; rubella

Note: The details for Scotland are broadly similar (see Ashley et al., 1991).

Source: McCormick (1993)

Data on other infectious diseases not notifiable under statute are collected through voluntary laboratory reporting by microbiologists (e.g. salmonella infections, influenza and HIV) and voluntary confidential clinical reporting systems (e.g. for AIDS). Details of cases reported by laboratories include age, sex, diagnosis, time and place of diagnosis. AIDS case reports include data on risk factors for HIV infection and clinical status of the patient at the time of diagnosis (McCormick et al., 1987). These data are collected by the Communicable Disease Surveillance Centre for England and Wales, and the Scottish Centre for Infection and Environmental Health in Scotland.

Notification of infectious diseases is recognised as being far from complete, especially for those conditions considered to be less severe or of lesser public health importance (Haward, 1973). Tuberculosis notifications were accurate to within 10 per cent (Davies et al., 1981). Clarkson and Fine (1985) estimated that for measles some 40–60 per cent of cases were reported, whereas for pertussis only between 5 and 25 per cent were. Significant under-reporting has also been found with notifications of meningitis (Goldacre and Miller, 1976). Tillett and Spencer (1982) found that influenza was under-reported as the underlying cause of death until there was an epidemic, when it tended to become over-reported.

In England and Wales the Royal College of GPs (RCGP, 1968; Fleming et al., 1996) collects data on patients with infectious diseases via a group of 'spotter' general practices that report on cases encountered. A similar scheme operates in Scotland.

2.3.5 Cancer registrations

Availability and scope

A system of cancer registration was introduced in the 1920s in several parts of England and Wales after the introduction of radium treatment, in order to follow the outcome in treated patients. In 1947 the GRO (later OPCS, now ONS) took over, from the Radium Commission, analysis of data supplied by local and regional registries under voluntary arrangements. However, it was not until 1962 that all regions in England and Wales were incorporated into a comprehensive national cancer registration scheme. Cancer registration in Scotland evolved from a scheme similar to that in England and Wales (Kemp et al., 1985). Complete coverage was achieved in 1947 when reports were obtained from cancer treatment centres, but the scheme was reorganised and computerised in 1958. Standard procedures for cancer registration are now widely established.

Since 1948 registration in England and Wales has been carried out by population-based regional registries, of which there are currently twelve. Most patients with cancer are likely to be admitted to hospital for diagnosis and/or treatment, so cancer registrations stem largely from information supplied to the registries on a voluntary basis by hospitals providing secondary and tertiary care. The registries record identification particulars, date of diagnosis and site of cancer for newly diagnosed cases in their defined population and aim to update the record, when relevant, with the date of death. All registries make use of diagnostic information generated by NHS hospital discharge data, but the extent to which this is supplemented with information from, for example, pathology and radiotherapy departments, hospices and private clinics, is variable (OPCS, 1990a). ONS provides the registries with copies of death drafts (Form 310) mentioning cancer. A generally small proportion of cases (which varies by registry and cancer site and over time) are registered only from the information obtained at death, in order to supplement hospital sources of data. A standard dataset is submitted by the registries to ONS.

ONS is also responsible for the flagging at the NHSCR of cases submitted by registries, the provision to regional registries of death drafts of flagged cases dying of other causes, and the editing, processing, analysis and publication of national statistics on cancer registration and survival. For a full description of the system in England and Wales, see OPCS (1994). In Scotland, a similar system of cancer registration is based on five regional registries and coordinated by the Information Services Division of the Scottish Health Service Common Services Agency.

Prior to 1971, registration data were published in the Registrar General's Statistical Review of England and Wales, Supplements on Cancer. Since 1971, cancer registration statistics have been published annually by ONS in the MB1 series of reports. The 1994 publication includes trends for 1979–89 and a commentary on the major cancer sites (OPCS, 1994), and a Monitor series on survival is planned. Trends for earlier time periods are presented in ONS's publication on cancer registration surveillance 1968–1978 (OPCS, 1982b, 1983a) and by the Cancer Research Campaign's publication for Great Britain (CRC, 1982). Data for Scotland are published by the Scottish NHS (Black *et al.,* 1993; Sharp *et al.,* 1993).

Validity of cancer registration statistics
There have been three reports by the advisory committee on cancer registration which have examined, among other things, the validity of cancer registration data (OPCS, 1970, 1981, 1990b). Consideration has been given to three aspects – completeness of ascertainment, accuracy of the items registered and the effectiveness of follow-up from which survival statistics are calculated. Since 1948, the number of registrations in England and Wales has risen, but it is unclear to what extent this is due to extension of the scheme, improvements in completeness of registration or an increase in the incidence of malignant disease. Using various sources of records, Alderson (1974) concluded that about 10 per cent of patients might not be registered, a result comparable with that obtained by Gillis (1971) in an examination of Scottish data. Of the items recorded, diagnosis was found to be relatively accurate, but errors and omissions occurred with date of registration, place of birth, histology and occupation (Alderson, 1974; West, 1976). More recent studies of selected groups have indicated a high degree of completeness of ascertainment (Stiller *et al.,* 1991; Swerdlow *et al.,* 1993).

The 1970 report recommended that the registration data should be linked with information on deaths in the NHS Central Registers (OPCS, 1970). The implementation of this procedure in England, Wales and Scotland in 1971 permitted automatic identification of the fact of death, thereby facilitating calculation of survival statistics, and relieving the cancer registries of *ad hoc* follow-up through hospitals and general practitioners. Differences in survival are related to the type of cancer, the stage in development at which it is diagnosed and the efficacy of treatment. This national system for linking cancer registration with subsequent death is the only way to make available unbiased data on cancer survival, which enable factors which determine prognosis to be monitored.

In 1990 it was found that the quality of cancer registration had considerably improved since the 1980 review, but there were persisting differences between registries in completeness and timeliness of registration, in respect of methods of data collection and items collected, and staffing and cost (OPCS, 1990a). The development and implementation of new computer technology, both at regional and central level, was expected to result in further improvements in the quality and completeness of cancer registration data. A recent major change is that cancer registration, which had been conducted on a voluntary basis since its inception, became mandatory with obligations on hospitals and other provider units to supply a 'minimum dataset for cancer registration' to the regional registries, and on the registries to send these data to ONS (Department of Health, 1995).

Cancer registries are uniquely able to provide information on the burden of cancer in the population at regional or national level. The data permit a wide variety of descriptive studies of cancer incidence to be carried out. For example, an important starting point in research into causes of cancer is often the study of trends of incidence with time. In addition, cancer registration data are increasingly used in evaluation of services and investigations of equity in health care. Rapid developments in screening and treatment require accurate information on cancer occurrence and survival for their planning and evaluation, and for estimates of their cost-effectiveness. The national cancer registration system has now become vital for management of the preventative and curative services, especially for service purchasers and providers.

In addition to cancer registers there are a number of other registers which have been set up for specific purposes (see Chapter 5).

2.3.6 Congenital anomalies

Partly as a result of the thalidomide epidemic of 1960 a national notification scheme was started in England and Wales in 1964, whereby doctors and midwives notified the local Medical Officer of Health about any congenital anomaly identifiable at birth or within 7 days, later extended to 10 days. This time limit has recently been removed. These data are forwarded to ONS for analysis (Weatherall, 1978; Botting, 1995). The validity of these data has been reviewed (Ashley *et al.*, 1991; OPCS, 1995b). Although there is under-notification and evidence of potential biases in notification, this varies according to the malformation; the most easily recognised ones have the most complete recording. The data were judged to be of sufficient quality to expose any increase in incidence.

2.3.7 Abortions

Abortion data when combined with data on births can provide information on teenage pregnancies and other important health issues relating to women and their babies, for example, on the occurrence of neural tube defects (Hey *et al.*, 1994). Statistics on 'conceptions' are produced combining abortion data with data on live and still births, based on the estimated year of conception. Reducing the number of conceptions to mothers under age 16 is a 'Health of the Nation' target. Similar data are processed for Scotland by the Information and Statistics Division. The concern about rising maternal mortality in the 1930s drew attention to the consequences of illegal abortion since at that time between 16 and 20 per cent of pregnancies ended in abortion (Report, 1936). The Abortion Act 1967 came into operation in Britain in April 1968, and requires notifications of termination of pregnancy to be made to the Chief Medical Officers within 7 days. ONS processes these data on behalf of the Department of Health. Limited abortion data were available, from 1949, from the Hospital In-Patient Enquiry (HIPE). Information is available on the woman's age, marital status, place of residence, number of previous children, length of gestation, statutory grounds for termination and methods used. Botting (1991) has reviewed the trends since 1968. The rapid increase between 1968 and 1972 is likely to be largely due to transfer of abortions from the illegal to the legal sector, and changing patterns of abortions to non-residents of England and Wales. In more recent years, however, the increase may have been influenced, at least in part, by changing fertility patterns, the changing age structure of the population of fertile women, changing contraception patterns and changing attitudes towards abortion.

2.3.8 Health service records

There is a vast amount of data stored in GP and hospital records. The availability of these data and their strengths and limitations for measuring population morbidity are discussed in Chapter 5.

2.3.9 Linked routinely collected data

The ONS Longitudinal Study is based on a 1 per cent sample of the usually resident population of England and Wales, and commenced with a sample taken from the 1971 decennial census. This consists of all individuals born on four specific days in the year. Data are linked to this sample from different routine sources. The study relies to a large extent on tracing individuals through the NHSCR. New births occurring on the four days in the year, and immigrants who register with the NHS who were born on these days, are added to the sample so that it continues to represent 1 per cent of the population. For each individual the following events are linked: live and stillbirths to women in the sample; deaths under 1 year of age of these children; immigration and emigration; death of a spouse; cancer registrations; death; and census data from subsequent years. The main value of this study is that it is possible to analyse changes over time using data on individuals, and it is relatively easy to perform exploratory analyses quickly in response to specific questions that arise from time to time, free from numerator/denominator biases. It has made significant contributions in the field of occupational mortality (Fox and Goldblatt, 1982) because the occupation of women is not always recorded on the death certificate, and men and women change occupations over time. It is particularly valuable in analysing socioeconomic data in relation to mortality.

Since the 1970s all cancer notifications have been sent to the NHSCR and subsequently linked to death records (OPCS, 1970). Another use that has been made of the NHSCR has been to link data on various kinds of exposure to subsequent mortality, for example in occupational mortality studies (Acheson, 1967; OPCS, 1993c). An early example of this was when a relationship was found between exposure to dyestuff of workers in the chemical industry and bladder tumours (Case and Pearson, 1954). The Oxford Record Linkage Study (Acheson, 1967) links hospitalisation records of individuals together, and to birth, death and cancer registration records. The Scottish Record Linkage System is somewhat different (Kendrick and Clarke, 1993).

2.3.10 Sickness Benefit Statistics

These nationally collected data are discussed by Fenton Lewis (1979). A major drawback in using these statistics from the Department of Social Security is that they are based on sickness benefits claims. Thus they only relate to those in work who can claim sickness benefit, and changes to the rules from time to time result in corresponding changes in the statistics that do not reflect morbidity. Given the provisos, they do give some measure of common conditions that are severe enough to cause time off work in the population in employment. Major changes affecting the statistics have occurred in September 1980, January 1982 and April 1983, and more recently when self-certification of short periods of sickness absence were introduced (DHSS, 1963–94).

2.3.11 Survey data

Surveys provide subjective information on health from the point of view of individuals in the population, as well as more objective information if physical examination is combined with the interview. A number of surveys that have been cited in Health of Adult Britain are discussed below.

General Household Survey (GHS)

This is an ongoing annual household survey of some 17,000 individuals that has been conducted by ONS since 1971 (OPCS, 1995c). It includes some core questions on general health and socioeconomic conditions. Questions on health-related behaviours such as smoking and drinking are included every other year. Additional health-related questions are included from time to time. It includes questions on longstanding illnesses and whether these limit the respondent's activities (a measure of disability). The 1989 survey included detailed questions on the causes of longstanding illness (Breeze *et al.*, 1991) and similar analyses were undertaken in the 1994 survey.

The Health Survey for England (HSFE)

This is an annual survey (from 1991) undertaken on behalf of the Department of Health, with a health interview and a physical examination, initially of only some 3,000 individuals, but now with a sample size similar to the GHS (16,600 individuals aged 16 and over in 1993 and 1994) (Bennett *et al.*, 1995; Colhoun and Prescott Clark, 1996). To date the questions have concentrated on cardiovascular disease and its risk factors, but the 1995 survey has broadened coverage to include asthma, accidents and disability.

The ONS Omnibus Survey

This is a monthly survey sampling some 2,000 individuals aged 16 and over in private households every month. Different organisations commission questions which run for however many months they are required. For example, in 1995 the Department of Health commissioned questions on general health, including the EuroQol (a quality of life measure).

The ONS Disability Surveys

The most recent disability surveys were carried out in 1985–88, and give information on the type and severity of disabling conditions, by age and sex (Martin *et al.*, 1988). They cover private households and communal establishments, but do not provide information on the prevalence of the conditions causing the disability.

Labour Force Survey (LFS)

This covers the population eligible for work, and includes prevalence information on reasons for sickness absence. It also asks about health problems that affect work. Data have been collected biennially since 1973, annually since 1984 (OPCS, 1992).

ONS Psychiatric Morbidity Surveys

These give a measure of prevalence of minor and severe mental health problems in the general population, as well as the population in institutions and the homeless (Meltzer *et al.*, 1995a, b). Analyses by socioeconomic characteristics were undertaken.

Health in England 1995

This was the first in a series of surveys of adults aged between 16 and 74, carried out by ONS on behalf of the Health Education Authority (Bridgwood *et al.*, 1996); 4,672 adults were interviewed. The aim was to monitor what people know, think and do in relation to healthy lifestyles, in order to measure progress towards Health of the Nation targets. Also included were questions on self-reported general health, whether they led a healthy life, stress and self-reported morbidity.

Dental Health Surveys

ONS conducted a survey of Adult Dental Health in 1968 which showed that 29 per cent of all adults had no natural teeth, with worse dental health in the North than the South. When the survey was repeated in 1978 dental health had improved – to different extents in different parts of the country (Todd and Walker, 1980; Todd and Dodd, 1982). Further surveys were undertaken in 1988 and subsequently (Todd and Lader, 1991; Todd *et al.*, 1994). Children's dental health has also been surveyed (Todd, 1974, 1975, 1988; Todd and Dodd, 1985; Todd and Lader, 1991; O'Brien, 1994; Hinds and Gregory, 1995).

British Food Surveys

Data have been collected from the middle of the nineteenth century, initially to monitor the nutrition of the less well-off. Early data sources may not be strictly comparable with later surveys, and were often based on small samples. Larger, more recent surveys were:

- Orr (1936): a survey of working class diets (sample size 1,152 households).

- Carnegie (1951): survey of urban working class in 1938–39 (sample size 1,111 households).

- Ministry of Food (1951): survey of wartime working class households (sample size 4,795).

- MAFF (1994): the National Food Survey (sample size 8,000–12,000 households, from 1950 onwards). Household information is provided by a main diary keeper who records all food consumed for one full week.

- The Dietary and Nutritional Survey of British Adults (sample size 2,197): carried out by ONS (Gregory *et al.*, 1990). Examined, among other measures, nutritional status through the use of a 7-day weighed diary and monitored food and beverages consumed within the household and outside the home. This provided the opportunity to observe both individual and household characteristics for persons aged from 16 to 64 years, allowing a comparison of nutritional status for age and sex as well as household characteristics.

- The National Diet and Nutrition Survey: children aged from 1.5 to 4.5 years (sample size 2,101), July 1992–June 1993. Examined the nutrition of children taken both inside and outside the home (Gregory *et al.*, 1995). This consisted of a weighed dietary record of a period of 4 days, which included Saturday and Sunday. A similar survey was carried out during 1967–8.

Surveys of height and weight

ONS Surveys have provided measurements over time of heights and weights of adults that in addition allow obesity trends to be monitored (Knight, 1984; Bennett *et al.*, 1995).

More recently the Health Survey for England has provided similar information for monitoring trends.

Other surveys relating to health

These include: People Aged 65 and Over (Goddard and Savage, 1994); Smoking Among Secondary School Children in England (Dobbs and Marsh, 1983, 1985; Goddard and Ikin, 1987; Goddard, 1989; Lader and Matheson, 1991; Thomas *et al.,* 1993; Bolling, 1994; Diamond and Goddard, 1995); Dental Crowns (Todd *et al.,* 1994); Survey of the Physical Health of Prisoners (Bridgwood and Malbon, 1995); Adolescent Drinking (Marsh *et al.,* 1986); Drinking in England and Wales (Wilson, 1980; Goddard, 1991); Scottish Drinking Habits (Dight, 1976); The Allied Dunbar National Fitness Survey (Allied Dunbar *et al.,* 1992). In addition ONS has a Health Survey Advice Centre to help NHS bodies to conduct their own health surveys.

2.3.12 Syntheses of survey and other health data

ONS has examined health expectancy on behalf of the Department of Health (Bone *et al.,* 1995). This combines data from the GHS and disability surveys with life tables to produce tables giving estimates of life expectation without disability. Other syntheses of datasets have been produced, for example, data from the Morbidity Statistics from General Practice Survey have been combined with data from the Census Sample of Anonymised Records to produce local estimates (Charlton and Heady, 1995).

2.4 Definitions of important concepts used in this book

2.4.1 Incidence

The rate at which new events occur in the population, i.e. the number of new cases of a disease in a specified period, divided by the population at risk of getting the disease during the period. Often expressed as rates per million population.

2.4.2 Prevalence rate

The number of people with a disease at a given time (point prevalence), or at any time in a specified period (period prevalence), divided by the number of people at risk from that disease. Often expressed as rates per million. Lifetime prevalence is another form of period prevalence.

2.4.3 Crude death rate

The number of deaths during a specified period, divided by the number at risk during the period. Usually expressed as a rate per million, it provides an estimate of the proportion of the population dying during the specified period (typically per year). It does not take into account the ages of the individuals in the population studied, and can be misleading when examining long-term trends because the age structure of the population may vary over time.

2.4.4 Age-specific rate

A rate for a specified age-group. The numerator and denominator refer to the same age-group, for example, number of deaths among ages 15–24 in a year, divided by the population at risk aged 15–24, multiplied by 1,000,000, gives the death rate per million.

2.4.5 Age-standardised rates and ratios (SMRs)

A procedure for adjusting rates to take account of differences in age composition when comparing rates for different populations, for example, at different dates or between different countries. There are two approaches used in this book: (1) direct standardisation (usually to the standard European population – see below); and (2) indirect standardisation, usually expressed as a standardised ratio (for example, standardised mortality ratio). Both methods are based on weighted averaging of rates specific for age, sex and sometimes other potential confounding variables.

- The direct method averages specific rates in a study population using as weights the population distribution of a specified population (see European population below). This standardised rate represents what the crude rate would have been in the study population if the population had the same distribution as the standard population with respect to the variables for which the adjustment or standardisation was carried out.

  Age-standardised rate = $(\sum P_k m_k)/\sum P_k$,
  where P_k is the standard population in sex/age group k,
  m_k is the observed mortality rate (e.g. deaths per million persons) in sex/age-group k
  and k = sex/age-group (e.g. 0, 1–4, 5–9,...,85 and over) for males and females.

- The indirect method is used to compare study populations for which the specific rates are either statistically unstable or unknown. The specific rates in the standard population are averaged, using as weights the distribution of the study population, to obtain an expected number of events such as deaths. The ratio of the observed events to expected events for the study population is the standardised mortality (or morbidity) ratio, or SMR. In studying trends, the standard population would typically be one of the years studied, often the first.

  SMR = 100 x (observed deaths/expected deaths),
  where expected deaths = $\sum p_k m_k$ and
  where p_k is the population in sex/age-group k in a year,
  m_k is the mortality rate (deaths per person) in sex/age-group k for the standard population/year
  and k = sex/age-group (e.g. 0, 1–4, 5–9,....,85 and over).

  The indirectly standardised rate is the product of the SMR and the crude rate for the standard population.

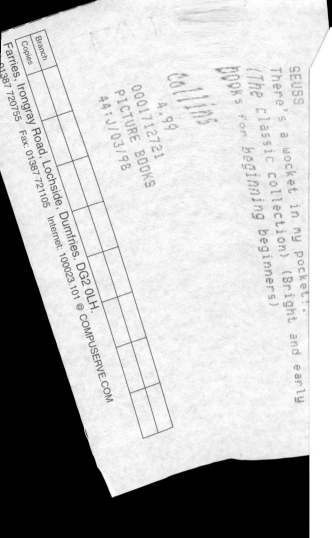

Another method of adjusting mortality data to take account of the age distribution of a population is the life table – see below (for methods see Armitage, 1971).

2.4.6 Sex ratio

The ratio of male to female rates, usually expressed as a percentage. For example, if the mortality sex ratio for a particular age range is 200 then males are twice as likely to die in that age range as females.

2.4.7 European standard population

An artificial population (WHO, 1991) used for direct standardisation of rates. It is in fact reasonably similar to the 1991 England and Wales population (although the age distribution is the same for men and women). The population figures are simplified to make calculations easier.

The standard European population distribution is:

Age-group	Standard European population	Population England and Wales 1991 (Total=100,000)		
		Persons	Males	Females
0	1,600	1,400	1,400	1,300
1–4	6,400	5,300	5,600	5,100
5–9	7,000	6,300	6,600	6,000
10–14	7,000	6,000	6,300	5,700
15–19	7,000	6,400	6,700	6,100
20–24	7,000	7,700	8,100	7,400
25–29	7,000	8,200	8,500	8,000
30–34	7,000	7,300	7,500	7,100
35–39	7,000	6,600	6,700	6,400
40–44	7,000	7,200	7,500	7,100
45–49	7,000	6,200	6,400	6,000
50–54	7,000	5,300	5,600	5,200
55–59	6,000	5,100	5,100	5,000
60–64	5,000	5,000	5,000	5,100
65–69	4,000	4,900	4,600	5,100
70–74	3,000	4,000	3,500	4,400
75–79	2,000	3,300	2,600	3,900
80–84	1,000	2,200	1,500	2,800
85 and over	1,000	1,600	800	2,300
All ages	100,000	100,000	100,000	100,000

2.4.8 Life table

A summarising technique used to describe the pattern of mortality and survival in populations. It describes: (1) out of an initial population of 100,000 live births, how many persons survive to age x (l_x); (2) the average number of further years of life remaining to persons who survive to age x (e^0_x); and (3) the proportion alive at age x who die between age x and x+1 years (q_x). Life expectation at birth is often used as a general health status measure for a population. One advantage of this measure is that it is readily understood by the general public. The survival data relate to a specific time, and it is assumed that the individuals in the table are subject throughout life to the age-specific death rates in question. Two types of life table exist:

- Current or period life tables are a summary of mortality experience over a brief period (e.g. 1-3 years), and the population data relate to the middle of that period. It represents the combined mortality experience by age of the population over the short period.

- Cohort or generation life tables describe the actual survival experience of a group, or cohort, of individuals born at about the same time. Theoretically, the mortality experiences of the persons in the cohort would be observed from their moment of birth through each consecutive age in successive calendar years until all of them die. In practice actuarial techniques are used to project future mortality based on changing patterns in the past.

Life tables are also classified according to the length of age interval in which the data are presented. A complete life table contains data for every single year of age from birth. An abridged life table contains data by intervals of 5 or 10 years of age. It should be noted that survival is cumulative, for example, the value of l_{40}, survivorship by age 40, is determined by the cumulative age specific death rates for all ages below 40.

A basic assumption that is made in constructing the life table is that the death rates used are applicable throughout the period. If there is significant in- or out-migration of healthy or unhealthy individuals this could affect the interpretation of the life table. Life tables for England and Wales are described in detail elsewhere (Devis, 1990).

2.4.9 Potential years of life lost (PYLL)

A measure of the relative impact of various diseases on premature mortality. PYLL highlights the loss to society as a result of early deaths (for example, below age 65 or 75). The figure is the sum, over all persons dying from that cause, of the years that those persons would have lived had they survived to the stated age (e.g. 65).

2.4.10 Age-period cohort analysis

Cohort
A group of people defined by a selected attribute, in these volumes usually the period in which they were born. This is so that its characteristics can be ascertained as it enters successive time and age-periods.

Cohort analysis
The tabulation and analysis of morbidity and mortality rates in relationship to the birth cohorts of the individuals concerned.

Cohort effects (generation effects)
Variations in health status that arise from the different causal factors to which each birth cohort in the population is exposed, as the environment and society change. Each cohort is exposed to a different environment that coincides with its life span.

Cohort slopes in graphs
Figure 2.3 illustrates this technique using mortality from a cause with a strong cohort effect, namely lung cancer. Most

deaths from this cause are due to cigarette smoking, which gained in popularity during the first half of the twentieth century and reached a peak for men in the 1940s, and some 20 years later for women. Cigarette smoking has declined considerably since the 1960s (see Chapter 9). Mortality rates have been plotted against year of birth for each age-group. People born at the turn of the century would have experienced the greatest exposures to cigarette smoke, and the graph shows that these people also have the highest mortality rates in all age-groups. Amongst women, smoking became popular some 20 years later, and thus the mortality peak was delayed. Those born after 1930 have had less and less exposure, and hence for them mortality has been declining. Men and women alike started giving up cigarette smoking from the 1960s (when those who were born in the 1930s were in their 30s), and hence both men and women experienced similar falls in mortality.

Period effects

Morbidity and morbidity rates could vary as a result of changes in: the way diseases are recognised and classified by doctors; incidence of disease; efficacy of treatment; or changes in coding rules. Such changes are likely to relate to specific periods of time and to affect different generations at the same time. These effects are known as period effects.

Age-period cohort analyses

These try to disentangle the influences operating over the individual's lifetime from those operating at a specific time on all generations, such as around the date of death. Published mortality tables, for example, give rates by 5-year age-groups and year of death, and it is thus possible to calculate the period of birth (year of death minus age at death). Data can thus be plotted against period of death, period of birth or both. There is, however, an identifiability problem in trying to pin down the observed changes to one or the other, since once age of death is known, year of birth and year of death are related by a simple arithmetic formula. If there is a linear decline in mortality it would be impossible to say whether the reason was a period or cohort effect. Various statistical regression based models have been proposed in attempts to estimate the non-linear effects of period and cohort separately (Clayton and Schifflers, 1987; Lee and Lin, 1995). All these models make certain simplifying assumptions in order to produce unique parameter estimates, and these need to be checked for biological plausibility.

2.4.11 Demographic transition

The transition from high to low fertility (and mortality) rates in a country, formerly thought to be related to technological change (including improved sanitation) and industrialisation but probably more directly related to female literacy and the status of women than to any other factors (Last, 1995).

2.4.12 Dependency ratio

The ratio of children and older people in a population to all others, i.e. the proportion of those assumed to be 'economically inactive' to the 'economically active'.

2.4.13 Odds ratio

The ratio of two odds, usually used when comparing risks among cases and controls. It measures the ratio of the odds in favour of exposure among the cases, to the odds in favour of exposure among the controls.

Figure 2.3

Lung cancer mortality – birth cohorts

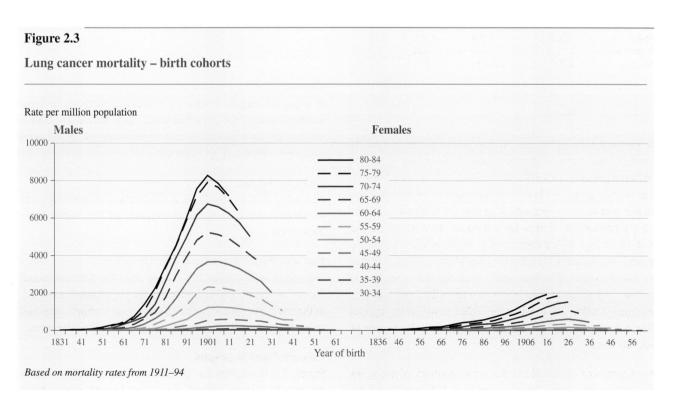

Based on mortality rates from 1911–94

2.4.14 Proportional mortality ratio (PMR)

The proportion of observed deaths from a specified condition in a defined population (e.g. an occupation), divided by the proportion of deaths expected from that condition in a standard population with that age/sex composition. The calculation is essentially the same as that for SMRs (see section 2.4.5), but the number of deaths from all causes replaces the population figures in the calculations. Thus the m_ks in the SMR formula become the proportion of all deaths in the reference population that are due to a specified condition in the PMR formula, and the number of deaths from all causes in the study population become the p_ks. Note that in any segment of the population a high PMR is compatible with a low underlying death rate.

2.4.15 International classification of diseases

This classification of specific medical conditions and groups of conditions is determined by an internationally representative group of experts who advise the World Health Organisation (WHO), which publishes periodic revisions. The ninth revision is currently in use in Britain for mortality, but for some morbidity conditions the tenth (published 1990) is used. Every disease is assigned a code number, and in the ninth revision these are grouped into 17 chapters. In addition there is a classification of injury and poisoning by the external causes of injury, for example, type of accident or suicide.

2.4.16 Correlation

The degree to which variables change together. A correlation coefficient is a measure of that association, where plus 1 indicates a perfect positive linear relationship and minus 1 represents a perfect negative linear relationship.

2.4.17 Regression analysis

Given data on a dependent variable y and one or more independent variables x_1, x_2,..., regression analysis involves fitting the 'best' mathematical model (within some restricted class of models) to predict y from the xs. Most common in epidemiology are ordinary linear models, logistic, Poisson and proportional hazards models.

Chapter 3

Trends in all-cause mortality: 1841–1994

By
John Charlton

Summary

- In 1841 life expectancy at birth was 41 years for men and 43 for women. Of babies born, only 68 per cent of boys survived to adulthood, and 71 per cent of girls. Males aged 15 could expect a further 44 years of life, females 45 years.

- As a result of reduced mortality, the population has changed from a predominantly young one in 1841 (36 per cent aged under 15, 4 per cent 65 and over) to an older one by 1991 (19 per cent under 15, 16 per cent 65 and over).

- Improvements in survival in the nineteenth century were confined to children and young adults. Reductions in mortality began first with younger age-groups. It was only from around 1950 that life expectancy of those aged 75 and over began to improve.

- Between ages 35 and 84, female mortality has fallen more than male mortality – most of this change has occurred during the twentieth century and is in part due to lung cancer and circulatory disease mortality in men – but since the 1970s the ratio of male to female mortality at ages 60–70 has fallen from over 2 to 1.7.

- Although mortality has fallen, the actual number of deaths per year has remained relatively constant, due to population growth and postponement of death.

- Generally each birth cohort has experienced lower age-for-age mortality than the previous one. The largest changes have occurred in childhood, especially for those born between 1911 and 1951. A comparison of expectation of life based on period and cohort life tables shows that the cohort experience was better than the expectation based on mortality rates prevalent at the time.

- In the last 20 years the smallest reductions in mortality have occurred among those aged 20–35. The greatest improvements were in those aged under 10. Between ages 45 and 75 the reduction in men's mortality has exceeded that of women.

- The composition of the population will continue to change, with the proportion of older people increasing, especially at higher ages.

3.1 Introduction

This chapter describes trends in overall mortality over a 150-year period, and examines the effects that these trends had on life expectancy and population structure. The different trends for men and women are compared. 'Cohort' and 'period' effects are examined, namely, the extent to which the mortality trends are related to factors associated with the life-long experiences of different birth cohorts or generations, or with the period around the time of death. Overall mortality is clearly important to study in its own right, but to understand the reasons behind the trends (not considered in this chapter) it is also necessary to study the different diseases comprising it, each of which has different influences and trends. Chapter 4 reviews mortality trends both by broad cause grouping and some major causes of death. Chapters 6 to 14 show trends for a selection of factors that may influence mortality, such as nutrition, smoking, alcohol and drug use, household composition, environment and medical advance, by way of background material to the health trends described in this and other chapters. The chapters in Volume 2 discuss specific diseases. The figures in this chapter refer to England and Wales unless otherwise stated.

Registration of deaths in England and Wales began in 1837, when the first Registrar General appointed William Farr to prepare a statistical account of mortality. Although earlier reports described mortality, the first detailed analysis was for 1841 (Registrar General, 1843). This was a census year, and thus relatively reliable denominator data became available.

3.2 Mortality in 1841

By 1841 Britain was an industrialised society, living with the effects of migration from the country to overcrowded towns. Jenner had published his research on smallpox vaccination in 1798, and the Factory Act of 1833 had banned any employment of children under the age of nine, restricted the working hours of older children, appointed factory inspectors and made its first grant to education. Conditions for the poorer sectors of the economy were still bleak, as described by Dickens in *Hard Times*, written in 1854. In the commentary to the Registrar General's Fifth Report for 1841 William Farr presented the first English Life Table, based on 1841 mortality rates (Registrar General, 1843). He also wrote a chapter explaining the life table, invented by Halley, discoverer of the comet:

Table 3.1

Life expectancy based on 1841 mortality rates – expected further years of life

At age:	0	5	15	35	55	75
Men	41	51	44	30	17	6
Women	43	52	45	32	18	7

By this simple and elegant table the mean duration of human life, uncertain as it appears to be ... can be determined with the greatest accuracy in nations, or in still smaller communities.

Life tables were in demand by Friendly Societies who were beginning to provide guaranteed life cover for families or their members in return for regular contributions. They needed reliable estimates of how much longer people of different ages were likely to live. Farr's table was not the first, but it related to the total population for the first time, and was more accurate than its predecessors.

Table 3.1 shows how many further years of life people in England and Wales of different ages could expect to live, based on the mortality rates prevailing in 1841. Life expectancy at birth was 41 years for men and 43 for women. If the initial particularly hazardous years of infancy could be survived, life expectancy was better – at 5 years of age boys and girls could expect to live a further 51 and 52 years respectively. By the age of 15 men and women could expect a further 44 and 45 years of life. By age 75 further life expectancy was 6 and 7 years respectively. At all ages women enjoyed at least a slight advantage over men in terms of life expectancy, but there was usually less than one year's difference between men and women for a given age.

Figure 3.1 shows that out of every 100,000 born only 73,000 boys survived to age 5, and 68,000 to age 15 (this volume's definition of the start of adulthood). For girls the figures were better: 76,000 to age 5, and 71,000 to adulthood. Also shown are the improvements that have occurred up to the present day – whereas most deaths occurred in early life in 1841, deaths in childhood are now comparatively rare, with the majority of deaths occurring at older ages, making the survival curve more 'rectangular'.

Table 3.2 shows mortality by age and sex in the period 1841–45. The death rate in the first year of life was 16 per cent for

Figure 3.1

Survivorship out of 100,000, 1841–1991

At stated age – current mortality

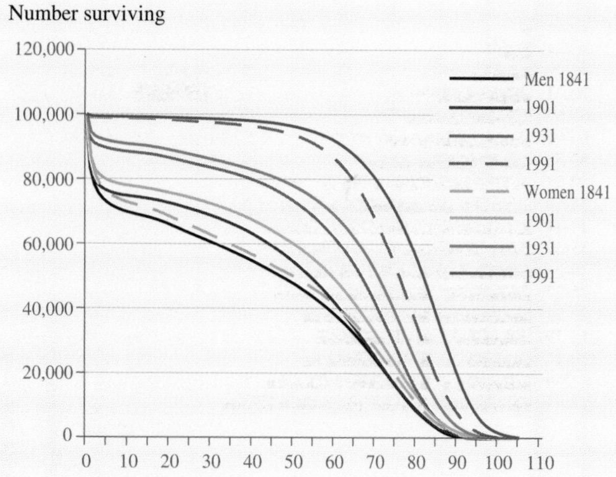

Table 3.2

Mortality rates per 10,000 population, 1841–45

Year	<1	1–4	5–14	15–24	25–34	35–44	45–54	55–64	65–74	75–84	85 & over
Male rates	1,620	332	68	79	94	122	172	303	655	1,437	3,051
Female rates	1,330	322	69	82	99	121	151	272	591	1,318	2,886
Ratio M:F rates (%)	122	103	99	96	95	101	114	111	111	109	106

Source: DH1 No 25

Figure 3.2a

Population distribution 1841, England and Wales

Standardised to a total population of one million

Total population = 15.9 million

Age

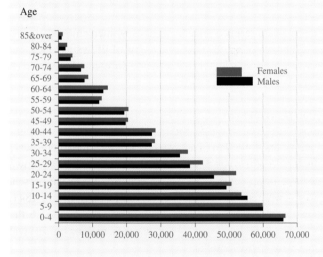

Figure 3.2b

Population distribution 1911, England and Wales

Standardised to a total population of one million

Total population = 36.1 million

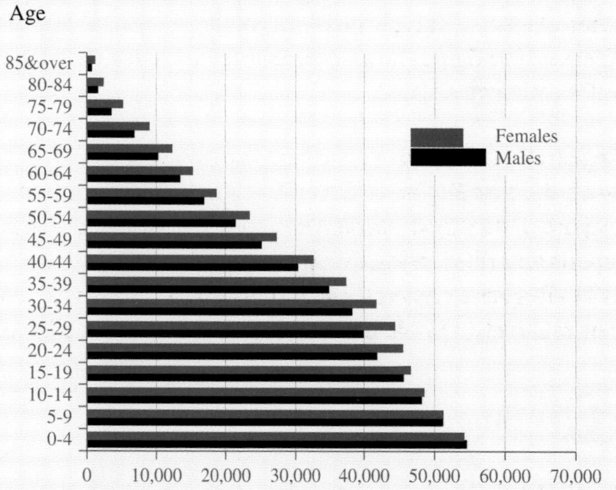

Age

Figure 3.2c

Population distribution 1951, England and Wales

Standardised to a total population of one million

Total population = 43.8 million

Age

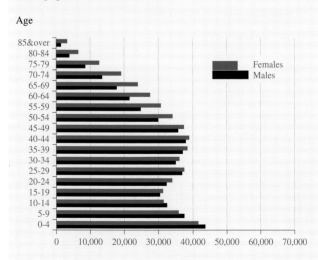

Figure 3.2d

Population distribution 1991, England and Wales

Standardised to a total population of one million

Total population = 50.9 million

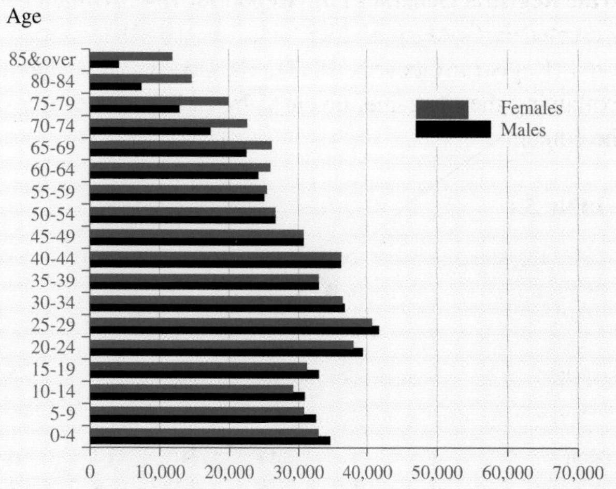

Age

boys and 13 per cent for girls. At age 1–4 this was much lower, at 3 per cent for both sexes. Death rates were at a minimum (0.7 per cent) in the age-group 5–14, thereafter rising in each successive age-group. Between ages 5 and 34 females had higher death rates than males, but otherwise male death rates were higher. These differences, and their trends, will be discussed later.

In 1841 the population was predominantly young (36 per cent were children under 15), and growing rapidly. Figure 3.2a shows the population distribution by age and sex in 1841, the result of previous high fertility and high death rates (Wrigley and Schofield, 1989). A substantial proportion of those born did not reach adulthood – 45 per cent of all deaths occurred among individuals aged under 15, and only 20 per cent among individuals aged 65 and over. It is also possible to see at a glance with this type of graph the imbalances between the sexes at different ages with, for example, relatively large deficits of men in the age range 20–34. The population were the survivors of people born during the previous 80 years or so, and the epidemics, wars, food shortages and other influences during that period, would have affected fertility, health status, and the risk of death.

3.3 Trends in life expectancy, 1841–1991, based on period mortality

Figure 3.1 showed how the proportion surviving different ages changed since 1841. Figure 3.3 shows the gains in further life expectancy for people at different ages. Immediately after 1841 life expectancy at birth decreased because mortality deteriorated during the 'hungry forties' (see Chapter 7). The improvement over the 60-year period between 1841 and 1901 was modest compared with the improvements during the twentieth century (see Table 3.3). In the nineteenth century nearly all the improvement in life expectancy was due to improvements in childhood and early adult survival. In fact life expectancy for those aged 35 and over did not improve at all until the twentieth century. It was only from around 1950 that life expectancy for those aged 75 and over began to improve. Improvements in life expectancy of women have outstripped those of men. Differences between male and female survivorship have been widening.

Although in 1841 the average expectation of life at birth was 41 for men and 43 for women nationally, there were

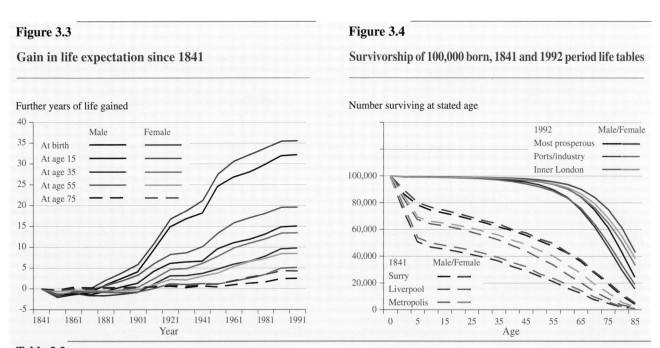

Figure 3.3

Gain in life expectation since 1841

Figure 3.4

Survivorship of 100,000 born, 1841 and 1992 period life tables

Table 3.3

Life expectancy at stated age, England and Wales

Expected further years of life

At ages:	0		5		15		35		55		75	
Year	M	F	M	F	M	F	M	F	M	F	M	F
1841	41	43	51	52	44	45	30	32	17	18	6	7
1901	45	49	54	56	46	48	29	32	16	18	6	7
1931	58	62	60	62	51	54	33	36	18	20	6	7
1961	68	74	65	71	55	61	36	41	19	23	7	9
1991	73	79	69	74	59	65	40	45	22	26	9	11

considerable variations between different parts of the country. William Farr produced life tables for Liverpool, Surrey and the Metropolis (London) to show the stark variations that existed in 1841 (Registrar General, 1843). He believed that if some parts of the country could achieve lower death rates then all other parts should aspire to these lower rates – anything higher must be avoidable. Average life expectation at birth was 45 in Surrey, 26 in Liverpool and 37 in the Metropolis. In Surrey, men and women aged 15 could expect to live a further 45 years. In Liverpool the figures for men and women were 37 and 38 years, respectively, and in the Metropolis 40 and 43, respectively. In Liverpool only 47 per cent of babies survived to age 15, whereas in Surrey 73 per cent did, and in the Metropolis 64 per cent did. Differences in survivorship are shown in Figure 3.4, which also shows variation by type of local authority for 1992 (Charlton, 1996). The pecking order of the three types of local authority areas was the same in 1992 as in Farr's day, but the degree of variation below age 65 was much less by 1992. However, the difference by age 85 between men in ports and industry and

women in most prosperous areas, was as great as the difference in 1841 between 5-year-old girls in Surrey and boys in Liverpool. In relative terms there is even greater variation at advanced ages.

3.4 Trends in mortality 1841–1994 by age-group

Figures 3.5–3.8 and Table 3.4 show the trends in mortality rates per 10,000 population for different age-groups and by sex, and the changes that have occurred in the ratio of male to female death rates – the mortality disadvantage of males relative to females.

Immediately after 1841, mortality levels actually rose slightly; thereafter death rates began to fall. Generally, declines in mortality began earlier for females than males, and the fall commenced at different times for different age-groups, starting with ages 5–24 from around 1860. From the early 1880s

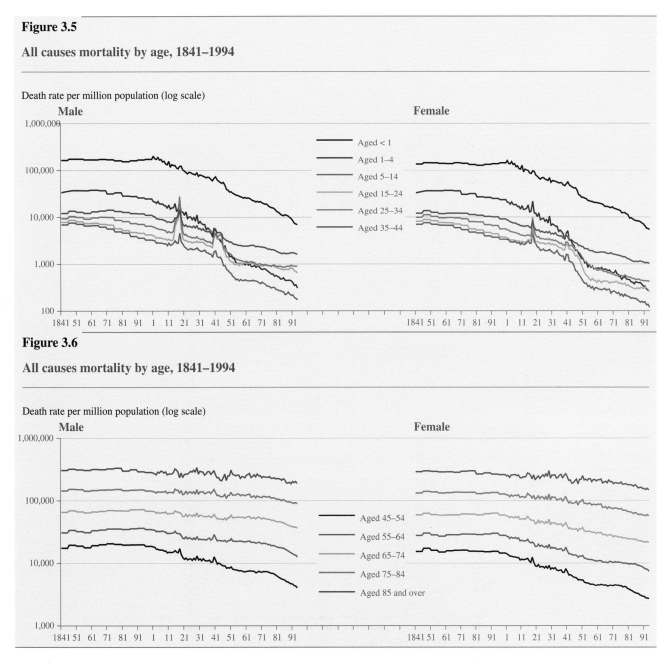

Figure 3.5

All causes mortality by age, 1841–1994

Death rate per million population (log scale)

Male / Female

Aged < 1
Aged 1–4
Aged 5–14
Aged 15–24
Aged 25–34
Aged 35–44

Figure 3.6

All causes mortality by age, 1841–1994

Death rate per million population (log scale)

Male / Female

Aged 45–54
Aged 55–64
Aged 65–74
Aged 75–84
Aged 85 and over

mortality in the two adjacent age-groups, 1–4 and 25–34, began to fall (some 10 years earlier for females), followed by falls in mortality at ages 35–44 from the early 1890s onwards (again some 10 years earlier for females). These staged declines suggest that for those above age 15 there was a generation (or cohort) effect. Above age 45 mortality rates rose during the nineteenth century apart from a slight fall among ages 85 and over.

In all age-groups apart from the oldest and youngest there were peaks during the two World Wars. This was due in part to influenza epidemics, but also because the wartime rates refer to the civilian population, and this population was depleted of healthy individuals.

Infant death rates began to fall steadily only from the beginning of the twentieth century. There was a marked

acceleration in the decline immediately after the Second World War, and since 1970 the rate of improvement has accelerated again. These death rates have fallen from around 150 per thousand in 1841–45 to under 7 in 1991–94 (Table 3.4). For ages 1–14 mortality fell particularly sharply during the 1950s and since the 1970s. The marked improvement during and immediately after the Second World War may be associated with better nutrition, the use of antibiotics, or other improvements in social conditions (see Chapters 6, 7, 11 and 14).

Those aged 15–34 were the most severely affected by the 1918 influenza epidemic and the two World Wars. Men, and to a lesser extent women aged 15–34 suffered a setback in the early 1930s, the time of the 'Great Depression'. The 1947 influenza epidemic did not have much impact on ages 15–64. There was an accelerated fall in mortality after the Second World War. Since the 1980s there has been little further improvement in mortality among men aged 25–34, although rates for women have continued to decline. The mortality decline among ages 15–24 also stagnated during the 1980s, but the most recent data for 1991–94, show that the decline has now recommenced. However there has still been very little improvement for men aged 20–24.

Mortality among ages between 35 to 44 has not declined as sharply as in the younger age-groups – the decline that began in the 1890s began to reverse in the late 1950s, rose to a small peak in the 1960s, and then fell again to reach a plateau in the 1990s. The most recent data suggest that mortality may again have started to decline.

At ages 45 and above (Figure 3.6) mortality in 1901 was similar to that of 1841. Reductions in mortality began first with the younger age-groups. Ages 45–54 saw reductions from the beginning of the century, a plateau during the 1960s until the mid-1970s, and a continuous decline since. Mortality in ages 55–74 began to decline in the 1920s. The major decline in mortality above age 74 began around the time of the Second World War, the greatest declines in all these older age-groups

Figure 3.7

Male:female mortality sex ratios, ages 0–44, England and Wales, 1841–1994

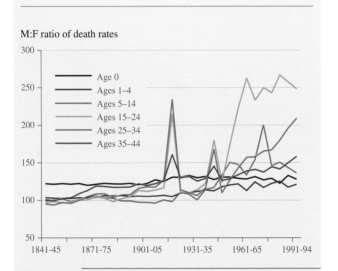

Figure 3.8

Male:female mortality sex ratios, ages 45 and over, England and Wales 1841–1994

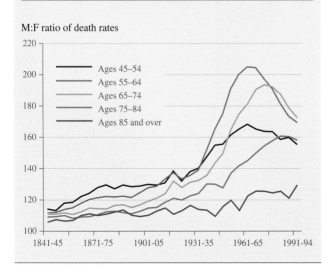

Figure 3.9

The ratio of male:female death rates

Table 3.4

Trends in mortality, 1841–1994

Rates per 10,000 population

Year	<1	1–4	5–14	15–19	20–24	25–34	Age 35–44	45–54	55–64	65–74	75–84	85&over
Males												
1841–45	1,620	332	68	68	90	94	122	172	303	655	1,437	3,051
1851–55	1,720	365	70	70	92	100	129	186	316	667	1,509	3,109
1861–65	1,660	373	66	64	87	98	132	189	328	664	1,459	3,166
1871–75	1,670	310	56	57	81	100	143	203	348	701	1,496	3,233
1881–85	1,520	279	46	45	60	82	128	193	342	688	1,454	2,979
1891–95	1,650	255	36	40	52	71	119	195	358	725	1,492	2,908
1901–05	1,510	201	29	35	47	59	97	170	324	653	1,376	2,746
1911–15	1,210	167	28	31	38	52	82	149	302	641	1,392	2,816
1921–25	860	106	22	28	36	41	65	116	249	582	1,355	2,727
1931–35	700	69	18	26	33	33	54	112	236	567	1,352	2,789
1941–45	560	37	14	29	56	42	48	99	231	517	1,216	2,261
1951–55	300	12	6	9	14	14	27	79	225	546	1,267	2,659
1961–65	230	9	4	9	11	11	25	74	217	540	1,213	2,532
1971–75	190	7	4	9	9	10	22	72	201	511	1,151	2,371
1981–85	110	5	3	8	8	9	17	57	174	452	1,035	2,208
1991–94	74	4	2	6	8	9	17	43	132	373	914	1,966
Females												
1841–45	1,330	322	69	77	86	99	121	151	272	591	1,318	2,886
1851–55	1,410	357	69	78	89	103	126	158	278	597	1,372	2,921
1861–65	1,360	362	66	69	82	98	121	155	279	591	1,338	2,879
1871–75	1,380	299	53	59	74	92	120	159	287	613	1,353	2,939
1881–85	1,250	264	45	47	59	79	109	152	281	591	1,290	2,655
1891–95	1,350	244	37	40	48	66	101	152	295	630	1,343	2,640
1901–05	1,240	192	30	32	38	50	81	131	254	548	1,199	2,494
1911–15	970	157	28	27	33	41	65	114	227	517	1,175	2,454
1921–25	660	97	20	27	32	36	50	88	187	455	1,129	2,412
1931–35	540	62	18	24	29	31	43	80	170	428	1,089	2,450
1941–45	440	33	12	23	28	25	33	64	140	360	935	2,066
1951–55	230	10	4	6	9	11	21	49	118	331	924	2,220
1961–65	180	8	3	4	5	7	18	44	106	298	836	2,067
1971–75	150	6	2	4	4	6	16	44	102	264	745	1,889
1981–85	90	4	2	3	3	5	12	36	96	241	644	1,759
1991–94	58	3	1	3	3	4	11	27	78	216	578	1,518
Ratio of male to female death rates (%)												
1841–45	122	103	99	88	105	95	101	114	111	111	109	106
1851–55	122	102	101	90	103	97	102	118	114	112	110	106
1861–65	122	103	101	93	106	100	109	122	118	112	109	110
1871–75	121	104	106	97	109	109	119	128	121	114	111	110
1881–85	122	106	102	96	102	104	117	127	122	116	113	112
1891–95	122	105	99	100	108	108	118	128	121	115	111	110
1901–05	122	105	97	107	122	118	120	130	128	119	115	110
1911–15	125	106	100	112	117	127	126	131	133	124	118	115
1921–25	130	109	110	106	110	114	130	132	133	128	120	113
1931–35	130	111	100	109	114	106	126	140	139	132	124	114
1941–45	127	112	117	129	198	168	145	155	165	144	130	109
1951–55	130	120	150	138	152	127	129	161	191	165	137	120
1961–65	128	113	133	238	215	157	139	168	205	181	145	122
1971–75	127	117	200	233	221	165	138	164	197	194	154	126
1981–85	122	125	150	254	239	180	142	158	181	188	161	126
1991–94	128	121	136	222	261	209	158	155	169	173	158	130

Source: DH1 No 25

having occurred since the 1970s. Mortality rates in the oldest ages have declined the least in relative terms, although because the death rates at these ages are high, the decline in *absolute* terms is greatest (Table 3.4). The difference in mortality rates between ages 45–54 and 85 and over is now greater than it was in the nineteenth century. Mortality levels of women have declined more than those of men, most of this relative improvement occurring after the Second World War. For women there was less of a plateau than for men in the post war period.

Figures 3.7 to 3.9 summarise how the differential rates of improvement affected the ratio of male to female death rates. A ratio of 150 means that male rates are 50 per cent higher than female rates. Throughout the nineteenth century there was virtually no change in the ratio of male to female mortality rates below age 35, which were similar (apart from infants). Male infant mortality has been some 25 per cent higher than

female throughout the 150-year period. The male–female mortality gap widened by 1991–94 to a ratio of 250 per cent by 1991–94 for ages 15–24, over 200 per cent for ages 25–34, and over 150 per cent for ages 35–44 (Figure 3.7). Between ages 35 and 84 female mortality fell faster than male, but male rates have subsequently been catching up (Figure 3.8), with different trends for different age-groups suggesting a cohort or generational effect (see Section 3.6). This is in part due to reductions in circulatory disease and lung cancer mortality in men (see Chapters 4, 9, 17 and 18 and Figure 2.3 of Chapter 2).

Figure 3.9 shows by single year of age the ages most affected. Male:female differences were relatively modest in 1841–43, with female mortality exceeding male mortality at most ages between 9 and 35 (Figure 3.9). At no stage was the difference between male and female mortality greater than 20 per cent.

Figure 3.10

Number of deaths, by age group, England and Wales, 1901–1991

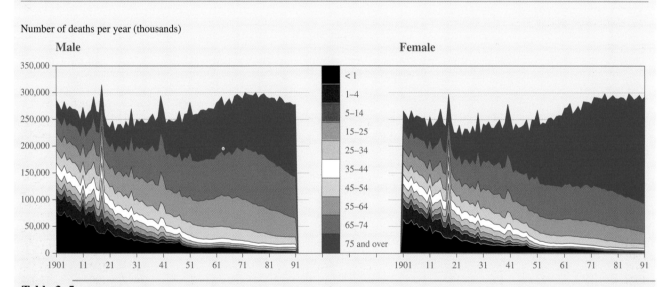

Number of deaths per year (thousands)

Table 3. 5

All cause mortality by age

Percentage of total deaths in each age group

Year	<1	1–4	5–14	15–24	25–34	35–44	45–54	55–64	65–74	75+	Total
1841	22	17	8	7	7	6	6	7	9	10	100
1881	23	14	6	5	6	7	8	10	11	10	100
1901	25	11	4	4	5	7	8	11	12	12	100
1911	22	10	4	4	5	7	9	11	15	14	100
1921	15	6	4	4	5	7	10	13	18	19	100
1931	9	4	2	4	4	6	10	16	22	24	100
1941	7	2	2	3	4	5	9	16	24	28	100
1951	4	1	1	1	2	3	8	15	27	39	100
1961	3	0	0	1	1	2	7	16	26	43	100
1971	2	0	0	1	1	2	6	15	27	45	100
1981	1	0	0	1	1	2	5	13	27	51	100
1991	1	0	0	1	1	2	4	10	23	59	100

Subsequently, peaks developed around age 18, and ages 60–70. The excess at older ages is now reducing, but the excess at younger ages continues to increase, so that men aged 18 are now three times more likely to die than women of the same age. Men are currently at 70 per cent greater risk of dying at age 65 than women – in 1971–73 they were more than twice as likely.

Figure 3.11

Population, England and Wales 1841 - 1991

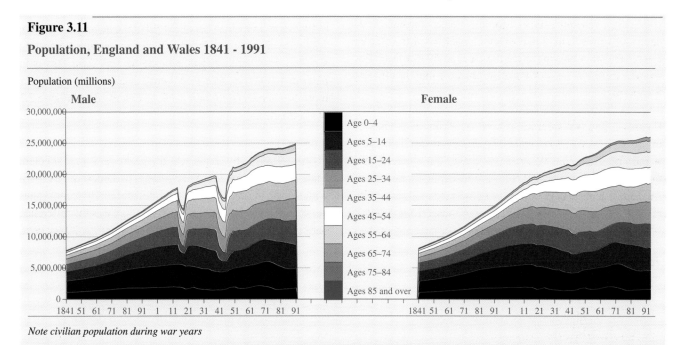

Note civilian population during war years

Table 3. 6

Population distribution and sex ratios, England and Wales, 1841–1991

Year	0–4	5–14	15–24	25–34	35–44	45–54	55–64	65–74	75–84	85&over	%	Number (thousands)
Total population (% distribution)												
1841	13	23	20	15	11	8	5	3	1	0	100	15,914
1851	13	22	19	15	11	8	6	3	1	0	100	17,928
1861	13	22	19	15	12	9	6	3	1	0	100	20,066
1871	14	23	18	15	11	9	6	3	1	0	100	22,712
1881	14	23	19	15	11	8	6	3	1	0	100	25,974
1891	12	23	19	15	11	9	6	3	1	0	100	29,003
1901	11	21	20	16	12	9	6	3	1	0	100	32,612
1911	11	20	18	16	14	10	6	4	1	0	100	36,136
1921	9	19	18	15	14	12	8	4	2	0	100	37,932
1931	8	16	17	16	14	12	9	5	2	0	100	39,988
1941	7	15	13	14	16	13	11	7	3	0	100	38,743
1951	9	14	13	15	15	14	10	7	3	0	100	43,815
1961	8	15	13	13	14	14	12	8	4	1	100	46,196
1971	8	16	14	13	12	12	12	9	4	1	100	49,152
1981	6	14	16	14	12	11	11	9	5	1	100	49,634
1991	7	12	14	16	14	11	10	9	5	2	100	50,955
Males as a percentage of the total population (%)											**All ages**	
1841	50	50	48	48	49	49	48	46	46	41	49	
1851	50	50	49	48	49	49	48	46	44	40	49	
1861	50	50	48	47	48	49	48	46	44	39	49	
1871	50	50	49	48	48	48	48	46	44	38	49	
1881	50	50	49	48	48	48	47	46	44	38	49	
1891	50	50	48	48	48	48	46	45	43	37	48	
1901	50	50	48	47	48	48	47	44	42	37	48	
1911	50	50	49	48	48	48	47	45	40	35	48	
1921	51	50	48	45	47	48	47	44	39	33	48	
1931	51	51	49	48	46	47	47	45	40	32	48	
1941	51	51	39	38	46	46	46	45	39	32	44	
1951	51	51	49	49	49	48	44	42	39	30	48	
1961	51	51	50	51	50	49	47	40	35	30	48	
1971	51	51	51	51	50	49	48	42	33	26	49	
1981	51	51	51	50	50	50	48	44	35	23	49	
1991	51	51	51	50	50	50	49	45	37	26	49	

3.5 Numbers of deaths

The actual number of deaths per year has remained fairly constant over the course of the years, as Figure 3.10 for period 1901–1991 shows. This is a result of the combination of population growth and postponement of death. There has been a marked shift in the distribution of age at death from younger to older age-groups. The changes between 1841 and 1901 were more modest than the changes occurring in the twentieth century. In 1841, 45 per cent of deaths occurred below age 15, and 20 per cent above age 64, compared with 40 and 24 per cent in 1901 and 1 and 82 per cent in 1991 (Figure 3.10 and Table 3.5). In 1901, deaths in the first year of life accounted for a quarter of all deaths, and those aged 75 and over accounted for only 12 per cent, whereas by 1991 the under ones accounted for less than 1 per cent of deaths, while those 75 and over accounted for 59 per cent.

3.6 Effect of mortality trends on population make-up

Figures 3.2 a–d and Table 3.6 show how, as a result of changes in birth rates, death rates, and migration into and out of the country, the age–distribution of England and Wales has changed. In all four graphs the size of the total population has been scaled to one million so that the different distributions can be more readily compared. The population had been growing rapidly: 2.8 million in 1541; 8.6 million in 1800; 16 million in 1841 (Wrigley and Schofield, 1989). It has continued to grow over the period 1841–1991, apart from reduced figures during the two World Wars, to 51 million by 1991 (Figure 3.11). The rate of growth has slowed down in the last 20 years. During this period the number of 0–4s has remained practically constant – the growth in population has come about largely through people living longer. Changing birth and migration rates have also affected the proportion of individuals in each age-group. Thus in 1841, 36 per cent of the population were under the age of 15, in spite of high childhood mortality rates, and a mere 4 per cent were over the age of 65, but by 1991 the number of children had fallen to 19 per cent of the population, while those 65 and over comprised 16 per cent of the population. Table 3.6 also shows the proportion of the population that is male, for each age-group. Largely because the mortality rates for women have fallen faster than those for men, the percentage of men in the 75-plus age-group has fallen from 45 to 35 per cent, and in the 85-plus group from 41 to 26 per cent. Other contributing factors include emigration/immigration and the effects of the Second World War.

Figure 3.12 shows the trends in crude mortality rates and also in rates that have been adjusted for the changing distribution of the population, by calculating what the death rate would be if the age-distribution of the population had not changed over the period (using the European standard population, and the 'direct' method – see Chapter 2). The crude death rate

---

Figure 3.12

Crude and age standardised death rates, England and Wales, 1901–91

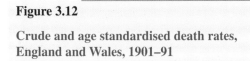

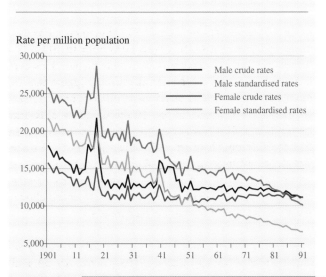

Figure 3.13

Male cohort mortality rates, year of birth, 1841–1981

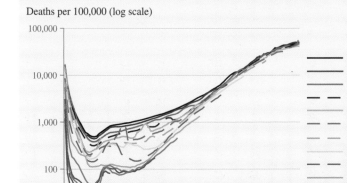

Figure 3.14

Female cohort mortality rates, year of birth, 1841–1981

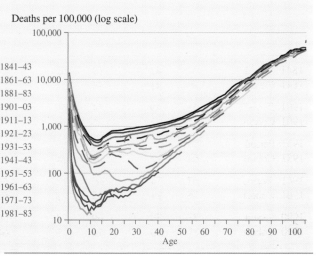

gives a false impression of trends, suggesting that there has been little reduction in mortality since 1950. This is due to the the growing proportion of the population at higher ages. Since older people have higher death rates, the crude rate under-estimates the improvements that have occurred. Because the age-distribution of the British population has varied over time, the trend data in the age-groups described here and in most other chapters have been 'age-standardised'.

3.7 Cohort mortality trends

It is often helpful to analyse mortality data by year of birth, since individuals born at the same time will be subjected to similar environmental and lifestyle influences throughout their lives. This type of analysis may shed light on possible causes of trends and suggest future trends. Figures 3.13 and 3.14 show mortality rates by birth cohort for males and females born between 1841–43 and 1981–83 respectively. For the nineteenth century birth cohorts, 20-year intervals have been plotted, whereas for the twentieth century, 10-year intervals

were chosen. Each line shows the mortality experienced by a particular birth cohort as they aged (for example, those born 1841–43). It can be seen that generally each birth cohort had lower age-for-age mortality than the previous one, although certain transient (period) effects show up, such as the 1918 influenza epidemic (affecting different birth cohorts at ages 10 years apart).

The largest changes have occurred in childhood, especially for those born between 1911 and 1951. During this period the state was taking increasing steps in providing welfare services for the less privileged and there were general improvements in the economy (see chapters 6 and 7). The 1931–33 cohort made considerable gains between ages 15 and 30 compared with those born 1921–23. The 1921–23 cohort would have been affected to a greater extent by the Second World War (Section 3.4), wheras the 1931 - 33 cohort would have been too young to be involved. The greatest gain in childhood mortality was made by the 1941 cohort. From 1951 onwards successive cohorts have made more modest gains. Around age 18, however, the pattern of improvement has not held up. For example, for men aged 18 the 1961–63 cohort had higher mortality than the 1941–43 and 1951–53 cohorts. For women mortality has also risen at this age, but to a lesser extent than for men.

In the age range between 40 and 50 the greatest gains were made by successive birth cohorts born prior to 1931–33 – subsequent improvements have been more modest. However, the most recent data for ages above 40 suggest that the mortality gap between successive birth cohorts is now widening. For example, at age 50 the mortality difference between the 1941–43 cohort and the 1931–33 cohort is greater than the difference between 1931–33 and 1921–23. Whether this degree of improvement will continue with subsequent cohorts remains to be seen. If so it could lead to a further increase in the number of elderly survivors over and above a simple forward extrapolation of past trends.

Figure 3.15 shows trends in the male/female mortality sex ratio by year of birth. In each age-group above age 54, male mortality rose relative to that of female for each successive

Figure 3.15

Trends in the M:F mortality sex ratio, cohort analysis by year of birth

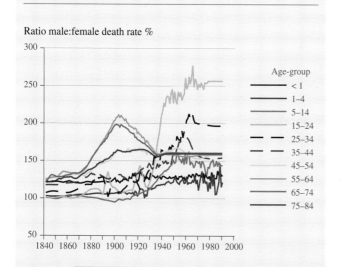

Ratio male:female death rate %

Age-group
— < 1
— 1–4
— 5–14
— 15–24
– – 25–34
– – 35–44
— 45–54
— 55–64
— 65–74
— 75–84

Table 3.7

Based on period and cohort tables, expected further years of life at ages

		0		5		15		35		55		75	
		M	F	M	F	M	F	M	F	M	F	M	F
1841	Period	41	43	51	52	44	45	30	32	17	18	6	7
1841	Cohort	40	43	49	51	43	45	29	31	16	18	6	7
1901	Period	45	49	54	56	46	48	29	32	16	18	6	7
1901	Cohort	51	57	60	66	52	58	35	42	19	25	8	10
1931	Period	58	62	60	62	51	54	33	36	18	20	6	7
1931	Cohort	68	72	68	74	59	65	41	46	23	27	10	12
1961	Period	68	74	65	71	55	61	36	41	19	23	7	9
1961	Cohort	76	81	73	78	63	68	44	49	26	30	11	13
1990	Period	73	79	69	74	59	65	40	45	22	26	9	11
1990	Cohort	77	83	74	79	64	69	45	50	26	30	11	14

birth cohort, until around 1905, since when the differences between men and women have been decreasing; this is clearly a strong cohort effect. It may be related to cigarette smoking, whose popularity increased rapidly among men from the 1890s, peaked in the 1940s to 1960s, and declined subsequently (see Chapter 9). For women, cigarette smoking began later (1920s) and peaked in the 1980s, but never achieved such high levels of consumption. The increases in the sex ratio among those aged 15–34 appears to be more of a period effect, beginning after the Second World War (compare Figures 3.7 and 3.15).

3.8 Cohort effects on life expectancy 1841–1991

Farr's life table, based on the age-specific mortality rates that prevailed at that time, is called a 'period life table'. In reality the actual mortality risks turn out to be different, since the environment, personal risk-taking and access to effective medical interventions change over time. 'Cohort life tables' can be constructed, based on the actual mortality experience of a group of people as they age. The Chester Beatty Research Institute, and subsequently the Government Actuary's Department (GAD, 1996), have reworked the original figures for the period 1841 to 1991 to provide both period life tables (based on 'current' mortality) and cohort life tables (based on the actual and projected mortality of a cohort born in that year) for single years of age (GAD, 1996 forthcoming). It is these reworked figures that are used extensively in this chapter. The more recent cohort-based life expectations have had to be based on assumptions regarding likely future mortality. Data such as that shown in Figures 3.13 and 3.14 would have informed the choice of assumptions. Past experience suggests that projection makers in Western countries have been

Figure 3.16a

Average life expectancy at birth

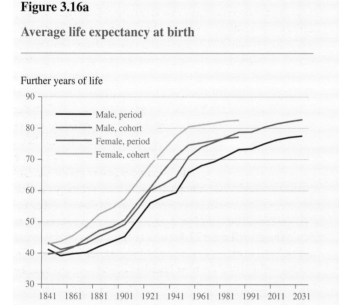

Figure 3.16b

Average life expectancy at 15

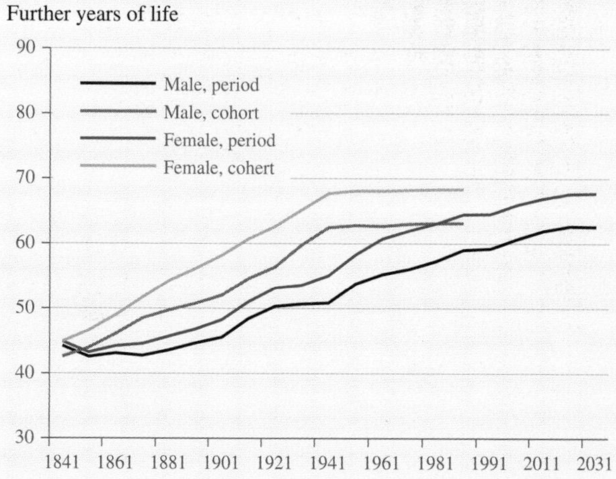

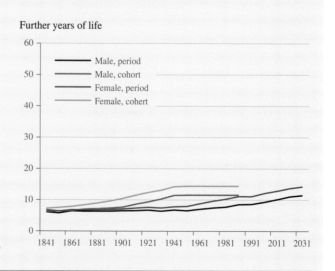

Figure 3.16c

Average life expectancy at 55

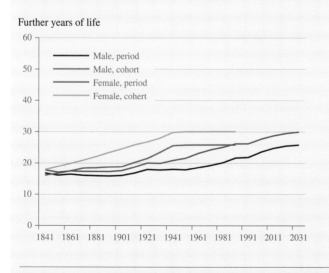

Figure 3.16d

Average life expectancy at 75

Cohort life expectancy based on GAD mortality projections for recent years. Period life expectancy projected to 2031.

overcautious in their assumptions, but projections made in the 1990s have adopted considerably more optimistic assumptions (Shaw, 1995). The period life tables, based on mortality rates prevalent at a particular time, make no assumptions about mortality rates changing in the future.

As a result of falling mortality rates, life expectancy has improved, and Figures 3.16 a–d compare improvements in life expectation at birth, and ages 15, 35, 55 and 75, based on period and cohort life tables. It can be seen that for men and women at each age, actual (cohort) experience was better than the expectation based on the mortality rates prevalent at the time, with the exception of those born in 1841. Table 3.7 summarises these differences.

Figure 3.17

Percentage change in mortality, 1991–94 compared with 1971–74

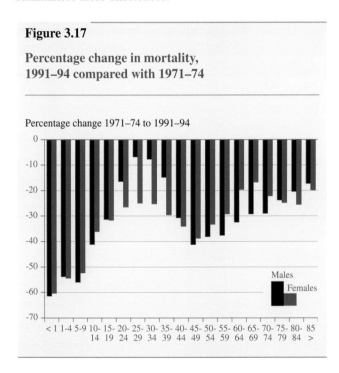

Percentage change 1971–74 to 1991–94

3.9 Recent trends: mortality in 1991 compared with 1971

Figure 3.17 summarises the changes that have occurred from 1971–74 to 1991–94. There has been least improvement in mortality rates between ages 20 and 35, and in this age-group men have fared worse than women. The greatest improvements have occurred below age 10, but there also have been substantial improvements in the age-range between 45 to 54. Between ages 45 and 74 the reduction in men's mortality has exceeded that of women. The reasons for this are discussed in Chapters 4 (Trends by cause) and 26 (Are we healthier?).

3.10 Conclusions

There have been very considerable falls in mortality, especially during the twentieth century. The trends for different age-groups have been different, and there is evidence that people born at different times have had different risks of mortality, some of which are more related to period of birth than period of death. The rate of decline continues, and it is not clear from the data if and when this decline might level off in the future. Careful analyses of reliable international data shows that the upper tail of the age-distribution of deaths has been moving steadily higher for more than a century, suggesting that there may be no limits to human longevity (Wilmoth and Lundstrom, 1996). One implication of these changes is that the composition of the population will continue to change, with the proportion of older people increasing, especially at very high ages (Chapter 27 discusses centenarians). The extent to which these older people might be a burden or a boon for society will depend on how healthy they are in old age, an issue which is discussed in some depth in Chapter 26.

Chapter 4

Trends in causes of mortality: 1841–1994 – an overview

By
John Charlton and Mike Murphy

Summary

- In the period 1848–72 the main causes of death (in order) were: infectious, respiratory, nervous, digestive and circulatory diseases. Infectious diseases accounted for one death in every three, and a third of these deaths were due to respiratory tuberculosis. Cancers formed only a small proportion of all deaths, but their rates had increased by more than threefold for men and twofold for women by 1901–10.

- During the twentieth century the decline of infectious disease mortality has been the most important cause of increased life expectation. Infectious diseases now only account for around 0.5 per cent of all deaths. The decline in respiratory disease mortality was second in importance. There have also been major declines in death rates from diseases of the digestive, genitourinary and nervous system. Counterbalancing these, there have been increases in mortality from circulatory diseases and cancers, especially in men.

- The number of deaths from cancer rose from 37,700 in 1911 to 146,000 by 1992 (from 7 to 26 per cent of all deaths). Currently the most common sites recorded on death certificates are: lung (23 per cent); colon and rectum (11 per cent); female breast (9 per cent); prostate (6 per cent); and stomach (6 per cent).

- The number of deaths from diseases of the circulatory system increased from 83,000 in 1911 (16 per cent of all deaths) to 293,000 in 1971 (52 per cent of all deaths), falling to 255,000 by 1992 (46 per cent of all deaths). Most of these deaths (57 per cent) are due to ischaemic heart disease, but 26 per cent are due to stroke. The increase in mortality has been more marked in men than in women.

- In 1992, 36 per cent of the 17,300 deaths due to injury and poisoning were due to suicide, 24 per cent to motor vehicle accidents, 20 per cent to accidental falls, 4 per cent to accidental poisoning, 3 per cent to fires, and 2 per cent each to homicides and drownings. For men these constituted 5.3 per cent of all deaths, for women 3.9.

- Although diseases of the circulatory system account for most deaths below age 65 (72 per cent of male deaths), they account for only half of the years of life lost below age 65. Accidents and suicides, on the other hand, account for only 12 per cent of male deaths below 65 but 19 per cent of years of life lost, because these deaths occur at younger ages.

- Reductions in fatalities from circulatory diseases, cancers (especially lung cancer), and injury and poisoning offer the greatest scope for increasing life expectancy in the present era.

4.1 Introduction

Chapter 3 described trends in overall mortality. This chapter examines how the different causes of death, each with their own trends, have contributed to the overall figures. The analysis gives further insights into the underlying processes behind the decline in mortality, and pointers to future trends. The major causes of death are covered in depth by other authors in this volume.

It is not easy to track trends by underlying cause over such a long period because there have been changes over time in the way causes of death have been reported, as well as improvements in the accuracy of diagnosis and reporting. The way that diseases are described and classified has also varied (see Chapter 2). In order to get round some of these difficulties we describe trends for the periods 1841–1910 and 1911–92 separately. For the earlier period we rely on the tables produced by Logan (1950). For the latter period we have matched cause data to the ICD chapters used in the ninth revision of the ICD, based on d'Espaignet *et al.* (1991), and ONS past and present coding practices.

Generally, over the period from 1841 to 1994 the number of deaths from infectious diseases declined dramatically while the number of deaths from degenerative diseases increased. Degenerative diseases may have been less well reported in the past (Gage, 1993), or have arisen through modern lifestyle (Trowell and Burkitt, 1981). They are more common now because more people survive to older ages at which such problems become manifest, but even at younger ages diseases such as heart disease have increased. Another problem in determining the causes of mortality decline is the fact that diseases may interact (Kunitz, 1983). For example, influenza may precipitate other infections, and infections can precipitate cardiovascular disease (Chapter 18), leading to death (Davenport, 1984). There also tends to be 'convergence' towards the common cardiovascular and respiratory causes of death, with conditions that are regarded as avoidable causes of death being less likely to be certified (Goldacre, 1993).

4.2 Trends in death rates by cause: 1841–1910

In this section we rely on Logan's (1950) tables. In describing death rates by cause from 1848 to 1947, Logan selected diseases and disease groups that were important causes of death, and:

> *had not undergone such great changes in classification that they could not be followed through the records, [and] which had not seriously changed their meaning or identity from the point of view of the certifying medical practitioners, and which appeared in the mortality tabulations by sex and age for the relevant periods.*

Logan's tables did not meet all the above criteria and there were some compromises. He did not spell out the constitution of each disease group, but it is clear that he followed the convention of the time in including stroke mortality in the category 'nervous system', rather than with circulatory diseases as is now current practice. Typhus and typhoid were not distinguished in the early data, nor were diphtheria and scarlet fever, so these pairs of diseases, although different, have to be taken together when comparing rates with 1901–10. He chose the periods 1848–72 and 1901–10 for comparison because the figures had previously been tabulated. His disease categories are not all-inclusive, so the death rates do not sum to the all-cause death rate.

4.2.1 Changes in crude mortality rates

Figure 4.1 shows crude death rates for the major disease groups in 1848–72 and 1901–10, and Table 4.1 compares these in greater cause detail. For all ages taken together, the order of importance of the five leading cause groups in 1848–72 was the same for both sexes: infectious, respiratory, nervous, digestive and circulatory diseases. Infectious diseases formed by far the largest group – crude rates for all ages were 7.5 per thousand for males and 7.2 for females, accounting for one death in every three. Among the infectious diseases, respiratory tuberculosis accounted for 11 per cent of all male deaths and 12 per cent of female, followed by diphtheria/scarlet fever (6 per cent of all deaths), typhus, typhoid and paratyphoid (4 per cent) and other tuberculosis (4 per cent for male and 3 per cent of female deaths). A third of infectious disease deaths were attributed to respiratory tuberculosis. Cancers formed only a small proportion of all deaths, but the rates had increased more than threefold for men and twofold for women by 1901–10.

Figure 4.1

Breakdown of crude mortality rate per million, by cause and sex

1848–72 compared with 1901–10

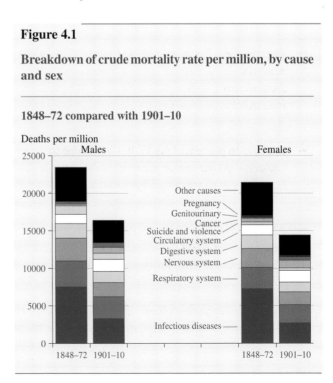

Table 4.1

**Mean annual crude death rates per million
All ages, 1848–72 and 1901–1910**

	Males		Females	
	1848–72	1901–10	1848–72	1901–10
All causes	23,448	16,373	21,418	14,404
Infectious diseases	7,517	3,282	7,232	2,703
Resp. tuberculosis	2,532	1,367	2,629	968
Other tuberculosis	900	535	690	453
Scarlet fever/diptheria	1,341	289	1,236	279
Typhus/typhoid	899	110	888	75
Smallpox	299	16	242	10
Measles	435	328	403	290
Whooping cough	471	255	553	279
Influenza	68	216	71	212
Cholera	231	0	218	-
Dysentry	81	9	68	7
Syphilis	63	58	57	43
Cancer	220	773	481	1,027
Diabetes	38	103	18	90
Diseases of the nervous system	3,029	1,909	2,502	1,702
Diseases of the circulatory system	1,254	1,606	1,351	1,578
Diseases of the respiratory system	3,469	2,917	2,864	2,409
Bronchitis	1,557	1,176	1,439	1,156
Pneumonia	1,325	1,467	994	1,056
Disease of digestive system	1,936	1,484	1,817	1,304
Diarrhoea and enteritis	1,102	874	991	713
Genitourinary system*	333	608	132	435
Nephritis	107	431	69	347
Pregnancy and childbirth etc.	-	-	217	211
Suicide and other violence	1,138	827	381	333
Other	4,552	2,967	4,441	2,702

*Note: * Excludes venereal diseases.*

Source: Logan (1950)

4.2.2 Trends by age-group and sex, 1848–72 to 1901–10

Figure 4.2 shows the proportion of total mortality due to each cause in each age-group in each period. Some of Logan's age-groups have been combined for simplicity, using direct age-standardisation and the European standard population (see Chapter 2). In 1848–72, between ages 1 and 44, infectious diseases accounted for almost three deaths out of every five. Diseases of the respiratory system were the second most important cause of death for all age/sex groups apart from men aged 15–44, where injury and poisoning was most important, accounting for 11 per cent of all deaths. For infants the most important category was 'developmental and wasting' diseases, which included prematurity, congenital anomalies, congenital debility, asphyxia, atelectasis and haemolytic disease of the newborn (27 per cent), followed by nervous system (20 per cent, mostly 'infantile convulsions'). For those aged 65 and over 'other causes' was the largest category, consisting mostly of ill-specified conditions such as 'old age'.

Table 4.2 shows, for each age-group, changes in death rates between 1848–72 and 1901–10. It also shows the percentage change for each cause, and the contribution of each cause towards the decline in overall mortality (change in each cause as a percentage of overall mortality for 1848–72). Interestingly, rates for infectious diseases in girls aged 1–14 were higher than those for boys in 1848–72 and 1901–10. The greatest declines generally occurred between ages 1 and 44, where infectious diseases were particularly important (more than 50 per cent reduction in ages 1–24, and around 40 per cent in ages 25–44). In contrast, infant mortality declined by only 18 per cent and mortality over the age of 64 by 8 per cent.

Infectious diseases made the greatest contribution to the fall in overall mortality – for example, among males aged 15–24 they accounted for some 40 per cent of the 52 per cent fall in overall mortality. Factors responsible included public health measures (Chapter 6), nutrition (Chapter 7), housing (Chapter 10) and awareness of hygiene (Chapter 14), but it is not possible with the available data to quantify the relative contribution of each.

The greater part of the decline in infectious disease mortality was due to falling rates for tuberculosis – for example, a third of the decline in infectious diseases in the under ones, and two thirds in the 15–24s (see Table 4.2). Tuberculosis primarily attacks the lungs, but can develop in other parts of the body. Non-respiratory tuberculosis (usually transmitted via cows' milk) was the most common form in the under ones. Respiratory tuberculosis is spread primarily from person to person by droplet infection – thus overcrowding and housing standards are important factors in its transmission (see Chapter 10), as is nutrition (see Chapter 7). The next most important infectious diseases in 1841 were scarlet fever and diphtheria (it has been estimated that two thirds of deaths in this group were due to scarlet fever (Logan, 1950)). Smallpox showed a considerable decline, impacting in particular on overall mortality under the age of 45. The decline in whooping cough deaths also made an important contribution to childhood mortality decline. Typhus deaths (including an unknown number of typhoid deaths) showed a very considerable decline (between 80 and 100 per cent in all age-groups). These deaths are strongly associated with insanitary living conditions. The period 1848–72 included severe cholera epidemics in 1849, 1854 and 1866, whereas during 1901–10 the death rate from cholera was practically zero (see Chapter 15). It is difficult to interpret the syphilis figures since syphilis has never been fully reported on death certificates, especially if the diagnosis was at all in doubt (Logan, 1950) – see Chapter 16.

Respiratory disease mortality hardly changed for the under ones, but declined between ages 1 and 64, more for women than for men.

Most deaths from diseases of the digestive system occurred under age one, where mortality increased by 30 per cent (mostly from enteritis). In the other age-groups there were falls of from 20 to 50 per cent. A major part of the fall was due to a reduction in deaths from diarrhoea and enteritis, which could be due to a number of different causes including gastro-intestinal infection, diet, food adulteration, or another undiagnosed condition.

Diseases of the nervous system declined more for younger people than older people – above age 64, female rates increased and male rates remained unchanged. In the 'diseases of the nervous system' category the reduction in infantile convulsions accounted for 11 per cent of the overall 18 per cent fall in infant deaths. In adults the fall was due to a reduction in deaths from cerebral haemorrhage.

Mortality for some causes rose markedly. For example, among males aged 45–64, cancer mortality rose by 246 per cent, diabetes by 183 per cent, while suicide rose by 130 per cent – the changes in these three conditions together added some 9.1 per cent to the overall mortality rate.

Cancer mortality increased in all age–groups, partly as a result of more complete certification by doctors. In adults, diabetes increased considerably, especially in older adults. Above age 44, mortality from diseases of the circulatory system, especially heart disease, rose.

Mortality from diseases of the genitourinary system rose in all age-groups under age 65, the low rates in 1848–72 being due to some extent to the fact that all deaths from dropsy were then assigned to the circulatory group, and some of this dropsy would have been renal in origin (Logan, 1950). Chronic nephritis deaths were largely due to streptococcal acute nephritis progressing, which is now uncommon.

Usually death rates due to complications of pregnancy, childbirth and the puerperal state are expressed relative to the number of live and still births, but in order to show how these deaths contributed to all-cause mortality they have been expressed here as population rates (Chapter 14 shows maternal mortality in relation to the number to births). The rates were high, and there were only modest declines; for example in age-group 25–44 from 0.62 per thousand to 0.59 (i.e. by 9 per cent). This contributed 0.5 per cent to the 45 per cent reduction in mortality among women aged 25–44.

Death rates from suicide in 1901–10 were more than double those of 1848–72, but death rates from other forms of violence had declined. Rates from injury and poisoning as a whole declined in ages 1–24 and for males aged 25–44, but increased in the other age and sex groups.

Figure 4.2

Mortality 1848–72 and 1901–10, by cause of death

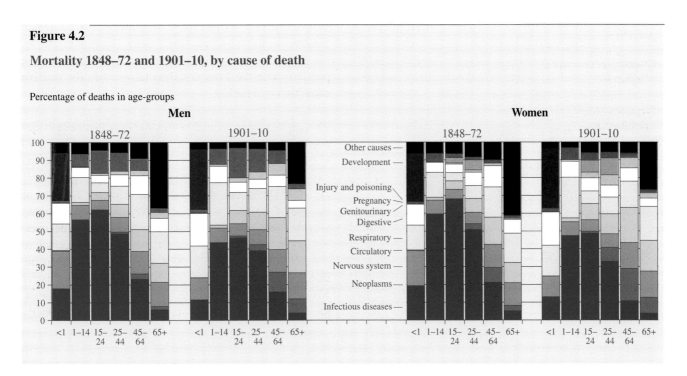

Table 4.2

Mortality rates in 1848–72, 1901–10, and changes in mortality rates for major causes of death as a percentage, and as contributions to change in all-cause mortality

Change in mortality rates for major causes of death as a percentage of all cause mortality in 1848–72

Mean annual death rates per million living

Cause	Ages <1 Males 1848–72	1901–10	%change	Contribution to % overall change*	Females 1848–72	1901–10	%change	Contribution to % overall change*
All causes	202,655	167,097	-18	-17.5	162,281	132,998	-18	-18.0
Infectious diseases	36,103	19,295	-47	-8.3	31,289	17,351	-45	-8.6
Typhus, typhoid and paratyphoid	1,010	11	-99	-0.5	841	8	-99	-0.5
Smallpox	2,035	49	-98	-1.0	1,859	59	-97	-1.1
Measles	2,877	3,249	13	0.2	2,421	2,767	14	0.2
Scarlet fever and diphtheria	4,056	606	-85	-1.7	3,178	499	-84	-1.7
Whooping cough	6,902	5,426	-21	-0.7	7,489	6,083	-19	-0.9
Influenza	486	506	4	0.0	384	366	-5	-0.0
Cholera	693	0	-100	-0.3	562	0	-100	-0.3
Dysentery	643	42	-93	-0.3	450	33	-93	-0.3
Respiratory tuberculosis	2,254	507	-78	-0.9	1,979	424	-79	-1.0
Other tuberculosis	10,661	6,287	-41	-2.2	8,045	4,941	-39	-1.9
Syphilis	1,541	1,623	5	0.0	1,319	1,324	0	0.0
Cancer	20	34	70	0.0	23	25	9	0.0
Diseases of the nervous system and sense organs	42,636	20,571	-52	-10.9	31,762	15,385	-52	-10.1
Cerebral haemorrhage, apoplexy, etc.	562	44	-92	-0.3	417	32	-92	-0.2
Infantile convulsions	40,058	16,828	-58	-11.5	29,897	12,579	-58	-10.7
Diseases of the circulatory system	809	144	-82	-0.3	690	110	-84	-0.4
Heart diseases (excluding diseases of the coronary arteries, etc.)	238	125	-47	-0.1	196	91	-54	-0.1
Diseases of the respiratory system	30,446	29,724	-2	-0.4	22,832	22,880	0	0.0
Bronchitis	11,972	13,587	13	0.8	9,192	10,650	16	0.9
Pneumonia (all forms)	16,394	14,830	-10	-0.8	12,121	11,222	-7	-0.6
Diseases of the digestive system	23,554	30,714	30	3.5	18,990	24,907	31	3.6
Diarrhoea and enteritis	20,677	26,418	28	2.8	17,171	21,745	27	2.8
Genitourinary diseases	90	329	266	0.1	54	225	317	0.1
Nephritis	32	259	709	0.1	21	191	810	0.1
Injury and poisoning	2,595	3,077	19	0.2	2,195	2,732	24	0.3
Other violence								
Accidental burns	176	176	0	0.0	174	168	-3	-0.0
Rail, road and air transport accidents	–	13	–	–	–	9	–	–
Developmental and wasting diseases	53,895	56,383	5	1.2	43,720	44,086	0	0.2

Cause	Ages 1–14** Males 1848–72	1901–10	%change	Contribution to % overall change*	Females 1848–72	1901–10	% change	Contribution to % overall change*
All causes	16,001	7,847	-51	-51.0	15,644	7,634	-51	-51.2
Infectious diseases	9,047	3,397	-62	-35.3	9,319	3,595	-61	-36.6
Typhus, typhoid and paratyphoid	962	53	-94	-5.7	1,089	59	-95	-6.6
Smallpox	397	9	-98	-2.4	391	9	-98	-2.4
Measles	1,014	859	-15	-1.0	1,019	834	-18	-1.2
Scarlet fever and diphtheria	3,438	883	-74	-16.0	3,379	914	-73	-15.8
Whooping cough	771	429	-44	-2.1	1,051	595	-43	-2.9
Influenza	29	47	65	0.1	29	46	58	0.1
Cholera	188		-100	-1.2	170		-100	-1.1
Dysentery	53	2	-96	-0.3	45	2	-96	-0.3
Respiratory tuberculosis	685	203	-70	-3.0	868	286	-67	-3.7
Other tuberculosis	1,413	852	-40	-3.5	1,165	799	-31	-2.3
Syphilis	11	11	-2	-0.0	13	11	-14	-0.0
Cancer	12	24	105	0.1	11	19	76	0.1
Diseases of the nervous system and sense organs	1,296	650	-50	-4.0	1,205	597	-50	-3.9
Cerebral haemorrhage, apoplexy, etc.	96	8	-92	-0.6	84	8	-90	-0.5
Infantile convulsions	644	164	-74	-3.0	620	154	-75	-3.0
Diseases of the circulatory system	257	128	-50	-0.8	247	163	-34	-0.5
Heart diseases (excluding diseases of the coronary arteries, etc.)	130	126	-3	-0.0	142	160	13	0.1
Diseases of the respiratory system	2,236	1,868	-16	-2.3	2,185	1,743	-20	-2.8
Bronchitis	754	428	-43	-2.0	748	422	-44	-2.1
Pneumonia (all forms)	1,258	1,253	-0	-0.0	1,227	1,157	-6	-0.5
Diseases of the digestive system	919	728	-21	-1.2	900	680	-24	-1.4
Diarrhoea and enteritis	723	497	-31	-1.4	722	476	-34	-1.6
Genitourinary diseases	66	83	26	0.1	39	75	92	0.2
Nephritis	37	76	108	0.2	25	68	169	0.3
Injury and poisoning	1,133	684	-40	-2.8	742	524	-29	-1.4
Other violence	847	449	-47	-2.5	451	300	-33	-1.0
Accidental burns	285	158	-44	-0.8	291	192	-34	-0.6
Rail, road and air transport accidents	–	76	–	–	–	31	–	–

Table 4.2 (continued)

Mean annual death rates per million living

Cause	Ages 15–24 Males 1848–72	1901–10	%change	Contribution to % overall change*	Females 1848–72	1901–10	%change	Contribution to % overall change*
All causes	7,578	3,609	-52	-52.4	7,817	3,195	-59	-59.1
Infectious diseases	4,688	1,670	-64	-39.8	5,297	1,556	-71	-47.9
Typhus, typhoid and paratyphoid	839	158	-81	-9.0	872	100	-89	-9.9
Smallpox	222	9	-96	-2.8	150	6	-96	-1.8
Measles	8	3	-63	-0.1	11	4	-64	-0.1
Scarlet fever and diphtheria	152	42	-72	-1.5	167	36	-78	-1.7
Whooping cough	1	0	-70	-0.0	2	1	-50	-0.0
Influenza	9	61	578	0.7	9	46	411	0.5
Cholera	102	0	-100	-1.3	97	0	-100	-1.2
Dysentery	20	2	-90	-0.2	15	1	-93	-0.2
Respiratory tuberculosis	3,064	1,120	-63	-25.7	3,741	1,112	-70	-33.6
Other tuberculosis	217	233	7	0.2	175	226	29	0.7
Syphilis	13	6	-54	-0.1	21	5	-76	-0.2
Cancer	22	41	86	0.3	25	33	32	0.1
Diabetes mellitus	23	41	78	0.2	13	31	138	0.2
Diseases of the nervous system and sense organs	405	247	-39	-2.1	413	209	-49	-2.6
Cerebral haemorrhage, apoplexy, etc.	101	19	-81	-1.1	109	20	-82	-1.1
Diseases of the circulatory system	332	267	-20	-0.9	374	289	-23	-1.1
Heart diseases (excluding diseases of the coronary arteries, etc.)	265	261	-2	-0.1	289	279	-3	-0.1
Diseases of the respiratory system	415	366	-12	-0.6	360	227	-37	-1.7
Bronchitis	82	22	-73	-0.8	87	20	-77	-0.9
Pneumonia (all forms)	218	308	41	1.2	169	180	7	0.1
Diseases of the digestive system	316	208	-34	-1.4	374	235	-37	-1.8
Diarrhoea and enteritis	108	28	-74	-1.1	123	27	-78	-1.2
Genitourinary diseases	80	87	9	0.1	57	103	81	0.6
Nephritis	43	79	84	0.5	34	81	138	0.6
Diseases of pregnancy, childbirth and the puerperal state	–	–	–	–	233	216	-7	-0.2
Puerperal sepsis	–	–	–	–	167	112	-33	-0.7
Injury and poisoning	978	609	-38	-4.9	172	136	-21	-0.5
Suicide	26	62	138	0.5	19	40	111	0.3
Other violence	891	436	-51	-6.0	120	67	-44	-0.7
Accidental burns	61	10	-84	-0.7	33	22	-33	-0.1
Rail, road and air transport accidents	–	101	–	1.3	–	7	–	–

Cause	Ages 25–44 Males 1848–72	1901–10	%change	Contribution to % overall change *	Females 1848–72	1901–10	%change	Contribution to % overall change *
All causes	11,415	7,161	-37	-37.3	10,891	5,959	-45	-45.3
Infectious diseases	5,559	2,795	-50	-24.2	5,538	1,960	-65	-32.9
Typhus, typhoid and paratyphoid	711	164	-77	-4.8	640	93	-85	-5.0
Smallpox	185	20	-89	-1.4	104	11	-89	-0.9
Measles	4	2	-50	-0.0	7	3	-57	-0.0
Scarlet fever and diphtheria	59	15	-75	-0.4	72	18	-75	-0.5
Whooping cough	0	0	-50	-0.0	1	0	-40	-0.0
Influenza	15	130	767	1.0	15	97	547	0.8
Cholera	217	0	-100	-1.9	220	0	-100	-2.0
Dysentery	44	10	-77	-0.3	33	5	-85	-0.3
Respiratory tuberculosis	4,088	2,180	-47	-16.7	4,241	1,508	-64	-25.1
Other tuberculosis	132	185	40	0.5	111	169	52	0.5
Syphilis	29	28	-3	-0.0	32	19	-41	-0.1
Cancer	118	244	107	1.1	359	465	30	1.0
Diabetes mellitus	46	68	48	0.2	23	56	143	0.3
Diseases of the nervous system and sense organs	937	608	-35	-2.9	690	453	-34	-2.2
Cerebral haemorrhage, apoplexy, etc.	458	137	-70	-2.8	329	143	-57	-1.7
Diseases of the circulatory system	837	698	-17	-1.2	846	674	-20	-1.6
Heart diseases (excluding diseases of the coronary arteries, etc.)	638	610	-4	-0.2	610	636	4	0.2
Diseases of the respiratory system	1,166	954	-18	-1.9	793	560	-29	-2.1
Bronchitis	383	117	-69	-2.3	321	106	-67	-2.0
Pneumonia (all forms)	462	722	56	2.3	249	389	56	1.3
Diseases of the digestive system	725	374	-48	-3.1	812	400	-51	-3.8
Diarrhoea and enteritis	141	61	-57	-0.7	201	58	-71	-1.3
Genitourinary diseases	226	288	27	0.5	137	345	152	1.9
Nephritis	121	253	109	1.2	79	246	211	1.5
Diseases of pregnancy, childbirth and the puerperal state	–	–	–	–	624	569	-9	-0.5
Puerperal sepsis	–	–	–	–	290	240	-17	-0.5
Injury and poisoning	1,194	934	-22	-2.3	178	190	7	0.1
Suicide	79	197	149	1.0	27	66	144	0.4
Other violence	1,050	585	-44	-4.1	127	96	-24	-0.3
Accidental burns	65	16	-75	-0.4	24	19	-21	-0.0
Rail, road and air transport accidents	–	136	–	–	–	9	–	–

Table 4.2 (continued)

Mean annual death rates per million living

Cause	Ages 45–64 Males 1848–72	1901–10	%change	Contribution to % overall change*	Females 1848–72	1901–10	%change	Contribution to % overall change*
All causes	23,936	22,331	-7	-6.7	20,618	17,477	-15	-15.2
Infectious diseases	5,549	3,551	-36	-8.3	4,374	1,884	-57	-12.1
Typhus, typhoid and paratyphoid	942	95	-90	-3.5	818	61	-93	-3.7
Smallpox	85	23	-73	-0.3	45	7	-84	-0.2
Measles	2	1	-50	-0.0	2	1	-50	-0.0
Scarlet fever and diphtheria	46	7	-85	-0.2	39	9	-77	-0.1
Whooping cough	0	0	-25	-0.0	1	0	-20	-0.0
Influenza	73	434	495	1.5	75	345	360	1.3
Cholera	346	0	-100	-1.4	324	0	-100	-1.6
Dysentery	93	15	-84	-0.3	90	13	-86	-0.4
Respiratory tuberculosis	3,622	2,607	-28	-4.2	2,708	1,204	-56	-7.3
Other tuberculosis	127	186	46	0.2	120	139	16	0.1
Syphilis	19	39	105	0.1	17	24	41	0.0
Cancer	715	2,473	246	7.3	1,701	3,162	86	7.1
Diabetes mellitus	92	260	183	0.7	39	221	467	0.9
Anaemia	–	148	–		–	157	–	0.8
Diseases of the nervous system and sense organs	3,014	2,824	-6	-0.8	2,665	2,539	-5	-0.6
Cerebral haemorrhage, apoplexy, etc.	2,092	1,684	-20	-1.7	1,985	1,769	-11	-1.0
Diseases of the circulatory system	2,960	4,015	36	4.4	3,167	3,457	9	1.4
Heart diseases (excluding diseases of the coronary arteries, etc.)	2,239	3,504	56	5.3	2,206	3,242	47	5.0
Diseases of the coronary arteries and angina pectoris	–	104	–	–	–	39	–	–
Diseases of the respiratory system	4,722	3,911	-17	-3.4	3,497	2,578	-26	-4.5
Bronchitis	2,410	1,490	-38	-3.8	2,152	1,294	-40	-4.2
Pneumonia (all forms)	1,037	1,911	84	3.7	535	1,026	92	2.4
Diseases of the digestive system	2,499	1,412	-43	-4.5	2,454	1,302	-47	-5.6
Diarrhoea and enteritis	458	201	-56	-1.1	468	180	-62	-1.4
Genitourinary diseases	688	1,470	114	3.3	293	1,034	253	3.6
Nephritis	263	1,195	354	3.9	149	846	468	3.4
Diseases of pregnancy, childbirth and the puerperal state	–	–	–	–	32	15	-53	-0.1
Puerperal sepsis	–	–	–	–	8	5	-38	-0.0
Injury and poisoning	1,616	1,642	2	0.1	379	427	13	0.2
Suicide	194	446	130	1.1	55	109	98	0.3
Other violence	1,368	954	-30	-1.7	275	245	-11	-0.1
Accidental burns	54	23	-57	-0.1	49	48	-2	-0.0
Rail, road and air transport accidents	–	219	–	–	–	25	–	–

Cause	Ages 65 and over Males 1848–72	1901–10	%change	Contribution to % overall change *	Females 1848–72	1901–10	%change	Contribution to % overall change *
All causes	95,625	88,135	-8	-7.8	86,269	78,312	-9	-9.2
Infectious diseases	5,725	3,561	-38	-2.3	4,455	2,933	-34	-1.8
Typhus, typhoid and paratyphoid	1,555	34	-98	-1.6	1,215	24	-98	-1.4
Smallpox	46	17	-63	-0.0	22	6	-73	-0.0
Measles	1	0	-70	-0.0	1	1	0	0.0
Scarlet fever and diphtheria	60	7	-88	-0.1	43	7	-84	-0.0
Whooping cough	1	1	0	0.0	1	2	100	0.0
Influenza	637	1,693	166	1.1	679	1,844	172	1.4
Cholera	491	0	-100	-0.5	462	0	-100	-0.5
Dysentery	344	37	-89	-0.3	309	36	-88	-0.3
Respiratory tuberculosis	1,864	1,268	-32	-0.6	1,175	638	-46	-0.6
Other tuberculosis	154	148	-4	-0.0	124	138	11	0.0
Syphilis	11	25	127	0.0	6	15	150	0.0
Cancer	1,825	7,000	284	5.4	2,548	7,026	176	5.2
Diabetes mellitus	145	728	402	0.6	44	544	1,136	0.6
Anaemia	–	–	–	–	–	187	–	–
Diseases of the nervous system and sense organs	12,941	12,884	-0	-0.1	11,078	11,511	4	0.5
Cerebral haemorrhage, apoplexy, etc.	10,784	9,815	-9	-1.0	9,620	9,193	-4	-0.5
Diseases of the circulatory system	10,189	15,793	55	5.9	9,735	13,510	39	4.4
Heart diseases (excluding diseases of the coronary arteries, etc.)	6,748	12,995	93	6.5	5,746	11,910	107	7.1
Diseases of the coronary arteries and angina pectoris	–	341	–	0.4	–	155	–	0.2
Diseases of the respiratory system	17,049	16,234	-5	-0.9	14,192	14,993	6	0.9
Bronchitis	11,155	10,405	-7	-0.8	10,244	10,447	2	0.2
Pneumonia (all forms)	2,201	4,235	92	2.1	1,521	3,343	120	2.1
Diseases of the digestive system	7,197	3,838	-47	-3.5	6,753	3,639	-46	-3.6
Diarrhoea and enteritis	2,605	930	-64	-1.8	2,479	923	-63	-1.8
Genitourinary diseases	3,145	5,680	81	2.7	544	2,307	324	2.0
Nephritis	395	2,980	654	2.7	212	1,897	795	2.0
Diseases of pregnancy, childbirth and the puerperal state	–	–	–	–	–	–	–	–
Puerperal sepsis	–	–	–	–	–	–	–	–
Injury and poisoning	2,201	2,413	10	0.2	1,426	1,439	1	0.0
Suicide	213	474	123	0.3	51	76	49	0.0
Other violence	1,881	1,557	-17	-0.3	1,095	1,131	3	0.0
Accidental burns	107	83	-22	-0.0	280	167	-40	-0.1
Rail, road and air transport accidents	–	299	–	–	–	65	–	–

The change in the number of deaths from the particular cause, divided by the number of deaths from all causes in 1848–72.
**Rates for age-group 1–14 created by standardising ages 1–4 and 5–14 to European population.*

Source: Calculations based on Logan (1950)

4.3   Trends in death rates by cause: 1911–94

4.3.1   Relative contributions of major causes of death to all-cause mortality

In order to make comparisons over time it is necessary to 'bridge' the various coding systems that have been used. We have chosen to convert historic data to their ICD 9 equivalents, and present data mostly at ICD 9 chapter level, highlighting a few important diseases as well. As a starting point in matching up codes we used the bridging adopted by the Australian Institute of Health (d'Espaignet *et al.*, 1991), and modified it to take into account practices in England and Wales. The codes used are listed in the Appendix.

Figure 4.3 shows in absolute terms (non-log scale) how changes in different causes of mortality have contributed to the overall decline. Sharp peaks in mortality occurred during the First World War, mainly affecting ages 15–44, and men more than women. Mortality and population statistics for the war periods refer to the civilian population, and therefore exclude those who died abroad, although they would be included if they were discharged on health grounds and died at home (see Chapter 2). The full height of these peaks has not been shown on the graphs because they would require a greatly extended scale – for example in 1918, mortality from all causes among men aged 15–24 was more than five times higher than the level in 1911–13. These sharp increases were

due mainly to respiratory diseases (which include influenza and pneumonia), infectious diseases, and injury and poisoning (see Table 4.3). There were major influenza epidemics in 1915 and 1918–19 (see Chapter 15).

Under the age of 65 the decline of infectious diseases was the most important cause of the decline in overall mortality between 1911 and 1992. Respiratory disease mortality, which was higher for men than for women, was second in order of importance. This declined for ages 0–14 throughout the period, and for ages 15–64 substantially since the Second World War. For older ages the major declines in respiratory diseases occurred later – for ages 65–74 in the 1970s (for men but less so for women), and ages 75 and over from 1984, when ONS reinterpreted WHO rule 3 and reassigned bronchopneumonia deaths to other causes where possible (see Chapter 2, and Chapters 12 and 20 regarding respiratory diseases). There were also important falls in death rates from diseases of the digestive, genitourinary and nervous systems, the last two disease groups particularly affecting those aged 45 and above.

Mortality from several causes rose over the period, counterbalancing the effect of falling rates for other diseases. Death rates from injury and poisoning increased in the 15-24 age-group after the Second World War, since when circulatory disease mortality for men aged 45 and above increased. Circulatory disease mortality has subsequently declined – from the 1970s below age 75, and from the 1950s for those aged 75 and over.

Figure 4.3

Mortality trends 1911–94

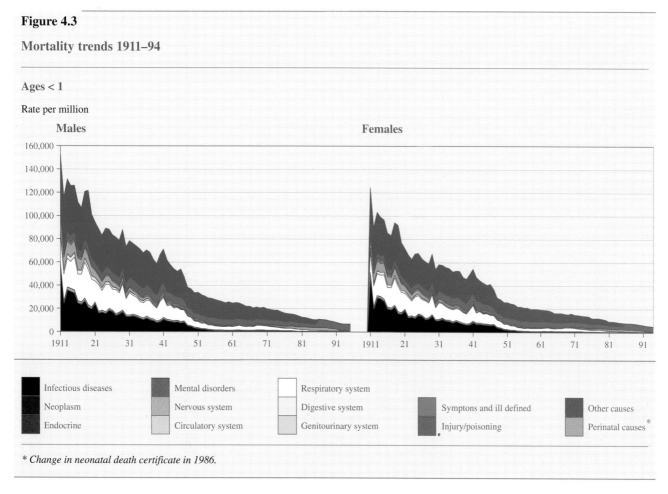

* *Change in neonatal death certificate in 1986.*

Figure 4.3 (continued)

Mortality trends 1911 – 94

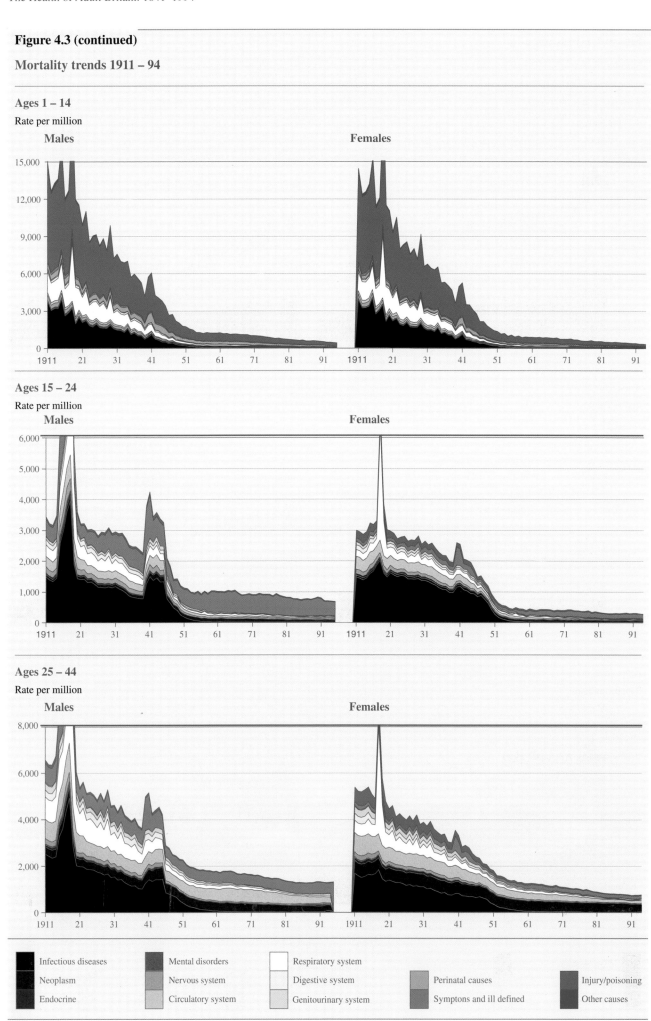

Figure 4.3 (continued)

Mortality trends 1911–94

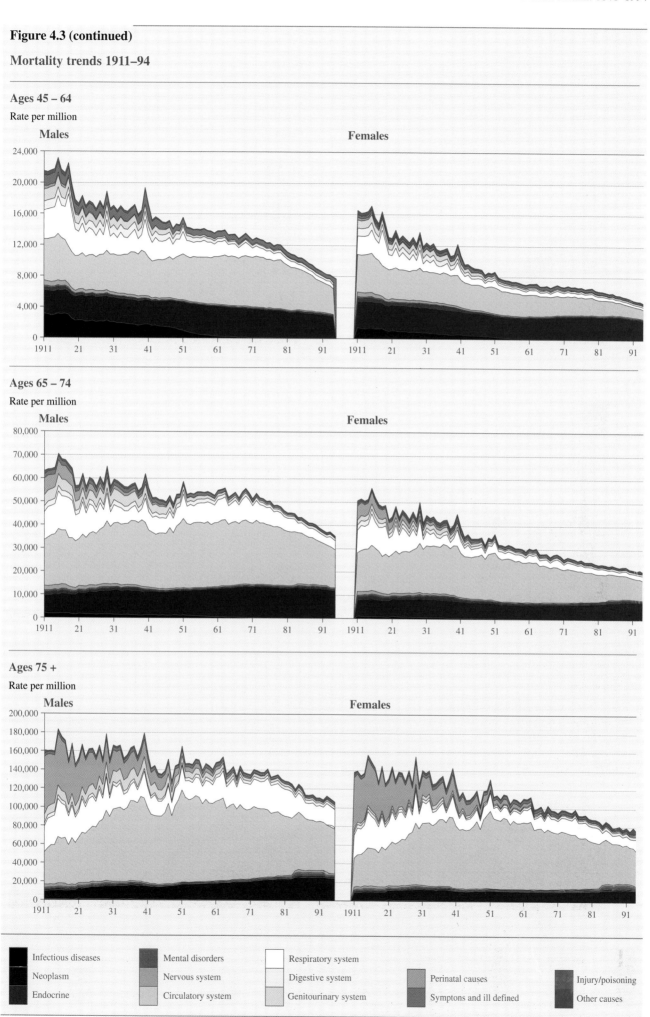

Ages 45 – 64
Rate per million

Ages 65 – 74
Rate per million

Ages 75 +
Rate per million

Table 4.3

Variations in mortality from infectious diseases, respiratory diseases, and injury and poisoning, around the time of the First World War

Year	Males 0–14	15–24	25–44	45–64	65–74	75 and over	Females 0–14	15–24	25–44	45–64	65–74	75 and over

Age-standardised mortality rates per 10,000 population

Infectious and parasitic diseases

Year	0–14	15–24	25–44	45–64	65–74	75+	0–14	15–24	25–44	45–64	65–74	75+
1912	46	14	24	31	20	11	45	14	16	13	11	7
1913	56	13	24	29	19	10	52	14	15	13	10	6
1914	55	14	24	30	19	12	52	14	15	13	10	8
1915	61	26	33	31	20	12	57	16	16	14	11	9
1916	42	30	36	30	21	12	40	17	16	13	10	8
1917	44	36	43	31	21	11	42	18	17	13	10	8
1918	50	40	49	30	20	11	48	20	18	13	10	7
1919	34	19	28	25	17	9	32	16	14	11	9	7
1920	38	14	20	22	16	9	36	15	13	10	8	6

Respiratory diseases

Year	0–14	15–24	25–44	45–64	65–74	75+	0–14	15–24	25–44	45–64	65–74	75+
1912	32	4	9	39	130	316	27	2	5	24	108	287
1913	33	4	10	39	126	304	28	2	5	24	99	273
1914	33	4	11	39	129	317	28	2	5	24	105	287
1915	42	8	15	49	163	413	34	3	6	30	136	391
1916	31	8	14	42	146	377	26	3	5	24	114	347
1917	33	10	17	43	145	347	27	3	5	22	103	315
1918	67	82	113	67	171	306	64	37	46	46	124	279
1919	45	18	35	51	158	351	37	11	17	34	121	331
1920	33	6	12	34	111	271	27	3	7	20	81	242

Injury and poisoning

Year	0–14	15–24	25–44	45–64	65–74	75+	0–14	15–24	25–44	45–64	65–74	75+
1912	6	5	8	14	18	27	4	1	2	3	8	24
1913	6	5	7	13	17	30	4	1	2	3	7	27
1914	6	6	9	14	18	27	4	1	2	4	7	26
1915	6	13	12	14	18	32	4	1	2	4	8	26
1916	6	22	17	13	20	33	4	1	2	3	8	28
1917	6	23	18	12	17	30	4	1	2	3	8	27
1918	6	30	21	11	16	26	4	1	2	3	6	22
1919	6	8	9	10	17	29	4	1	1	3	6	23
1920	5	5	6	11	16	27	3	1	1	3	6	24

Other causes

Year	0–14	15–24	25–44	45–64	65–74	75+	0–14	15–24	25–44	45–64	65–74	75+
1912	61	10	23	131	469	1,248	48	12	30	121	388	1,078
1913	65	10	23	135	476	1,261	52	12	30	123	388	1,036
1914	63	10	24	135	479	1,241	50	12	30	123	392	1,052
1915	61	17	28	138	505	1,378	48	12	29	124	406	1,142
1916	60	19	30	131	495	1,332	47	11	28	116	391	1,115
1917	55	21	33	127	495	1,325	44	11	26	111	370	1,080
1918	58	22	36	118	451	1,159	47	11	25	103	341	968
1919	62	13	26	112	448	1,295	49	10	24	101	351	1,089
1920	53	11	22	110	423	1,148	42	11	26	99	331	985

All causes

Year	0–14	15–24	25–44	45–64	65–74	75+	0–14	15–24	25–44	45–64	65–74	75+
1912	145	32	64	214	637	1,603	124	29	52	162	515	1,396
1913	160	32	64	216	639	1,604	135	29	52	162	505	1,343
1914	157	35	67	218	645	1,596	135	30	53	164	514	1,372
1915	170	63	88	232	705	1,835	143	32	54	171	562	1,568
1916	139	80	97	217	682	1,753	117	32	51	156	523	1,498
1917	139	90	112	213	677	1,712	118	33	49	149	491	1,430
1918	181	174	220	225	658	1,501	164	70	91	164	481	1,276
1919	146	58	99	198	640	1,684	122	38	58	148	488	1,450
1920	129	36	61	178	565	1,455	108	30	48	131	426	1,258

Source: ONS historic deaths database

In order to examine *relative* changes in mortality levels Figure 4.4 shows falls in age standardised rates (standardised to the old European population – see Chapter 2) on a logarithmic scale. The first year of each ICD revision is also indicated on the graphs. Data are shown for broad age-groups 15–74 and 75 and over. For completeness, Figure 4.4 also shows trends for ICD chapters which contribute relatively few deaths in ages 15–74 – these are shown on a non-log scale. Some caution needs to be taken in interpreting data for the 75 and over age-group, since it is open ended, and the tendency for people to live longer means that the average age of this group is increasing. Age standardisation does not fully adjust for this. The different revisions of the International Classification of Diseases (ICD) that were used for different years are shown in Appendix A. It can be seen from the graphs that the different revisions did not affect trends much at the ICD chapter level. However, ONS coding changes in implementing WHO rule 3 in 1984 (see Chapter 2) did reduce the figures for respiratory disease, while increasing the figures for diseases of the nervous system, mental disorders and, for ages 75 and over, diseases of the musculoskeletal system. The introduction of automatic cause coding by ONS in 1993 had effects that tended to reverse the effect of the 1984 decision, affecting, in particular, infectious diseases, endocrine and metabolic disorders, respiratory diseases, genitourinary diseases and diseases of the musculoskeletal system.

4.3.2 Trends for major disease groups by age and sex – 1911–94.

This section describes changes in mortality classified by each individual ICD 9 – chapter. Table 4.4 shows as a background the number of deaths in each ICD 9 chapter at different times, and the proportion of total deaths that these constituted. The causes of death presented in this chapter are those recorded as the underlying cause, and the concept of a single underlying cause may not be applicable to some deaths, particularly in

---

Figure 4.4

Mortality trends 1911–94

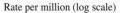

Ages 15–74 by major causes – (a) age standardised to European population

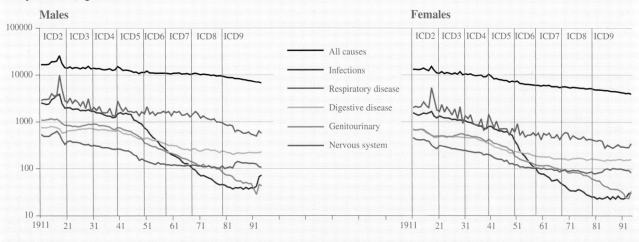

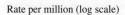

Ages 15 – 74 by major causes (b) age standardised to European population

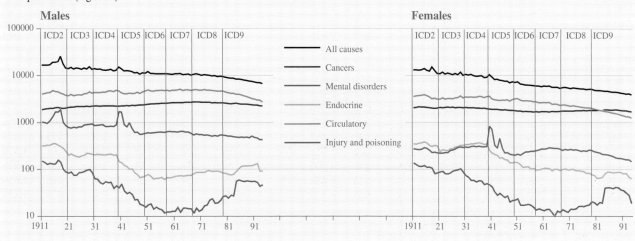

Figure 4.4 (continued)

Mortality trends 1911–94

Ages 75 and over, by major causes (a)

Rate per million (log scale)

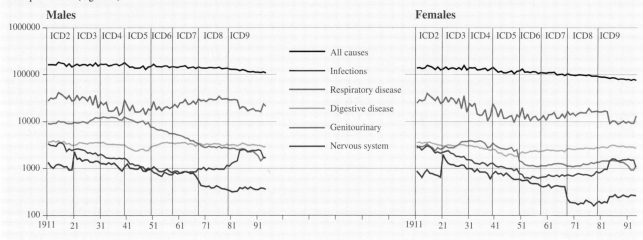

Ages 75 and over, by major causes (b)

Rate per million (log scale)

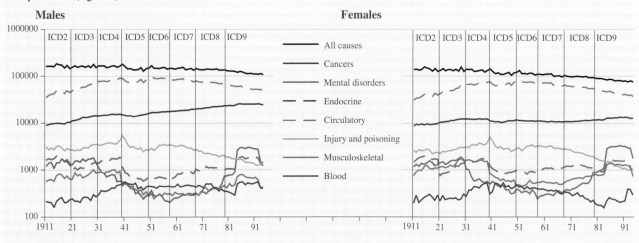

Other causes, ages 15 – 74

Rate per million

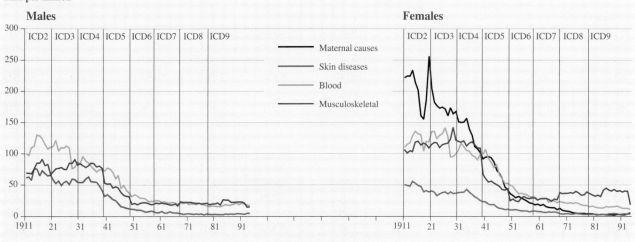

'Mortality trends - Other causes' chart on a normal scale (i.e. non-logarithmic).

Table 4.4a

Total deaths by ICD chapter, 1911-94

Year	All Causes	I Infectious diseases	II Neoplasms	III Endocrine	IV Blood	V Mental disorders	VI Nervous system	VII Circulatory system	VIII Respiratory system
Males									
1911	272,512	70,593	16,385	3,539	1,088	1,505	8,346	39,272	46,216
1931	249,717	32,677	29,660	3,200	1,267	1,032	5,649	71,875	41,731
1951	281,724	12,211	45,562	1,659	812	521	3,041	126,934	47,080
1971	288,359	1,958	63,570	2,395	680	480	3,000	142,728	42,026
1991	277,582	1,234	75,853	4,732	1,096	4,458	5,725	125,876	30,820
1994	267,555	1,913	73,792	3,383	869	2,747	4,377	116,119	37,652
Females									
1911	255,298	59,458	21,312	4,309	1,338	1,668	7,990	43,483	40,179
1931	241,913	25,876	33,801	5,602	1,701	1,491	5,180	79,001	37,601
1951	267,656	7,418	42,464	3,667	1,351	815	3,211	13,8803	37,034
1971	278,903	1,342	54,476	4,309	944	951	3,258	150,303	32,536
1991	292,462	1,172	69,502	5,806	820	9,042	6,164	135,958	32,453
1994	285,639	1,405	67,955	4,047	1,029	5,295	4,633	126,094	43,833
Persons									
1911	527,810	130,051	37,697	7,848	2,426	3,173	16,336	82,755	86,395
1931	491,630	58,553	63,461	8,802	2,968	2,523	10,829	150,876	79,332
1951	549,380	19,629	88,026	5,326	2,163	1,336	6,252	265,737	84,114
1971	567,262	3,300	118,046	6,704	1,624	1,431	6,258	293,031	74,562
1991	570,044	2,406	145,355	10,538	1,916	13,500	11,889	261,834	63,273
1994	553,194	3,318	141,747	7,430	1,898	8,042	9,010	242,213	81,485

Year	IX Digestive system	X Genito- urinary system	XI Maternal mortality	XII Skin	XIII Musculo- skeletal system	XIV Congenital anomalies	XV Perinatal period	XVI Symptoms ill defined	XVII injury and poisoning
Males									
1911	9,930	11,022	–	1,002	846	2,019	19,438	23,743	14,566
1931	10,805	14,001	–	1,006	1,495	2,199	9,803	8,744	14,573
1951	8,880	9,266	–	289	493	2,425	6,375	3690	12,486
1971	6,919	4,084	–	124	701	2,434	3,732	1,007	12,521
1991	7,923	2,964	–	242	1,294	859	1,346*	1,620	11,018
1994	8,059	3,006	–	273	850	672	–	1,922	10,246
Females									
1911	9,977	7,977	3,413	928	1,286	1,641	15,029	26,752	6,011
1931	8,806	9,370	2,601	882	2,520	1,712	6,997	11,745	7,027
1951	6,600	4,580	566	363	987	2,204	4,236	5,937	7,333
1971	7,762	3,615	133	274	1,878	2,097	2,430	2,214	10,103
1991	10,585	3,500	45	688	4,123	784	947*	3,588	6,268
1994	10,576	3,806	50	834	2,556	629	–	5,832	5,845
Persons									
1911	19,907	18,999	3,413	1,930	2,132	3,660	34,467	50,495	20,577
1931	19,611	23,371	2,601	1,888	4,015	3,911	16,800	20,489	21,600
1951	15,480	13,846	566	652	1,480	4,629	10,611	9,627	19,819
1971	14,681	7,699	133	398	2,579	4,531	6,162	3,221	22,624
1991	18,508	6,464	45	930	5,417	1,643	2,293*	5,208	17,286
1994	18,635	6,812	50	1,107	3,406	1,301	–	7,754	16,091

1985 figures for perinatal causes. Since 1986 underlying cause of death for deaths occuring in first 28 days has not been available.

Table 4.4b

Percentage of total deaths in each ICD chapter, 1911-94

Year	All causes	I Infectious diseases	II Neoplasms	III Endocrine	IV Blood	V Mental disorders	VI Nervous system	VII Circulatory system	VIII Respiratory system
Males									
1911	100.0	25.9	6.0	1.3	0.4	0.6	3.1	14.4	17.0
1931	100.0	13.1	11.9	1.3	0.5	0.4	2.3	28.8	16.7
1951	100.0	4.3	16.2	0.6	0.3	0.2	1.1	45.1	16.7
1971	100.0	0.7	22.0	0.8	0.2	0.2	1.0	49.5	14.6
1991	100.0	0.4	27.3	1.7	0.4	1.6	2.1	45.3	11.1
1994	100.0	0.7	27.6	1.3	0.3	1.0	1.6	43.4	14.1
Females									
1911	100.0	23.3	8.3	1.7	0.5	0.7	3.1	17.0	15.7
1931	100.0	10.7	14.0	2.3	0.7	0.6	2.1	32.7	15.5
1951	100.0	2.8	15.9	1.4	0.5	0.3	1.2	51.9	13.8
1971	100.0	0.5	19.5	1.5	0.3	0.3	1.2	53.9	11.7
1991	100.0	0.4	23.8	2.0	0.3	3.1	2.1	46.5	11.1
1994	100.0	0.5	23.8	1.4	0.4	1.9	1.6	44.1	15.3
Persons									
1911	100.0	24.6	7.1	1.5	0.5	0.6	3.1	15.7	16.4
1931	100.0	11.9	12.9	1.8	0.6	0.5	2.2	30.7	16.1
1951	100.0	3.6	16.0	1.0	0.4	0.2	1.1	48.4	15.3
1971	100.0	0.6	20.8	1.2	0.3	0.3	1.1	51.7	13.1
1991	100.0	0.4	25.5	1.8	0.3	2.4	2.1	45.9	11.1
1994	100.0	0.6	25.6	1.3	0.3	1.5	1.6	43.8	14.7

Year	IX Digestive system	X Genito-urinary system	XI Maternal Mortality	XII Skin	XIII Musculo-skeletal system	XIV Congenital anomalies	XV Perinatal period	XVI Symptoms ill defined	XVII Injury and poisoning
Males									
1911	3.6	4.0	–	0.4	0.3	0.7	7.1	8.7	5.3
1931	4.3	5.6	–	0.4	0.6	0.9	3.9	3.5	5.8
1951	3.2	3.3	–	0.1	0.2	0.9	2.3	1.3	4.4
1971	2.4	1.4	–	0.0	0.2	0.8	1.3 *	0.3	4.3
1991	2.9	1.1	–	0.1	0.5	0.3	0.5 *	0.6	4.0
1994	3.0	1.1	–	0.1	0.3	0.3	–	0.7	3.8
Females									
1911	3.9	3.1	1.3	0.4	0.5	0.6	5.9	10.5	2.4
1931	3.6	3.9	1.1	0.4	1.0	0.7	2.9	4.9	2.9
1951	2.5	1.7	0.2	0.1	0.4	0.8	1.6	2.2	2.7
1971	2.8	1.3	0.0	0.1	0.7	0.8	0.9 *	0.8	3.6
1991	3.6	1.2	0.0	0.2	1.4	0.3	0.3	1.2	2.1
1994	3.7	1.3	0.0	0.3	0.9	0.2	–	2.0	2.0
Persons									
1911	3.8	3.6	0.6	0.4	0.4	0.7	6.5	9.6	3.9
1931	4.0	4.8	0.5	0.4	0.8	0.8	3.4	4.2	4.4
1951	2.8	2.5	0.1	0.1	0.3	0.8	1.9	1.8	3.6
1971	2.6	1.4	0.0	0.1	0.5	0.8	1.1 *	0.6	4.0
1991	3.2	1.1	0.0	0.2	1.0	0.3	0.4	0.9	3.0
1994	3.4	1.2	0.0	0.2	0.6	0.2	–	1.4	2.9

* 1985 figures for perinatal causes. Since 1986 underlying cause of death for deaths occuring in first 28 days has not been available.

the case of older persons, where there may be multiple pathologies and less accurate diagnoses. There is considerable variability in positioning diagnoses in parts: I and II of the death certificate (Leitch, *et al., (*1987 see also Chapter 2). Thus, some caution is required in interpreting trends for those aged 75 and over. The data are presented separately for each sex in six standard age-bands, within each of which the original data for 5-year age-groups has been age-standardised to the European standard population (Chapter 2). For ICD chapters where mortality rates have been particularly high below age 1 these rates are shown separately.

Infectious and parasitic diseases

Figure 4.5 shows trends for infectious and parasitic diseases –most of the diseases that can be transmitted from one person to another, including tuberculosis, diphtheria and measles. It also includes food poisoning. Based on 1992 data the most common causes of death in this ICD chapter are: septicaemia (31 per cent); tuberculosis (16 per cent); viral infections (14 per cent); and intestinal infections (9 per cent). The following are not included in this ICD chapter: acquired immune deficiency syndrome (AIDS), through this has been included among infectious diseases from 1993 onwards; meningitis (except that meningococcal meningitis (036.0) and meningitis due to enterovirus (047) are included) and other infections of the nervous system (see nervous system); rheumatic fever (see circulatory diseases); acute respiratory infections, such as influenza and pneumonia (see respiratory system); infections of the kidney and bladder (see genitourinary system); infections following childbirth (see complications of pregnancy, childbirth and the puerperium); and infections of the skin (see diseases of the skin and subcutaneous tissue).

The number of deaths in this ICD chapter fell from 130,000 to 2,400 between 1911 and 1991. As a proportion of all deaths, deaths from infections have fallen from 25 per cent to around 0.5 per cent. Mortality differences between age-groups were

much smaller prior to 1950. Ages under 1, 15–24 and 25–44 have witnessed the sharpest declines since then – rates for oldest age-groups have declined least, but were lowest in 1911. Above age 45 mortality rates for women have fallen faster than those for men, with the result that the sex ratio (male:female mortality rates) rose from 2 to 3.5 by 1951. Male rates have subsequently fallen faster than female rates, with the result that by 1992 the ratio had reduced to 1.5. Apart from the war periods the M:F ratio for ages 25–44 drifted down from 1.5 in 1911 to 1.0 in the late 1960s, but has been rising since the mid-1970s and now stands at around 2.2. Although mortality from this ICD chapter has been falling until 1983 (2,000 deaths, 0.35 per cent), it has been rising subsequently (2,600 by 1992). The rises have occurred mainly among ages 15–44. Some of these deaths may be due to AIDS-related diseases associated with the AIDS epidemic. Although AIDS was not included with infectious diseases until 1993 some deaths from infections may be the result of an immune system weakened by AIDS.

Chapter 15 describes trends in the number of notifications and deaths for non-sexually transmitted diseases. Chapter 16 describes trends for sexually transmitted diseases, including AIDS.

Neoplasms

Neoplasms, described in Figure 4.6, involve the multiplication of abnormal cells, which may infiltrate and destroy other parts of the body, often leading to death. The most common of these in 1992 were: cancer of the lung (23 per cent); colon and rectum (11 per cent); female breast (9 per cent); prostate (6 per cent); and stomach (6 per cent). Breast cancer is the leading cancer for women (19 per cent), and lung cancer is the most common cancer among men (29 per cent).

The number of deaths rose from 37,700 in 1911 to 146,000 by 1992 (from 7 to 26 per cent of all deaths). Under the age

Figure 4.5

Mortality trends 1911–94

Infectious and parasitic diseases

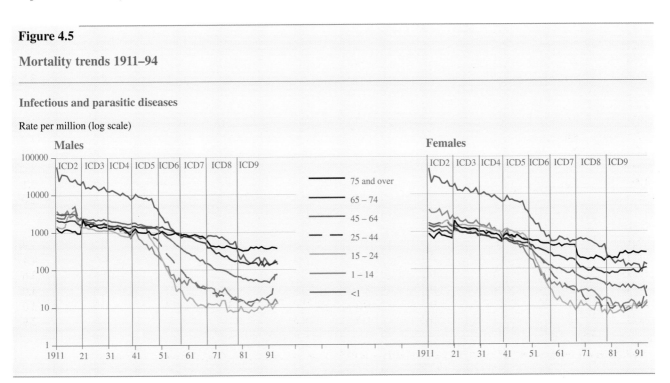

45

of 25 mortality rates rose up to the 1950s and subsequently fell. In ages 25–44 mortality for men has shown a similar pattern (but falling from the early 1940s), while rates for women fell throughout the period. In men aged 45–64 the rise was reversed in the 1960s, while at ages 65–74 this reverse occurred in the 1970s, and for those aged 75 and above rates have only recently levelled off. For women the trends have been different, with rates at older ages rising since the 1960s. In ages 25–44 mortality rates have been higher for women than for men (M:F ratio between 0.5 and 0.75) but at other ages the reverse is true. At ages 65 and over the ratio increased from 1 in 1911 to over 2 by 1970, and has since declined to 1.5, largely due to the rise and fall in lung cancer in men.

In order to understand these complex trends better it is necessary to analyse neoplasms by site. In Figure 4.7 data for 1911 to 1950, taken from McKensie, *et al.* (1957), are shown for ages 15 and above. Lung cancer has increased enormously since 1911, and has been falling for men since the late 1970s, but has only recently begun to level off for women; and cancers of the colon, rectum and stomach have been falling since the 1930s. Prostate cancer in men has been rising steadily, as has ovarian cancer in women, although the latter has now begun to fall. There have also been major changes in pancreatic and oesophageal cancer over the century. Coggan and Inskip (1994) have argued that the slowly evolving epidemic of cancer is largely attributable to cigarette smoking, which is the major cause of lung cancer. Chapter 9 reviews smoking-related deaths, and Chapter 17 describes cancer trends in detail for the most recent 25 years. Oesophageal cancer is strongly associated with alcohol consumption, the effects of which are dealt with in Chapter 8.

Figure 4.6

Mortality trends 1911–94

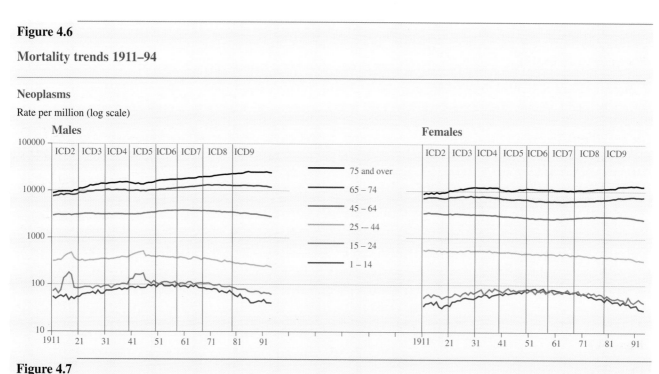

Neoplasms

Rate per million (log scale)

Figure 4.7

Cancer deaths 1911 – 94

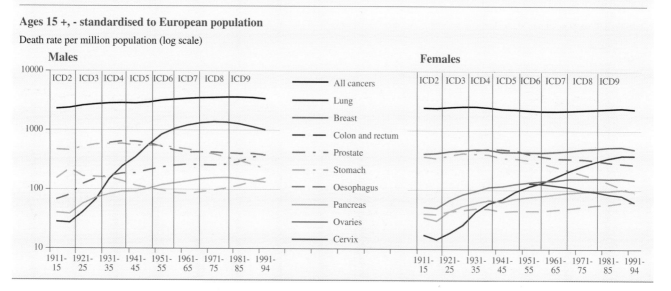

Ages 15 +, - standardised to European population

Death rate per million population (log scale)

Endocrine, nutritional and metabolic diseases, and immunity disorders

Figure 4.8 shows the trends for this ICD chapter, of which the two most important causes of death are diabetes and AIDS (until 1993 when AIDS was transferred to the infectious diseases chapter). AIDS was identified in the late 1970s and has had some impact on overall mortality trends since the early 1980s, especially for ages 25–44 (5 per cent of deaths in this ICD chapter in 1992); it is reviewed in detail in Chapter 16. The number of deaths in this ICD chapter fell from 7,800 in 1911 to 5,300 in the 1950s, rising by 1991 to 10,500 (1.5, 1.0 and 1.8 per cent of all deaths)

Diabetes mellitus (ICD250) is numerically by far the most important cause of death in this ICD chapter (76 per cent of the deaths in 1992), and Figure 4.9 shows trends since 1901. The numbers of deaths recorded as due to diabetes are likely to be underestimates because diabetes is not always recorded as the underlying cause on the death certificate, and when 'mentions' are taken into account the numbers are considerably higher (OPCS, 1988). A changed interpretation by ONS from 1984 to 1992 of WHO 'coding rule 3' increased the number of deaths attributed to diabetes, and these were reduced with the adoption of automatic cause coding in 1993 (Figure 4.9). There were peaks for younger men during the two World Wars, largely because many healthy men were removed from the civilian population, leaving a higher proportion of diabetics in the residual population. Above age

Figure 4.8

Mortality trends 1911–94

Endocrine system

Rate per million (log scale)

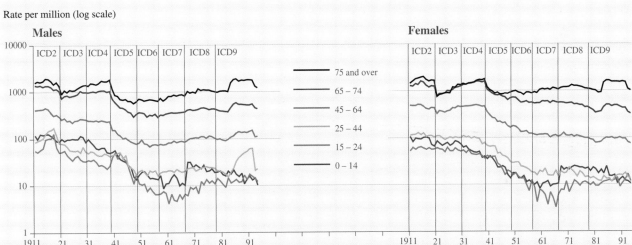

Figure 4.9

Diabetes mellitus 1901–94

Standardised to European population

Rate per million population (log scale)

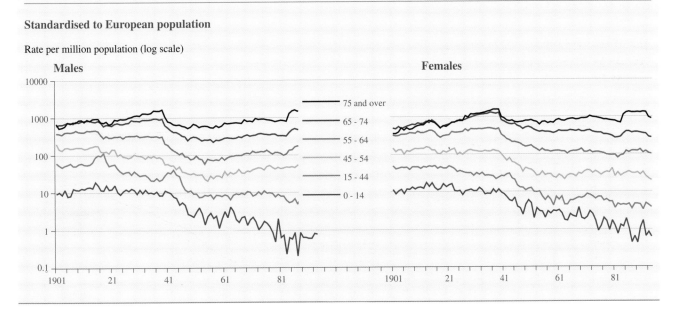

45 these trends to a large extent determine those of the entire ICD chapter. Below age 55 diabetes mortality has been falling since the 1920s, and more steeply after the Second World War. Most diabetes at younger ages is insulin-dependent (as opposed to late-onset) diabetes. Insulin was first isolated as a pancreatic extract in 1921. Slower acting insulins were introduced in the period 1936–45. Other improvements in management over the same period included better control of infections, which were particularly hazardous in diabetics, through antibiotics, sulpha drugs and penicillin (Dublin *et al.*, 1949). The advent of the National Health Service after the war made health care (hence early detection and treatment) freely available to everyone.

Diseases of the blood and blood-forming organs

This ICD chapter includes bone marrow, the spleen and other lymphoid tissue, such as the lymph nodes. In 1992 41 per cent of the deaths in this ICD chapter were due to anaemias. The diseases have disparate causes including nutrition and environment. Mortality levels changed dramatically during the Second World War, from a high plateau of around 75 per million (ages 15–74) to a lower plateau of around 25 per million during and after the war (Figure 4.4e). Part of the explanation may be due to the change from the 4th to 5th revision of the ICD, when there was a rule change for determining the underlying cause of death. They account for some 0.4 per cent of all deaths currently.

Mental disorders

This ICD chapter includes all psychiatric disorders, as well as drug abuse, drug dependency, mental retardation, and dementia (mainly at the older ages). Suicide, however, is not included – it is classified under 'Injury and poisoning' (see later). Most of the diseases are not fatal. In 1992, 92 per cent of the deaths were due to psychoses (72 per cent to senile and presenile organic psychotic conditions). The trends for mortality from mental disorders (Figure 4.10) follow a U-shaped curve for men and to a lesser extent for women, with peaks for young men during the two World Wars. In 1911 they constituted 0.6 per cent of all deaths, in 1951 0.2 per cent, and in 1991 2.4 per cent of all deaths (13,500 deaths). This ICD chapter was affected by ONS's revised interpretations of rule 3 in 1984 and 1993, especially for the older age-groups. The recent rise for young adults is in part due to rising drug-related death rates - (see Chapter 8). However, many drug-related deaths are likely to be classified in a different ICD chapter (e.g. alcoholic cardiomyopathy, accident, or suicide). In 1992, 1 per cent of this ICD chapter's deaths were attributed to alcohol dependence syndrome, and 2 per cent to drug dependence.

Diseases of the nervous system and sense organs

This ICD chapter includes diseases of the brain and spinal cord, including infections such as meningitis (although some types of meningitis are included in ICD chapter I). It does not include cerebrovascular disease. Main causes of death in 1992 were: Parkinson's disease (33 per cent); multiple sclerosis (7 per cent); epilepsy (8 per cent); cerebral degenerations such as Alzheimer's disease (17 per cent) and motor neurone disease (11 per cent); and muscular dystrophies (2 per cent). Also included are disorders of the eyes and ears, which are now seldom fatal. Mortality trends for this ICD chapter were affected by ONS's reinterpretations of rule 3 in 1984 and 1993, especially for the older ages (Figure 4.11). These deaths constituted 3.1 per cent of deaths in 1911, 1.1 per cent in 1951 and 2.1 per cent in 1992. Apart from ages 75 and over the mortality trends have been downward; one exception is for men aged 25-44, where the most recent data show a small rise. Chapter 19 covers neurological diseases including Alzheimer's disease.

Figure 4.10

Mortality trends 1911–94

Mental disorders

Rate per million (log scale)

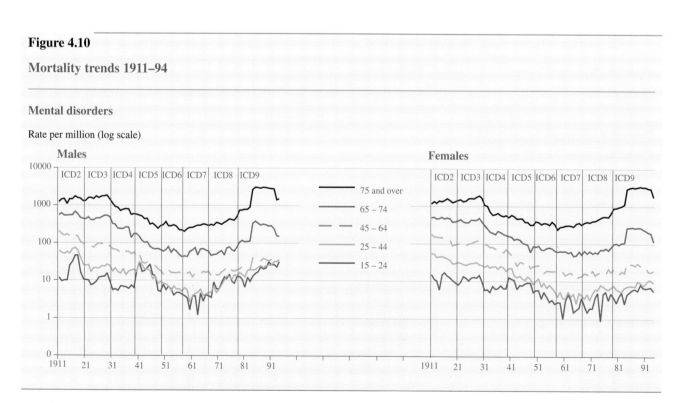

Diseases of the circulatory system

This covers diseases of the heart, arteries and veins. Rheumatic fever, which has fallen dramatically since 1911, is included. Hypertension remains a significant cause of death, particularly through strokes. Ischaemic heart disease is the most important cause of death in this group, but its importance as a cause of death was probably not fully appreciated at the beginning of the century.

Deaths from diseases of the circulatory system increased from 83,000 in 1911 (16 per cent of deaths) to 293,000 in 1971 (52 per cent of deaths), and have fallen to 255,000 by 1992 (46 per cent of deaths). The 1992 composition of this ICD chapter was: ischaemic heart disease (57 per cent); cerebrovascular disease (26 per cent); aortic aneurism (4 per cent); atherosclerosis (1 per cent); hypertensive disease (1 per cent); rheumatic fever almost entirely chronic (1 per cent). Figure 4.12a shows the trends since 1911 – these clearly show different patterns above and below age 25. The trends for those under age 25 reflect mainly changes in rheumatic fever, since ischaemic heart disease is very rare in this age-group. Differences in trends for men and women are striking. There has been a recent rise in death rates among women aged 25–44. M:F mortality ratios have increased since 1911 among ages 25–64 from less than 1.25 to 2.75 by 1992 (4.12b). For ages 65-74 the ratio has increased from a similar level to 2.0. Among those aged 75 and over there has been little change, and the ratio stands at around 1.25. Chapter 18 is devoted to cardiovascular diseases – IHD and stroke. Chapter 9 discusses the impact of smoking on these trends.

Diseases of the respiratory system

This ICD chapter includes infectious diseases such as pneumonia and influenza, as well as diseases that reflect long-term damage to the lungs such as asthma, chronic bronchitis and emphysema, and occupational diseases related to coal

Figure 4.11

Mortality trends 1911–94

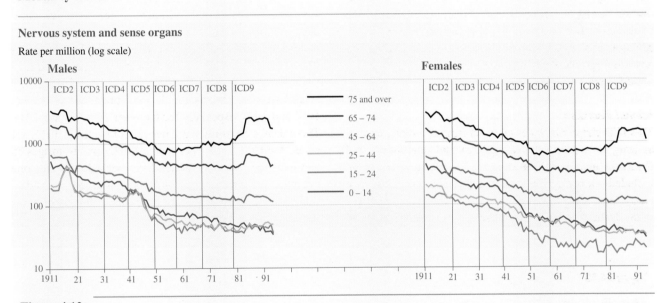

Figure 4.12a

Mortality trends 1911–94

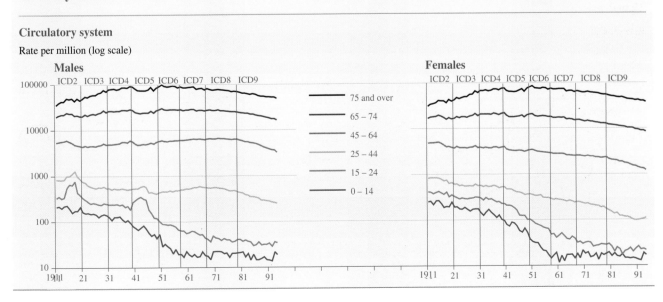

Figure 4.12b

Mortality sex ratio trends 1911–94

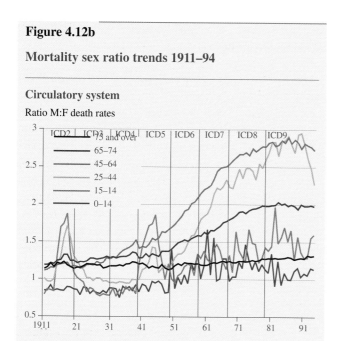

Circulatory system

Ratio M:F death rates

dust and asbestos exposure. It also includes many minor diseases such as the common cold. Deaths have declined from 16 per cent of all deaths (86,400) in 1911 to 11 per cent by 1992 (60,400), still constituting a sizeable proportion of all deaths. In 1992 pneumonia constituted 43 per cent of respiratory deaths, and chronic obstructive lung disease 47 per cent (asthma constituted 3 per cent), acute bronchitis constituted 1 per cent and influenza 0.4 per cent.

Figure 4.13 shows the trends in mortality rates since 1911. The trends at different ages are different, reflecting to some extent the different mixtures of constituent diseases at different ages. Under age 65 mortality has been falling. Ages 0–14 have experienced particularly dramatic falls from the Second World War period to the mid-1950s, and from the late 1960s onwards. Ages 15–24 reflect this first fall, but there is not quite such a sharp fall from the 1960s. In ages 25–44 rates fell, particularly after the war, but have been rising since the mid-1980s in men, and static in women. Among men aged

Figure 4.13

Mortality trends 1911–94

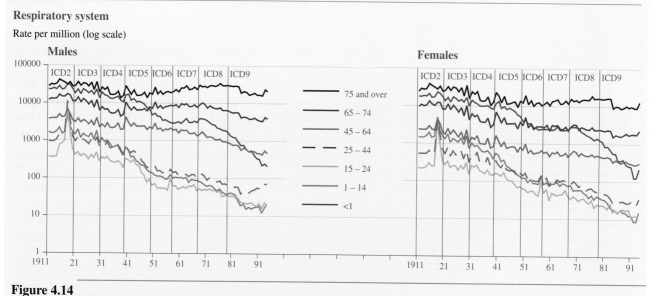

Respiratory system

Rate per million (log scale)

Figure 4.14

Influenza deaths 1901–92

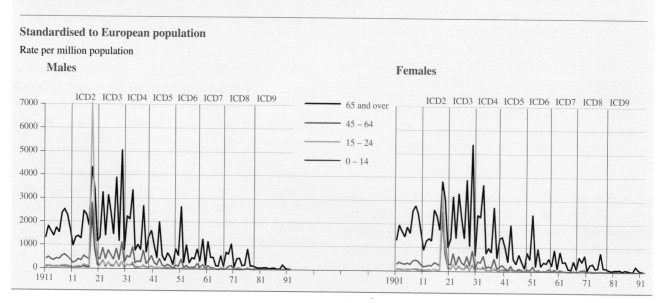

Standardised to European population

Rate per million population

65–74 death rates rose between the war and the mid-1960s, and have been falling since. The fall in ages 75 and over commenced some 10 years afterwards. The older age-groups are particularly influenced by influenza epidemics (Figure 4.14 and Chapter 13) which can affect overall mortality rates dramatically in epidemic years (note the spiky trends in Figures 4.3e and 4.3f). Unusually the 1918 influenza epidemic affected younger men (aged 15–44) more than any other group. This could reflect the fact that the healthiest young men had been removed from the civilian population as a result of the war effort, but also the fact that older men may have had previous exposure to a similar virus, and consequently had greater immunity. The general trend in influenza mortality has been downward. Above age 45 female rates for deaths due to respiratory disease have declined faster than male rates between 1931 and 1960, but since then the male rates have declined faster.

Chapter 20 covers respiratory diseases in detail. Other related chapters are 9 (smoking), 10 (housing), 7 and 8 (the environment), 15 (infectious diseases) and 5 (health service utilisation data).

Diseases of the digestive system
The diseases in this group which contributed most to mortality in 1992 were: cirrhosis of the liver (16 per cent) (related mainly to alcohol consumption – see Chapter 8); gastric and duodenal ulcers (19 per cent); enteritis and colitis (13 per cent); diverticular disease (8 per cent); and hernias (4 per cent). Deaths from diseases in this ICD chapter comprised 3.8 per cent of all deaths in 1911 (19,900 deaths) and currently comprise 3.4 per cent (18,700 deaths).

Figure 4.15 shows that there are different trends at different ages. Under age 24 there have been dramatic falls in mortality. In age-group 25–64 death rates have not fallen since the 1970s, and are now rising among ages 25–44. Part of this rise is due to rising rates of liver cirrhosis (see Chapter 9 - alcohol-related deaths). Chapter 22 discusses gastrointestinal diseases in depth.

Diseases of the genitourinary system
The majority of deaths in this ICD chapter in 1992 (39 per cent) were from kidney failure (nephritis, nephrotic syndrome and nephrosis) which has a range of causes. Chronic nephritis deaths were in the past largely due to streptococcal acute nephritis progressing, which is now uncommon – diabetes and hypertension are now the most common causes. Kidney infections accounted for a further 12 per cent, and urinary tract infections 27 per cent. Diseases in this ICD chapter comprised some 3.6 per cent of all deaths in 1911 (19,000 deaths), 2.5 per cent in 1951 and 1.0 per cent in 1992 (5,300 deaths).

Figure 4.16 shows that rates have been falling in all age-groups, although from the early 1970s to the late 1980s rates among those 75 and over did not fall and even rose for women. The greatest falls occurred after the Second World War. There was a small rise in rates from this cause from 1993 onwards due to the effects of automatic cause coding. Chapter 21 discusses kidney disease in some detail.

Complications of pregnancy, childbirth and the puerperium
The ICD chapter includes all maternal deaths related to pregnancy, from the earliest stages through to the puerperium, the period of adjustment after childbirth. In 1911 there were 3,413 deaths (1.3 per cent of all female deaths), but by 1992 there were only 45 deaths, a negligible proportion of total female deaths. Figure 4.4e shows the fall in age-standardised mortality. Since these are population death rates (i.e. not related to the number of births) there was a marked reduction during the the First World War, when few babies were born. Maternal mortality is discussed further in Chapter 14 (medical advance and iatrogenesis).

Diseases of the skin and subcutaneous tissue
The diseases in this ICD chapter include skin infections, a rare cause of death. In 1911 they comprised 0.4 per cent of all deaths (1,900 deaths), and in 1992, 0.2 per cent (907 deaths). In 1992, 27 per cent of deaths were due to infections and 59 per cent to skin ulcers. Figure 4.4e shows the trends in age-standardised rates for ages 15–74.

Diseases of the musculoskeletal system and connective tissue
Included here are inflammation and damage to joints, infections of bone, disorders of the spine, and acquired deformities of limbs and the vertebral column. These conditions cause much disability but rarely cause death. In 1911 they comprised 0.4 per cent of all deaths (2,100 deaths) and by 1992 0.2 per cent (907 deaths), where 58 per cent were due to arthropathies, 29 per cent to osteoporosis and 4 per cent dorsopathies. Figures 4.4d and e show trends in mortality from these causes, above and below the age of 75. Chapter 23 describes trends for diseases in this ICD chapter, including arthritis and rheumatism.

Congenital anomalies
Included here are structural birth anomalies such as spina bifida, cleft lip and chromosomal abnormalities such as Down's syndrome. They constituted 0.7 per cent of all deaths in 1911, 0.8 per cent of deaths in 1971 and 0.3 per cent by 1992, when 54 per cent of these deaths were due to abnormalities of the heart and circulatory system. Figure 4.4e shows trends in age-standardised death rates, which have been relatively stable over time, but were affected greatly by changes in the coding rules introduced in 1940. There has been a gradual decrease in rates since the 1950s.

Certain conditions arising in the perinatal period
The perinatal period covers labour and the first week after birth. The ICD chapter includes diseases of the unborn and newborn child other than the structural and chromosomal anomalies covered by the congenital anomalies ICD chapter. Infections specific to the perinatal period are included, as are

many conditions caused by complications of pregnancy and problems of childbirth. Deaths from this cause occur at all ages, but most commonly during the first year of life. Death rates for this underlying cause have not been available for neonatal deaths (first 27 days of life) since 1986 due to the introduction of new neonatal and stillbirth death certificates (see Chapter 2). The number of deaths have fallen from 34,500 in 1911 (6.5 per cent of all deaths) to 2,300 in 1985 (0.4 per cent of all deaths). Perinatal mortality is discussed in Chapter 14 (medical advance).

Symptoms, signs and ill-defined conditions

These are deaths whose cause could not be attributed to any of the preceding ICD chapters. Variations in death rates are thus more likely to reflect variations in diagnosis, certification and classification of cause of death than real changes in patterns of disease. To some extent they can be used as an index of the quality of death certification. In 1911 they accounted for 9.6 per cent of all deaths (50,500 deaths), by 1951, 1.8 per cent, and by 1992, 0.9 per cent (5,300 deaths). Rates vary considerably with age (Figure 4.17), with the highest rates at ages 75 and over, where they have been rising since the mid-1980s. There was an 'epidemic' of sudden infant deaths when this category was introduced into the ICD in 1969 (see trends for ages under 1), but rates have been falling since the mid-1980s. Rates at all ages fell from 1911 until the 1950s, but for ages 15–64 these have increased since then. For older age-groups rates have been increasing since the 1980s. In 1992, 81 per cent of deaths in this ICD chapter were attributed to 'senility without mention of psychosis' and 12 per cent to 'sudden death, cause uncertain'.

Figure 4.15

Mortality trends 1911–94

Digestive system

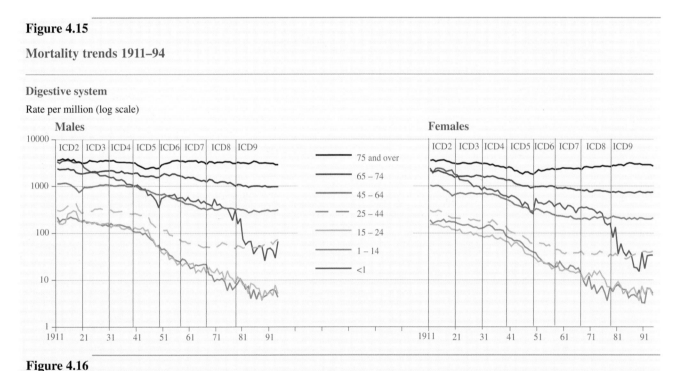

Figure 4.16

Mortality trends 1911–94

Genitourinary system

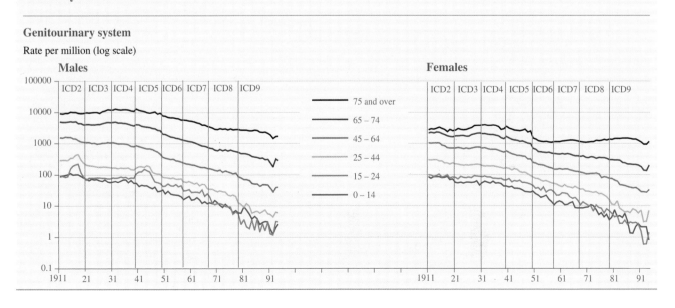

Injury and poisoning

The ICD chapter includes burns, drowning, fractures, wounds and other injuries, poisoning, and complications of medical and surgical treatment. Deaths are also classified as to whether the external cause was an accident, suicide, homicide, misadventure during treatment, injury from legal intervention or war, or undetermined whether accidentally or purposely inflicted. The ICD chapter accounted for 3.9 per cent of all deaths in 1911 (20,600 deaths), 4.4 per cent in 1931, 3.6 per cent in 1951 and 3.0 per cent in 1992 (17,300 deaths). The figures for men are higher than those for women: for men in 1911 and 1992 the percentages of all deaths that were due to injury and poisoning were 5.3 and 3.9; for women the corresponding figures were 2.4 and 2.1 per cent. In 1992, 36 per cent of these deaths were due to suicide, 24 per cent to motor vehicle traffic accidents and 20 per cent to accidental falls. Accidental poisoning accounted for 4 per cent, fires for 3 per cent, and homicide and drownings for 2 per cent each.

Figure 4.18a shows that the pattern by age has changed considerably since 1911. Mortality rates were sharply elevated during the two World Wars (in all age-groups in the Second World War). Rates for men aged 65 and over, and to a lesser extent for those aged 45–64, have fallen since the early 1940s, but rates for ages 15–24 have risen substantially, while those for ages 25–44 have also risen. Thus, what were previously very different rates among adults aged 15–74 converged by 1992. For women, on the other hand, rates in young adults showed a marked rise between the mid-1940s and the early 1960s, since when they have been falling and, although there has been some convergence of rates, the relative ranking of different age-groups has been preserved. Figure 4.18b shows the trends in mortality sex ratios and indicates a general pattern of male rates considerably exceeding those of females except for ages 75 and over.

Chapter 24 reviews trends for accidents. Suicides are another important component of this ICD chapter, particularly for young adults. Figure 4.19 shows trends in death rates for suicides plus deaths undetermined whether accidentally or purposely inflicted, a category that was introduced into the ICD in 1968. Nearly all undetermined deaths above age 15 are regarded as suicides. Suicide rates have fluctuated widely over time, and were at their highest around 1931, when rates for the oldest age-groups were considerably higher than those of the youngest. There has been a marked increase in suicide death rates in ages 15–24 since the end of the 1950s, although for women in this age-group there was a fall from the mid 1970s until the mid-1980s, following the replacement of carbon monoxide gas cooking by natural gas (gas poisoning was the principal method then used by women). Mortality among men aged 25-44 has risen since the 1950s, to a level higher than the older age-groups, which experienced declines. Suicide rates are strongly associated with mental health problems, such as depression, which in themselves are seldom fatal. Although there is no specific chapter in this book on trends in mental health, this topic is covered to some extent in several chapters of the volume: Chapters 8, 10, 25, and 26. ONS has published several reviews of suicide trends (Charlton, *et al.,* 1992; Charlton, *et al.,* 1993; Kelly, *et al.,* 1995).

4.4 The epidemiological transition 1911–94

During the twentieth century the causes of mortality have changed considerably, undergoing what Omran (1971) termed the final stage of the 'epidemiological transition'. For this transition three distinct stages were defined: (1) the age of pestilence and famine; (2) the age of receding pandemics; (3) the age of degenerative and man-made diseases. The term

---

Figure 4.17

Mortality trends 1911–94

Symptons, signs, ill defined

Rate per million (log scale)

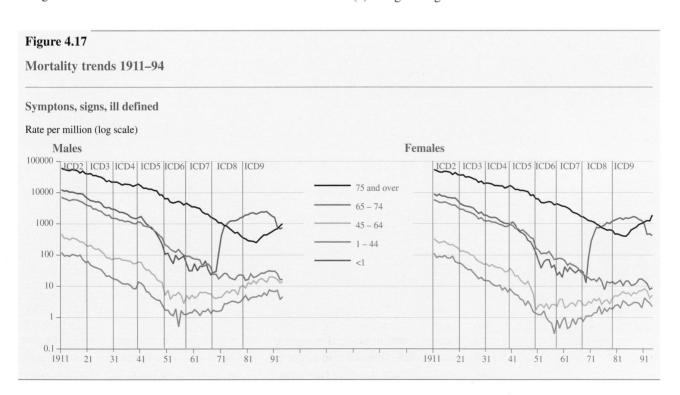

Figure 4.18a

Mortality trends 1911–94

Injury and poisoning

Rate per million (log scale)

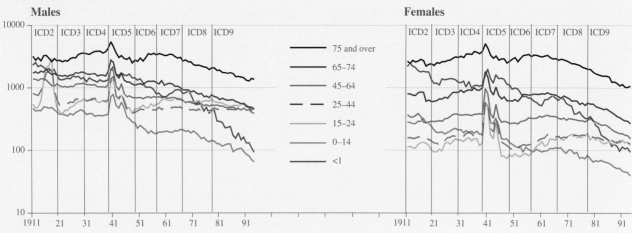

Figure 4.18b

Mortality sex ratio trends 1911–94

Injury and poisoning

Ratio M:F death rates

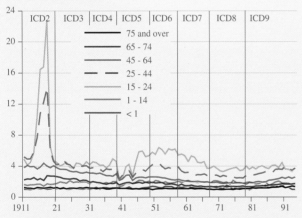

Figure 4.19

Suicide and undetermined deaths 1911–94

Standardised to European population

Rate per million population (log scale)

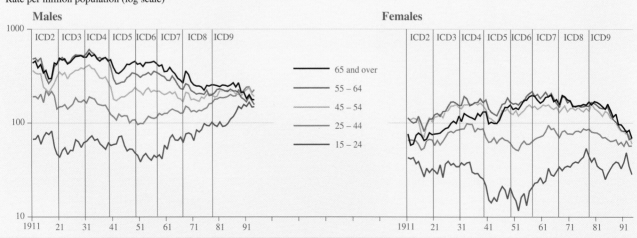

'degenerative and man made-diseases' has been criticised as misleading (Mackenbach, 1994), since cancer and cardiovascular diseases have complex aetiologies. Figure 4.20 shows the percentage breakdown of all cause mortality at different ages for males and females in 1911–15, 1951–55, and 1987–91. This shows clearly the decline in importance of infectious diseases and the increasing importance of injury and poisoning, cancers and circulatory diseases. Figure 4.21 shows the average annual number of deaths per ICD chapter (1990–92).

Table 4.5 summarises the proportion of deaths that occurred in 1992 that were due to a number of major disease groups, and their contribution to years of life lost below ages 65 and 75, which is directly related to life expectation. Thus, it can be seen, for example, that among men, diseases of the circulatory system and neoplasms account for most deaths below age 65 (72 per cent together) but only half of years of life lost below age 65. Accidents and suicides on the other hand account for only 3 per cent of deaths but 19 per cent of years of life lost below age 65, because these deaths occur at younger ages. For women they account for 10 per cent of years of life lost below age 65, still a substantial proportion. Thus, reductions in fatalities from injury and poisoning, circulatory diseases and cancers (especially lung cancer) offer the greatest scope for increasing life expectancy in the present era.

Figure 4.20

Mortality by cause and age

Male

Percentage of total deaths

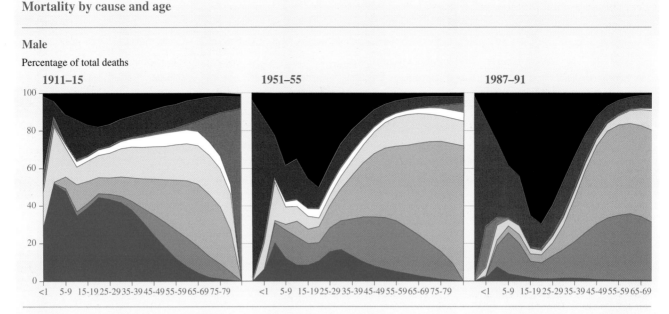

Female

Percentage of total deaths

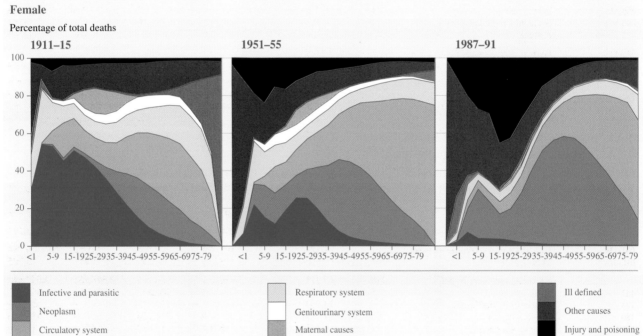

■ Infective and parasitic	▨ Respiratory system	▨ Ill defined
▨ Neoplasm	□ Genitourinary system	▨ Other causes
▨ Circulatory system	▨ Maternal causes	■ Injury and poisoning

Figure 4.21

Breakdown of average number of deaths per year, by ICD chapter, 1990–92

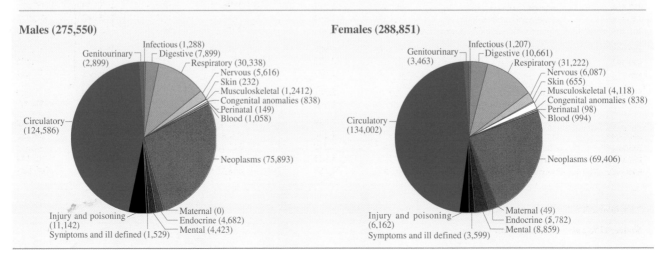

Table 4.5

Years of life lost and numbers of deaths in 1992, England and Wales

| | | Percentage of total deaths, 1992 | | Percentage of years of life lost, 1988–1992 | | | |
| | | | | Under age 65 | | Under age 75 | |
		Males	Females	Males	Females	Males	Females
	All causes	100	100	100	100	100	100
	Deaths under 28 days	1.0	0.7	6.9	8.5	6.4	7.8
001-139	Infectious and parasitic diseases	0.5	0.4	1.2	1.4	1.1	1.2
010-018	Tuberculosis	0.1	0.1	0.1	0.1	0.1	0.1
	All malignant neoplasms	28.1	24.3	22.5	37.6	24.5	37.3
162	Lung cancer	8.3	3.8	6.0	4.8	7.1	5.4
174	Cancer of female breast	–	4.8	–	10.9	–	10.0
180	Cervical cancer	–	0.6	–	2.3	–	2.0
201	Hodgkins disease	0.1	0.1	0.3	0.3	0.3	0.3
204-208	Leukaemia	0.7	0.6	1.3	1.5	1.2	1.3
250	Diabetes	1.3	1.6	0.8	0.9	0.8	1.1
345	Epilepsy	0.2	0.1	0.8	0.8	0.7	0.7
	Circulatory diseases	45.0	46.2	27.9	17.1	31.6	22.3
410-414	Ischaemic heart disease	29.1	23.3	20.6	8.8	23.2	12.3
430-438	Cerebrovascular disease	9.2	14.4	3.4	4.6	4.2	5.7
401-405, 430-438	Hypertension and CVD combined	9.7	15.1	3.8	4.9	4.6	6.1
480-486	Pneumonia	3.4	5.9	1.4	1.2	1.4	1.3
490-492	Bronchitis and emphysema	1.5	0.7	0.3	1.0	0.8	0.7
493	Asthma	0.3	0.4	0.6	0.9	0.6	0.9
531-533	Gastric, duodenal and peptic ulcers	0.7	0.8	0.4	0.3	0.4	0.4
571	Chronic liver disease and cirrhosis	0.6	0.5	1.4	1.5	1.3	1.4
	Accidents and suicides	3.9	2.0	19.3	9.6	15.9	7.9
E800-949	Accidents	2.3	1.5	11.5	5.7	9.5	4.7
E810-819	Motor vehicle traffic accidents	1.0	0.4	6.8	3.2	1.6	9.1
E880-888	Accidental falls	0.5	0.7	0.9	0.4	0.8	0.4
E950-959, E980-989	Suicide and undetermined*	1.6	0.6	7.8	3.9	6.4	3.2

| | | Total deaths in 1992 | | Years of life lost, 1988–92 | | | |
| | | | | Under age 65 | | Under age 75 | |
		Males	Females	Males	Females	Males	Females
	All causes	271,732	286,581	8,607,224	5,202,700	10,595,983	6,555,073
	Deaths under 28 days	2,606	1,933	590,632	443,055	681,602	511,295
001-139	Infectious and parasitic diseases	1,362	1,271	105,594	70,362	112,901	75,834
010-018	Tuberculosis	268	150	9,336	4,259	11,322	5,205
	All malignant neoplasms	76,248	69,715	1,934,516	1,958,764	2,596,933	2,447,670
162	Lung cancer	22,668	10,994	512,457	248,275	753,669	354,703
174	Cancer of female breast	–	13,663	–	569,247	–	657,299
180	Cervical cancer	–	1,647	–	118,206	–	130,206
201	Hodgkins disease	239	159	26,160	15,699	27,261	16,610
204-208	Leukaemia	1,969	1,647	108,744	75,462	122,532	84,647
250	Diabetes	3,565	4,502	65,017	47,233	88,615	69,380
345	Epilepsy	515	389	70,223	43,911	71,484	45,019
	Circulatory diseases	122,381	132,302	2,397,529	887,907	3,352,923	1,459,523
410-414	Ischaemic heart disease	79,182	66,722	1,773,987	458,101	2,454,159	805,670
430-438	Cerebrovascular disease	24,897	41,394	294,026	238,985	442,782	374,525
401-405, 430-438	Hypertension and CVD combined	26,274	43,161	325,527	255,355	486,902	401,159
480-486	Pneumonia	9,351	16,906	117,619	63,389	146,083	88,067
490-492	Bronchitis and Emphysema	3,943	2,127	29,469	50,283	88,783	47,526
493	Asthma	714	1,077	54,211	49,097	59,308	56,621
531-533	Gastric, duodenal and peptic ulcers	1,915	2,381	31,301	17,330	45,124	27,020
571	Chronic liver disease and cirrhosis	1,753	1,303	121,860	78,705	133,443	88,967
	Accidents and suicides	10,562	5,829	1,660,695	498,388	1,688,895	518,902
E800-949	Accidents	6,203	4,246	992,432	295,833	1,010,234	309,822
E810-819	Motor vehicle traffic accidents	2,848	1,210	587,141	168,553	173,262	593,633
E880-888	Accidental falls	1,327	1,941	77,636	20,503	83,451	25,444
E950-959, E980-989	Suicide and undetermined*	4,359	1,583	668,263	202,556	678,661	209,081

Excluding ICD 988.8 – inquest adjourned.

Source: ONS public health database

Chapter 5

Morbidity statistics from health service utilisation

By

Patricia Fraser, Douglas Fleming, Mike Murphy, John Charlton, Leceister Gill and Michael Goldacre

Summary

- The chapter describes the history, availability and features of GP- and hospital-based data, and describes some of the trends.

- Health service utilisation data do not necessarily measure morbidity directly, since they depend on: the patient recognising problems and seeking medical help; health professionals recognising the problem; and, for some data sources, on appropriate treatment being given. Such data can complement other sources, however, and in a number of instances do provide good measures of morbidity.

- The general practitioner is the gatekeeper to the health services in Britain, and thus data collected from this source could yield the most comprehensive information on health service utilisation.

- Sources of GP data include the national GP-based morbidity surveys undertaken at 10-year intervals, the Weekly Returns Service of the Royal College of GPs and the General Practice Research Database. Some examples of the data available from these sources are given.

- When the year commencing September 1991 is compared with 10 years previously there have been increases in the annual prevalence of most categories of disease presented to GPs, including serious illnesses. To some extent this may be measuring increased survival.

- Age-standardised hospital discharge ratios have been increasing in England and Wales and in Scotland since the 1960s, the earliest date from which data are readily available.

- Hospital discharge and episode data for England and Wales count episodes rather than patients. The Oxford Record Linkage Study and Scottish SHIPS data allow patient counts as well as episode counts. A comparison of the two types of data shows that the ratio of episodes per person has in fact been rising, but that there have also been increases in person-based rates.

5.1 Introduction

Mortality data are used most extensively in this volume, because they provide the most reliable information on long-term trends in health. However, for many diseases, mortality only represents the tip of a much larger 'iceberg of disease', and other sources need to be used to provide complementary information. Most illness is treated by the individuals themselves without contact with health services, with the health services treating only the illnesses deemed to be more severe. Population sample surveys can tap the base of the iceberg of disease, namely the symptoms and diseases recognised by the interviewee, and biomedical measurements such as blood pressure, height, weight and cholesterol, which provide more objective measures of health, can also be measured, as in the *Health Survey for England* (Bennett *et al.*, 1995). However, health surveys are expensive and designed to obtain specific types of information. Table 5.1 shows by ICD chapter how the main sources of *routine* morbidity data compare. The General Household Survey (GHS) data in this table come from the 1989 survey, and describe by ICD chapter the long-standing illnesses that are perceived by individuals to limit their activities. Each year the GHS provides information on limiting long-standing illness rates, but only occasionally asks about the illness responsible. Sickness benefit statistics relate only to the population who qualify for claiming sickness benefit, GP and hospital data relate to the uptake of medical services, which can depend on a number of factors other than level of illness. All these data sources have inherent flaws that the user needs to bear in mind when using them, but since there is no ideal health data source they are valuable because they help to piece together the complex health jigsaw. This chapter describes the history, availability, and features of GP and hospital data, and gives some trend data. Other data sources are described in Chapter 2.

Table 5.1

Comparison of morbidity data sources: patients consulting GP, hospital in-patient cases and mortality by ICD9 chapter

England and Wales

International Classification of Diseases chapter	Chapter headings*	Long-standing illness 1989 (1)	Days of certified incapacity by cause 1990/91 (2)	Patients consulting in general practice 1991/92 (3)	GP consultations by cause 1991/92 (3)	In-patient cases 1992/93 (4)	Deaths 1992
		(Rate per 100)	(%)	(Rate per 100)	(Rate per 100)	(%)	(%)
I	Infectious and parasitic diseases	0.2	0.7	14.0	20.0	1.2	0.5
II	Neoplasms	0.8	1.5	2.4	4.9	8.9	26.1
III	Endocrine and immunity disorders	2.5	2.9	3.8	7.1	1.3	1.9
IV	Diseases of blood	0.4	0.3	1.0	1.5	1.2	0.4
V	Mental disorders	1.8	18.2	7.3	17.6	3.2	2.3
VI	Diseases of the nervous system	2.4	7.0	17.3	28.5	5.3	2.1
VII	Diseases of the circulatory system	7.3	20.0	9.3	24.0	8.9	45.6
VIII	Diseases of the respiratory system	6.7	7.7	30.7	62.0	6.2	10.8
IX	Diseases of the digestive system	3.2	2.8	8.7	14.9	9.6	3.4
X	Diseases of the genitourinary system	1.3	1.4	11.3	20.5	8.2	1.0
XI	Complications of pregnancy	–	0.7	1.1	1.8	11.7	0.0
XII	Diseases of the skin	1.6	0.6	14.6	22.9	1.9	0.2
XIII	Diseases of the musculoskeletal system	11.6	26.4	15.2	30.7	5.4	1.0
XIV	Congenital anomalies	–	0.3	0.5	0.7	1.1	0.3
XV	Perinatal period	–	–	0.1	0.2	2.0	0.0
XVI	Signs, symptoms and ill-defined conditions	–	3.9	15.1	23.4	7.1	0.9
XVII	Injury and poisoning	–	5.6	13.9	19.5	7.0	3.0
XVIII	Supplementary classification**	0.1	–	33.5	47.6	9.8	0.0
	Total	100	78.0	347.8	100	100

Source: Based on table compiled by Department of Health as part of analyses of burdens of disease, from the following sources:
(1) Long-standing illness: GHS (1989)
(2) Incapacity: DSS (1990–91)
(3) Patients consulting: MSGP4 (1991–92), (OPCS MB5 No.3 England and Wales)
(4) Hospital Episode Statistics: DH (1992–93). (England, ordinary admissions and day cases combined)

* The mortality figures for individual chapters exclude deaths under 28 days.
** Includes factors influencing health status and contact with health services (e.g. screening, immunisation, antenatal and contraceptive care).

Health service utilisation data depend on: the patient recognising a health problem; bringing that problem to health care professionals; health care professionals recognising the problem and making appropriate diagnoses; and, to be counted in some statistical sources, treatment needs to be provided by the professional.

5.2 Morbidity data from general practice

The general practitioner is gate-keeper to health services (except for emergencies and genitourinary medicine), and thus utilisation data collected from this source should give us the most comprehensive picture of overall health service utilisation. In deciding whether to consult a general practitioner, however, a patient may be influenced by their perception of the severity of the problem, the expectation that they might be helped, the accessibility of the surgery premises, the need for sickness certification, and the availability of alternative sources of care such as accident and emergency departments and family planning clinics. The data thus measure individuals' expressed need for GP care. They can also be heavily influenced by organisational characteristics; for example a shift of routine care from hospitals to GP care (e.g. for diabetics – see later) could result in an artefactual increase in prevalence of the disease treated, according to the GP data, but a reduction according to the hospital data. In this section corresponding hospital data are referred to when appropriate.

5.2.1 General practice data

The first national GP-based morbidity survey was conducted by Logan and Cushion in 1955–56 (GRO, 1958). The second and third studies were conducted in 1970–76 (RCGP/OPCS/DHSS, 1974, 1979, 1982) and 1981–82 (RCGP/OPCS/DHSS, 1986, 1990). The two most recent morbidity surveys in 1981 and 1991–2 surveyed 300,000 and 500,000 persons respectively. Until 1991 the studies required GPs to record morbidity in the form of special manual records. The 1991–92 survey, however, recruited practices which routinely recorded all their consultation data on computers (McCormick et al., 1995). The survey covered 1 per cent of the population of England and Wales. The patients were similar in terms of age and socio-economic characteristics to the population of England and Wales, as recorded in the 1991 Census, although the practices tended to have larger lists and younger GPs than the average. The Weekly Returns Service (WRS) of the Royal College of General Practitioners monitors the incidence of new disease presented to general practitioners each week (Fleming et al., 1991). Ninety two practices with a combined population of approximately 700,000 persons record new episodes of illness and report the numbers in age- and sex-groups on each Wednesday for the previous week. The data are aggregated at the Research Unit in Birmingham. The practices are well distributed nationally and data are presented in three supraregional groups – North, Central and South. There are currently a number of other databases collecting data from general practices on a continuous basis, including

the General Practice Research Database (GPRD) (Hollowell, 1994). In addition, health authorities are working with GPs in their areas to collect data in order to assess local needs. GP morbidity data from national samples have also been used in conjunction with census data to produce estimates of local morbidity (Charlton et al., 1995).

Recording for both the morbidity surveys and the WRS is based on the assessment diagnosis of the general practitioner (Fleming, 1991). Information systems can be based on the presenting symptoms of patients, on assessment diagnosis, or on diagnoses confirmed by laboratory tests. Of these, the assessment diagnosis is the most useful for monitoring purposes. Presenting symptoms are often multiple and do not always link easily with the nature of the morbidity. For example, pain is commonly the reason which prompts consultation but tells little about the diagnosis. At the other extreme, recording that is limited to diagnoses confirmed by laboratory tests, depends on the availability, routine use and reliability of tests, but does not reflect the burden of disease in the community. Whilst for some conditions (e.g. hypothyroidism, glandular fever) most practices routinely base the diagnosis on test results, the majority of conditions are diagnosed on clinical grounds. The assessment diagnosis of the doctor has a particular advantage in that it is the basis for action, including therapeutic and referral interventions, and thus is the determinant of resource utilisation. By using the assessment diagnosis, we are able to describe the entire range of problems presented in primary care.

The quality of general practice data is sometimes criticised. Internal consistency is illustrated in regional analysis of data for allergic rhinitis presented in Figure 5.1 for 1992, a year in which incidence rates of allergic rhinitis were particularly high (Ross and Fleming, 1994). Comparability with specialist diagnosis is demonstrated in an examination of data for hospital discharges with a diagnosis of asthma and new episodes presenting to general practitioners (LAIA, 1993) (see Figure 5.2). Laboratory validation of general practitioner diagnoses is illustrated by comparing the incidence of influenzal illness with the results of virological investigation (Fleming et al., 1995) (see Figure 5.3). Although there may be a time lag for laboratory reports, it is valuable to use such different sources in conjunction to confirm validity.

5.2.2 Trends in morbidity as measured by general practice 1981–82 and 1991–92

Because there have been changes in the way morbidity has been recorded in successive surveys, trend data have only been presented from 1981 onwards (see McCormick et al., 1995). For some conditions accurate comparisons cannot be made because the disease classification used in the 1981–82 study was not entirely compatible with that used in the later study. Since 1982 there have been major changes in general practice; the number of practice nurses and the scope of their activities has increased substantially. Nurse activity was not recorded in MSGP surveys until 1991–92 and practice responsibilities in delivering preventive health care have

Figure 5.1

Hay fever by region: weeks 13–33, England and Wales, 1992

Rate per 100,000 population

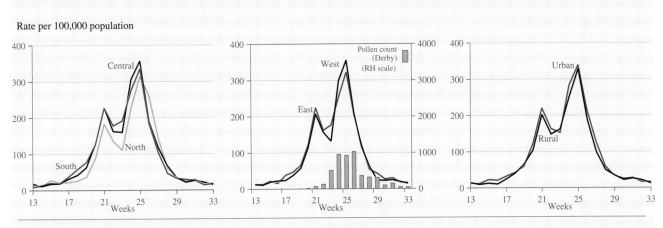

Source: RCGP Weekly Returns Service

Figure 5.2

Average 4-weekly percentage variation from the trend in hospital admissions for asthma and new GP episodes of asthma, by age

Average % variation from the trend

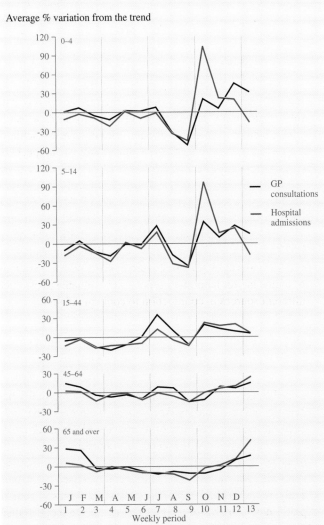

Source: HES and RCGP Weekly Return Service

Figure 5.3

Influenza and flu-like illness, six practices, all practices and positive swabs

Rate per 100,000 population

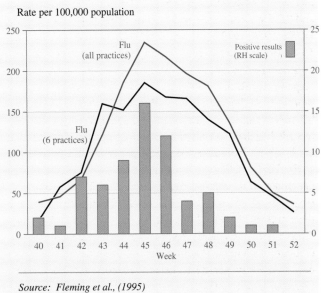

Source: Fleming et al., (1995)

increased. Selective reimbursement for health promotion clinics and the introduction of target payments influenced both practice activities and the quality of recording the appropriate data. Procedures for certification of sickness were simplified between the two surveys, leading to a reduced requirement for GPs to issue certificates. Only three fundholding practices were included in the sample, so the effect of this innovation on the results is likely to be small. Computerised information systems used for recording the data in all practices in 1991–92 led to greater accuracy of practice registers and reduced errors in morbidity recording.

Table 5.2 compares prevalence rates in the two periods for some disease groups for which comparisons were possible. Prevalence is defined as the number of people per 10,000 consulting at least once during the study year. This prevalence

rate may depend on the survival time following initial diagnosis, and may thus be increased by earlier diagnosis or successful treatment. For example, the incidence of breast cancer did not increase but the prevalence did, because survival has improved (see Table 5.3).

The proportion of patients consulting their GP during the year increased from 71 per cent to 78 per cent – the increase was greatest among the elderly, but occurred in every age-group and both sexes. There were also increases in the proportion of people who consulted for serious illness, and rates increased in every ICD chapter apart from mental disorders, and symptoms, signs and ill-defined conditions. For some conditions the increase in patients consulting their GP could be due to raised expectations of medical care. A few selected disease categories are discussed in some detail to present

Table 5.2

Changes in annual prevalence rates per 10,000 person years at risk, 1981–82 and 1991–92
Patients consulting their GP for selected conditions

Condition		1981–82	1991–92	% change	Condition		1981–82	1991–92	% change
All diseases and conditions	Persons	7,116	7,803	+10	Asthma (ICD 493)	Males	200	429	+114
						Females	159	422	+165
Serious illnesses	Persons	1,439	1,829	+27					
					Acute and unspecified				
Intermediate illnesses	Persons	4,160	4,741	+14	bronchitis, and	Males	578	676	+17
					bronchiolitis (ICD 466,490)	Females	584	834	+43
Trivial conditions	Persons	5,702	6,576	+15					
					Chronic bronchitis (ICD 491)	Males	81	54	-33
I Infectious and parasitic						Females	40	37	-8
diseases	Persons	1,172	1,339	+14					
					IX Digestive	Males	678	742	+9
II Neoplasms	Persons	135	239	+77		Females	758	1,009	+33
Malignant neoplasms	Males	64	77	+20	**X Genitourinary**	Persons	864	1,133	+31
	Females	71	95	+34					
					XII Skin	Persons	1,178	1,455	+24
Benign neoplasm of	Males	23	56	+143					
skin (ICD 216)	Females	33	94	+185	**XIII Musculoskeletal**	Persons	1,328	1,521	+15
III Endocrine	Persons	288	377	+31	Osteoarthritis (ICD 715)	Males	144	228	+58
						Females	318	398	+25
Diabetes (ICD 250)	Males	74	119	+61					
	Females	47	73	+40	Rheumatoid arthritis	Males	33	28	-15
					(ICD 714, 720.0)	Females	76	54	-29
IV Blood	Persons	78	97	+24					
					Back pain (ICD 720.1-.9,	Males	276	259	-6
V Mental disorders	Persons	854	728	-15	724.1,724.2,724.5-.9)	Females	304	339	+12
Serious mental illness	Persons	72	113	+57	Osteoporosis (ICD 733.0)	Males	1	2	+100
						Females	7	22	+214
VI Nervous system	Persons	1,409	1,732	+23					
					XVI Signs, symptoms				
Glaucoma (ICD 365)	Persons	12	21	+75	**and ill-defined**	Persons	1,595	1,510	-5
Cateract (ICD 366)	Persons	22	34	+55	**XVII Injury and poisoning**	Persons	1,135	1,390	+22
VII Circulatory system	Persons	850	931	+10	**XVIII Supplementary**				
					classification	Persons	2,003	3,348	+67
VIII Respiratory	Persons	2,696	3,070	+14					

Source: OPCS, Series MB5 no 3

features of GP data, based on MSGP4, the Weekly Returns Service and the GPRD.

Neoplasms

The prevalence of malignant neoplasms increased between the morbidity survey of 1981/82 and that of 1991/92 by 20 per cent in males and 34 per cent in females. Prevalence rates include persons who are continuing to receive treatment after initial diagnosis, and thus an increased prevalence does not mean more people are diagnosed with cancer or that cancer is more common. Indeed with constant incidence but improved survival, prevalence would increase. Table 5.3 compares the prevalence and incidence of two groups of cancers in 1981/82 and 1991/92.

Both the prevalence and incidence of cancers of the larynx, trachea, bronchus and lung decreased in men, whereas the equivalent figures for women showed increases in elderly women. For cancer of the female breast there was increased prevalence in all age-groups but incidence was only increased in the age-group 75 years and over. However, incidence data from the cancer registries show increases above age 50 (see Chapter 17). Three factors contribute to explaining these differences between incidence and prevalence:

- Increased breast cancer incidence is partly explained by more rigorous screening and clinical appraisal of the problems of older people.

- Reduced smoking has had a recognisable effect on the incidence of lung and related cancers, though this is not seen among older women (see Chapter 9).

- The fact that prevalence of breast cancer increased more than incidence suggests that persons with breast cancer are being diagnosed earlier and/or living longer. This

Table 5.3

Selected cancers: prevalence and first incidence rates per 10,000 persons

		All ages	0–4	5–14	15–24	25–44	45–64	65–74	75+
Cancer of the larynx, trachea, bronchus and lung (ICD 161,162): prevalence rates per 10,000 person years at risk, by sex									
Males	1971–72	14	1	–	–	2	28	68	60
	1981–82	14	–	–	–	2	24	66	66
	1991–92	10	–	–	0	1	16	51	67
	1981/91 change	–29%	–	–	–	–	–27%	–23%	+2%
Females	1971–72	3	–	–	–	1	6	13	4
	1981–82	4	–	–	–	0	10	18	7
	1991–92	5	–	–	–	0	10	17	17
	1981/91 change	+25%	–	–	–	–	–	–6%	+143%
Cancer of the larynx, trachea, bronchus and lung (ICD 161,162): first incidence rates per 10,000 person years at risk, by sex									
Males	1981–82	6	–	–	–	1	8	33	41
	1991–92	4	–	–	–	0	6	18	32
	Change	–33%	–	–	–	–	–25%	–45%	–22%
Females	1981–82	2	–	–	–	0	6	8	3
	1991–92	2	–	–	–	0	3	6	9
	Change	–	–	–	–	–	–50%	–25%	+200%
Cancer of breast (ICD 174): prevalence rates per 10,000 female years at risk, by sex									
	1971–72	19	–	–	1	8	35	51	67
	1981–82	23	–	–	–	8	44	72	69
	1991–92	30	–	–	–	10	61	81	88
	1981/91 change	+30%	–	–	–	+25%	+39%	+12%	+28%
Cancer of breast (ICD 174): first incidence rates per 10,000 female years at risk, by sex									
	1981–82	8	–	–	–	4	15	26	18
	1991–92	8	–	–	–	4	15	20	25
	Change	–	–	–	–	–	–	–23%	+39%

Sources: MSGP2, MSGP3 and MSGP4

situation contrasts with the data presented for lung and related cancers where male prevalence and incidence had decreased by similar amounts.

Asthma

Increasing prevalence of asthma during the last 30 years is widely acknowledged. A substantial increase in the prevalence of asthma was reported between the Second and Third Morbidity Surveys (Fleming and Crombie, 1987). There have also been marked increases in hospital admissions since the mid-1970s in Britain and elsewhere (Hyndman *et al.*, 1994), and the reasons for this are much debated (Strachan and Anderson, 1992). Between the Third and Fourth Morbidity Surveys prevalence again increased, by 114 per cent in men and 165 per cent in women. Many more people are being diagnosed as asthmatic, and this is reflected in the drug bill, where in the 10 years 1980 to 1990 the number of prescriptions issued for asthma rose from 15 million to 29 million. Prescribing data from the GPRD for 1991 to 1993 show an increase which is concentrated on people aged from 10 to 44 (see Figure 5.4) (Hollowell, 1994). Part of this increase in patients treated stems from the fact that we now have more effective remedies for asthma than 20 years ago. At the same time, more attention has been given to the management of asthma: it has become a target area for quality improvement in general practice. In Table 5.4 the proportion of cases with asthma in each of the five age-groups reported in the Weekly Returns Service data for the years from 1988 to 1994 is compared with hospital admission data reported in hospital episode statistics data (DoH 1994, 1995a). Among hospital admissions with asthma, 35 per cent are in age-group 0–4, while only 19 per cent of new asthma episodes in general practice are in this age-group; this difference is as expected. Above age 44 the proportions are similar. The mean weekly incidence of asthma reported in the Weekly Returns Service has changed little over the last 4 years and the numbers of hospital admissions did not increase between 1988/89 and 1993/94. There have been small increases in the reported incidence (Weekly Returns Service data) but these have been confined to the age groups 0–4 and 5–14 years. There has been no comparable increase during the last 5 years in hospital episode data though caution is needed when interpreting these data since persons treated in Accident and Emergency (A & E) departments are not admitted and thus not counted. In recent years it has become quite common for children with asthma to be treated in A & E departments with nebulisers and not admitted. The recent levelling off of the increase in incidence is encouraging, as is the fact that standardised mortality rates for asthma in both sexes have been falling since 1986, most especially in age-groups under 55 years (DoH 1995b).

Table 5.4

Asthma: the numbers per 10,000 population and the percentage distribution of hospital admissions and new episodes in general practice, by year and age-group

| | Rates per 10,000 population | | Percentage distribution | | | | | | | | | | | |
| | | | All ages | | 0–4 | | 5–14 | | 15–44 | | 45–64 | | 65+ | |
	HA	GP	HA	GP	HA	GP	HA	GP	HA	GP	HA	GP	HA	GP
1988/89	223	1,774	100	100	34	19	20	27	24	33	13	13	9	8
1989/90	196	1,843	100	100	33	17	19	25	26	33	14	15	10	10
1990/91	183	1,889	100	100	35	19	18	24	25	33	13	15	9	10
1991/92	195	2,613	100	100	32	21	19	24	26	32	13	13	10	10
1992/93	189	2,458	100	100	33	20	17	22	26	34	14	14	10	9
1993/94	202	2,624	100	100	31	19	17	24	26	33	14	14	11	10

Note: HA = hospital admission
GP = general practice new episodes (Weekly Returns Service)

Sources: Hospital admissions: HES, GP new episodes: RCGP Weekly Returns Service

Figure 5.4

Percentage of patients prescribed bronchodilator drugs, 1991–93

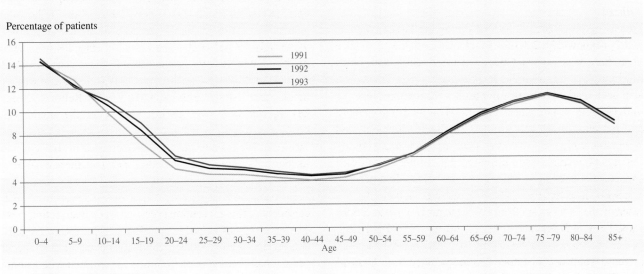

Percentage of patients

Legend: 1991, 1992, 1993

Age: 0–4, 5–9, 10–14, 15–19, 20–24, 25–29, 30–34, 35–39, 40–44, 45–49, 50–54, 55–59, 60–64, 65–69, 70–74, 75–79, 80–84, 85+

Source: GPRD, Hollowell (1994)

Measles, mumps and rubella

The mean weekly incidence of measles, mumps and rubella for each 4-week period since 1970 is given in Figure 5.5, based on data from the Weekly Returns Service. These diagnoses are generally made by general practitioners using clinical criteria rather than on serological or salivary immunoglobulin investigation. Though some cases of all conditions occur in adults, these illnesses predominantly affect children. In the last 5 years, of those who reported measles, mumps and rubella, 89 per cent, 70 per cent and 79 per cent respectively were aged 0–14 years.

In 1988 a combined vaccine for measles, mumps and rubella was introduced at a time when the incidence of mumps was in the trough of an approximately triennial cycle. In spite of that, a reducing incidence was evident within 6 months of its introduction. For measles, vaccination had been available since the early 1960s but uptake rates were poor in the early years. The rubella vaccination programme has been undertaken in three phases. In the early 1970s, vaccination of schoolgirls in their early teens was first introduced. A few years later this was extended to include postnatal women (after screening rubella titres had been obtained) and women receiving contraception. The figure shows the impact of the combined MMR programme directed towards universal coverage of the population at an early age which has been much more effective than previous, more limited, programmes for measles and rubella individually.

Hypertension and ischaemic heart disease

A major thrust in the prevention of stroke and, to a more limited extent, of ischaemic heart disease has been a more aggressive approach to the identification and treatment of persons with hypertension. The prevalence (persons consulting per 10,000 person years at risk) and incidence (new episodes per 100,000) reported in the third and fourth morbidity surveys for hypertension, acute myocardial infarction, angina pectoris and cerebrovascular disease are compared in Table 5.5.

Table 5.5

Comparison between the Third and Fourth Morbidity Surveys in prevalence and incidence per 10,000 persons of uncomplicated hypertension, acute myocardial infarction, angina pectoris and cerebrovascular disease

	Males		Females	
	Prevalence	Incidence	Prevalence	Incidence
Hypertension (ICD 401.1, 401.9)				
1981	314	86	427	115
1991	347	83	459	106
% change	+11	-3	+7	-8
Acute myocardial infarction (ICD 410)				
1981	55	34	29	19
1991	38	29	20	16
% change	-31	-15	-31	-16
Angina pectoris (ICD 413)				
1981	81	33	58	26
1991	130	55	98	49
% change	+60	+67	+69	+88
Cerebrovascular disease (ICD 430–438)				
1981	39	38	43	44
1991	64	47	67	56
% change	+64	+24	+56	+27

Sources: MSGP3 and MSGP4

Figure 5.5

Mean weekly incidence in 4-week periods, 1967–95

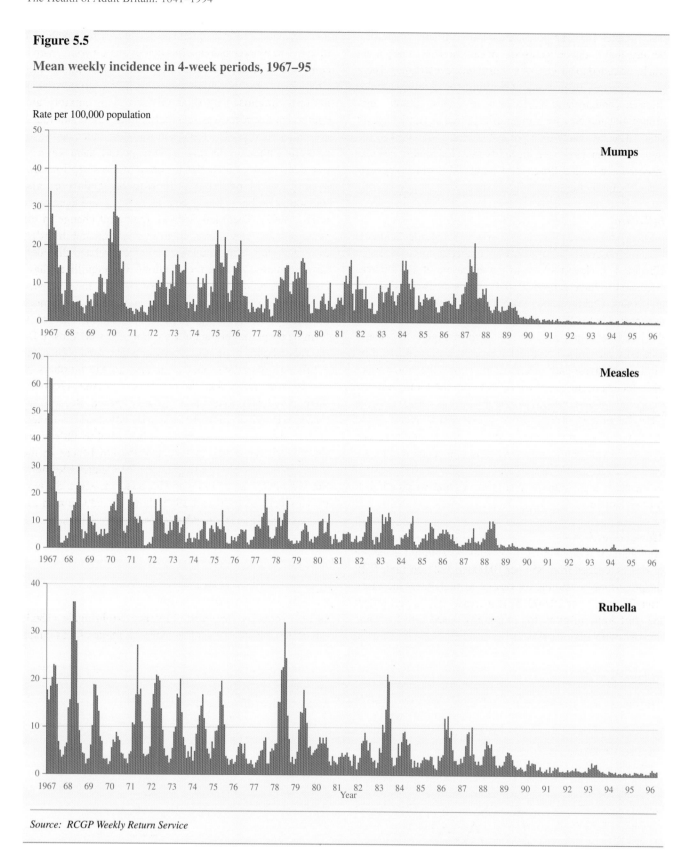

Rate per 100,000 population

Source: RCGP Weekly Return Service

There was a small increase in the proportion of patients consulting for uncomplicated hypertension, confined to men aged 45 and over and women aged 65 years and over, but the incidence of uncomplicated hypertension declined. There was a 31 per cent reduction in the prevalence of acute myocardial infarction, but a 60 per cent or more increase in the prevalence and incidence of angina pectoris. The proportionate reduction in acute myocardial infarction was largest in ages 25–44 (65 per cent), and smaller in each successive age-group. These data suggest that more people are recognised (and presumably treated) with angina pectoris. This may have contributed to the reduction in the number of persons experiencing acute infarctions. The 1993 Health Survey for England (OPCS, 1995) estimated that 13 per cent of adult males and 14 per cent of adult females were taking one or more cardiovascular drugs at the time of visit. Comparison of hospital admission data for England (HES) for 1988 to 1993 for ischaemic heart disease shows a rising trend, but mortality rates are falling (see Chapter 18). The hospital data are difficult to interpret because they count only episodes of care, and the same patient can be admitted to the care of a consultant several times. There were increases in persons consulting for cerebrovascular disease. Though these increases were seen in all adult age-groups, the numbers were insignificant in those under age 44 years. The incidence data presented alongside point in the same direction. However, mortality rates for cerebrovascular disease have been falling (see Chapter 18), which suggests that GPs are seeing more minor strokes.

Influenza

Influenza remains a problem which is perhaps underestimated because most cases of influenza are relatively minor (see also Chapter 13). Nevertheless, in the epidemic of 1989 it was estimated to have caused 25,000 excess deaths in England and Wales (Curwen *et al.*, 1990). The incidence of influenza as reported in the Weekly Returns Service of the RCGP over the last five winter periods is shown in Figure 5.6. These clinically recognised outbreaks have all been confirmed by virological investigation. The figure shows that some cases of influenza occur every winter but both the timing and the magnitude of the epidemic varies considerably. The antigenic character of the influenza virus is constantly changing and the threat of a major change and the consequent emergence of a worldwide pandemic is of continuing concern to health care planners. The most important factor in the fight against influenza is a programme of routine annual vaccination of 'at risk' persons.

Mental disorders

Although the total number of persons consulting for mental disorders reduced from 854 per 10,000 to 728 (see Table 5.2), the proportion consulting for *serious* mental illness increased from 72 to 113 per 10,000. This increase may in part reflect the shift from hospital- to community-based care for some persons with major psychiatric disease. There have been marked reductions in hospital bed occupancy for psychiatric illness. The marked increase in suicides among young men is consistent with an increase in serious mental illness (see Chapter 4). A substantial reduction in the proportion of patients diagnosed by their GP as having anxiety and depressive disorders was seen between the third and fourth morbidity surveys. The reduction was distributed across all ages and both sexes. During the same period, there was a 12 per cent reduction in the number of prescriptions for hypnotics, 54 per cent reduction for sedatives and tranquillisers, but a 30 per cent increase in antidepressants (OHE, 1992). There has been an important change in the general practitioner management of minor mental disorders in recent years. Consultations for anxiety-related disorders have decreased and the prescriptions of tranquillisers have been much reduced. It may be that patients have stopped presenting minor anxiety disorders because they are much less likely to receive tranquilliser medication. The habit-forming properties of tranquilliser drugs are well known. On the other hand, more antidepressants are used. Since the available prescribing data refer only to the numbers of prescriptions rather than the numbers of persons receiving them, their interpretation is necessarily limited. Because GP data for mental disorders are so heavily influenced by factors such as the above, the statistics probably tell us little about the underlying trends in levels of mental illness in the community, and surveys such as the Psychiatric Morbidity Survey (Meltzer *et al.*, 1995) provide better measures. Surveys by Goldberg in 1970 and 1995 show no reduction in the prevalence of mental disorders (Kisely *et al.*, 1995).

5.3 Hospital in-patient statistics

In her *Notes on Hospitals*, Florence Nightingale (1863) advocated the collection of an extended range of particulars

---

Figure 5.6

Influenza and flu-like illness, all ages, 1991/92 to 1995/96

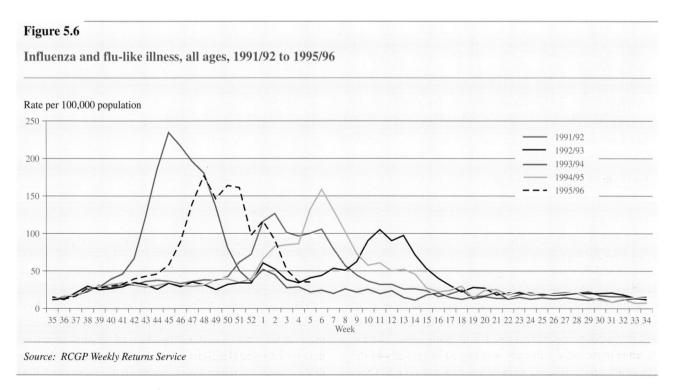

Rate per 100,000 population

	1991/92
	1992/93
	1993/94
	1994/95
	1995/96

Source: RCGP Weekly Returns Service

on hospital patients, and some hospital statistics were published in the nineteenth century (Statistical Society, 1842, 1844, 1862, 1866). However, it was not until 1929, when local health authorities took over the management of hospitals, and mechanical methods for tabulation of hospital records became widely available, that recording and reporting of hospital statistics on a large scale really began (Spear and Gould, 1937). The systems for collecting hospital in-patient data in the United Kingdom since then, and their uses, have been described in detail (Ashley, 1972; Ashley *et al.*, 1991) with particular reference to variations in practice between the different countries. This section includes data from the Hospital In-patient Enquiry (HIPE) and its successor Hospital Episode Statistics (HES); Mental Health Enquiry (MHE) in England and Wales; Scottish Hospital In-patient Statistics (SHIPS); and Oxford Record Linkage Study (ORLS).

5.3.1 Trends in HIPE discharge rates

One of the main purposes of the HIPE, HES and SHIPS systems was to provide information about illness among patients admitted to hospital, as a guide to morbidity occurrence in the community. However, patients admitted to hospital with a disease are not necessarily representative of all persons with that disease, numerically or in terms of severity. Those individuals and diseases which can be managed within the community and those who die without referral or before transfer to hospital are excluded. In addition, routine hospital data relate to admissions to hospital and not to individual patients, thereby limiting their usefulness in estimating the incidence of chronic diseases for which patients are often admitted more than once.

The pattern of hospital admissions may be complicated further by multiple pathology, resulting in the admission of a single patient several times for different conditions. The availability and accessibility of hospital in-patient services, beliefs about the effectiveness of treatments and perceived home conditions can also significantly affect how patients with the same condition are hospitalised in different localities. Thus an admission to in-patient care is the result of a complex interaction between a number of related factors (condition, individual, home conditions, hospital services and medical practice). Variation in one or more of these factors over time may have a marked effect on hospital morbidity patterns even when the true incidence of a particular disease has remained relatively unchanged (Paterson, 1988). For example, the introduction of a new treatment, or a change from medical treatment (as an out-patient) to surgical treatment (as an in-patient), or vice versa, may lead to a change in admission rates without there being any change in disease occurrence. Increased bed availability due to shorter lengths of stay, or decreased availability due to closure of hospital beds, will also influence admission rates (McPherson and Coleman, 1988). Changes in diagnostic fashion and variation in the completeness of data capture may further complicate the interpretation of trends in hospital admission data. With the introduction of HES, finished consultant episodes (FCEs) relate to care under each consultant and there can be multiple

FCEs in an admission episode, further complicating the interpretation of trends (Steering Group on Health Services Information, 1982a,b).

For all these reasons and because of the very important differences in data collection over time and between different parts of Britain, we present statistics from the earliest time available to the most recent (1993/4) only for general hospital admissions (minus maternity and psychiatric admissions). Figure 5.7 shows trends in indirectly age-standardised discharge ratios for ages 15–74 (all episodes in Scotland in 1984=100). Ratios cannot be compared between men and women because different standards have been used for each, but Scotland's index of admissions has clearly been higher than that for England and Wales. Of note is the recent levelling off of rates in England and Wales, compared with the continued increase in Scotland. For ease of presentation we hereafter discuss cause-specific admissions, using HIPE and ORLS data, to illustrate trends.

Figure 5.7

Age-standardised discharge ratios (age 15–74), by sex (Scotland, men and women=100)

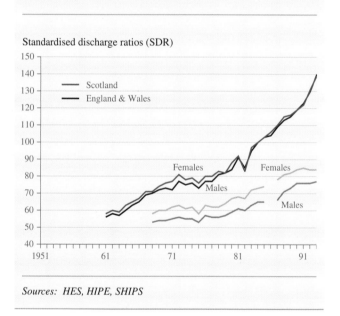

Sources: HES, HIPE, SHIPS

HIPE trends

Trends in HIPE discharge rates, i.e. the estimated number of discharges, including deaths, per head of population, over the period 1968–78, have been described in detail elsewhere (DHSS and OPCS, 1972, 1989; Fraser *et al.*, 1983). The trends in discharge rates for all adult (15 and over) admissions and for each ICD chapter as presented in the annual tabulations of HIPE are reproduced here, extended to 1985 (England only, 1982–85), and compared with episode-based and person-based data from the Oxford Record Linkage Study (ORLS) over the same 18-year period. The trends in discharge rates in both datasets were directly standardised using the standard European population (Waterhouse *et al.*, 1976). They exclude maternities and admissions to psychiatric hospitals.

Figure 5.8 shows how discharge rates varied by age and sex in 1985, the last year for which HIPE data were available. Between 1968 and 1985 the all-cause 5-year age-specific HIPE discharge rates increased at all ages in both sexes (see Figure 5.9). The increases were greater at older ages. In men, the age-standardised percentage change was 19 per cent at ages 15–44, 29 per cent at ages 45–64, 48 per cent at ages 65–74 and 69 per cent at ages 75 and over. The age-standardised percentage increases in female discharge rates were slightly higher in these broad age-groups – 20, 37, 57 and 73 per cent respectively. The age-standardised discharge rates over all age-groups increased by 35 per cent in men from 74 per 1,000 in 1968 to 99 per 1,000 in 1985, and by 38 per cent in women from 82 to 113 per 1,000 (see Figure 5.11). The age-standardised rate in women was 11 per cent higher than the male rate in 1968 and 14 per cent higher in 1985, giving a male/female rate ratio of about 0.9 throughout the study period. However, these summary statistics conceal the fact that, while female age-specific rates were higher than male rates in all 5-year age-groups under 55 years, the male rates were higher at older ages (see Figure 5.8).

Figure 5.8

Hospital discharges for all diagnoses per 1,000 population, by age and sex, 1985

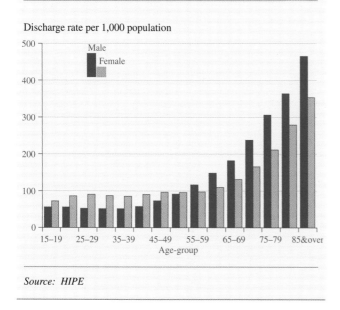

Discharge rate per 1,000 population

Source: HIPE

In 1968, the major causes of hospital admission among men were diseases of the circulatory system (17 per cent) and digestive organs (16 per cent), injury and poisoning (13 per cent), respiratory diseases (10 per cent) and malignant neoplasms (9 per cent). These five disease groups accounted for nearly two thirds (66 per cent) of all male admissions to hospital. In women in 1968, circulatory (13 per cent) and digestive (11 per cent) diseases, injury and poisoning (8 per cent), and malignant neoplasms (7 per cent) were also among the commonest causes of admission to hospital but they followed diseases of the breast and genito-urinary system which alone accounted for 17 per cent of all female admissions.

Figure 5.9

Percentage change in hospital discharges for all diagnoses per 1,000 population, by age and sex, 1968–85

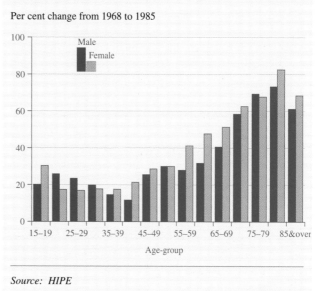

Per cent change from 1968 to 1985

Source: HIPE

Table 5.6

Annual percentage change in episode-based rates by ICD chapter, 1968–85 (ORLS and HIPE)

	ORLS		HIPE	
	Males	Females	Males	Females
Symptoms, signs XVI	4.4	4.7	6.6	6.8
Musculoskeletal XIII	4.0	3.6	4.4	4.3
All malignant II	1.4	2.7	3.2	3.7
Blood diseases IV	2.3	1.3	1.9	1.4
Nervous diseases VI	2.5	2.5	1.3	1.9
Genitourinary X	3.6	1.2	2.1	1.0
Injury, poison XVII	1.1	1.4	1.0	1.7
Circulatory VII	1.8	0.8	1.7	1.1
Endocrine III	2.9	–0.6	1.9	0.4
Skin diseases XII	3.5	3.4	0.6	1.5
Digestive IX	1.5	2.5	0.2	1.1
Congenital XIV	0.2	–0.1	0.3	0.3
Respiratory VIII	0.7	1.7	–0.2	0.7
Pregnancy XI	–	1.9	–	0.4
Mental disorders V	3.3	1.7	0.1	0.2
Benign neoplasms IIc	–0.1	–2.6	–2.1	–2.6
Infective diseases I	–1.9	–1.4	–3.4	–2.3

Sources: HIPE, ORLS

An increase in age-standardised discharge rates between 1968 and 1985 is seen for nearly all the broad disease groups represented by the ICD chapters (see Table 5.6). In both sexes, the greatest increases were seen for symptoms and ill-defined conditions, diseases of the musculoskeletal system and connective tissue, and all malignant neoplasms. The fact that symptoms and ill-defined conditions show the greatest increase is in large part due to a change in analysis practice. From 1973 the principal diagnosis as given was retained in the analysis where previously a definitive condition had been mandatory. In both sexes, discharge rates for infective and parasitic diseases, and benign neoplasms and neoplasms of unspecified nature decreased between 1968 and 1985. These negative trends reflect the decreasing importance of infection as a cause of adult admission to hospital, and the increasing tendency to manage many benign neoplasms as day cases.

Despite differences in the annual percentage change by ICD chapter, there were relatively few changes in the ranking of ICD chapters by frequency of admissions over the 18-year period. In 1968 and 1985 the same five disease groups accounted for over 60 per cent of all male admissions, but admissions for symptoms and ill-defined conditions,which increased from 7 to 14 per cent, ranked second to diseases of the circulatory system in 1985. Similarly, in women the same five disease groups accounted for more than half of all female admissions in 1968 and 1985 but symptoms and ill-defined conditions (13 per cent) occupied second place in 1985.

Although the general HIPE includes patients suffering from mental disorders in general wards, only 1 per cent of admissions fall into this category as the majority of mentally ill patients are treated in psychiatric hospitals covered by the Mental Health Enquiry (MHE). The report for 1974 describes the trends in admissions to mental illness hospitals and units in England from 1860 to 1974 (DHSS, 1977). For many years prior to 1945 the annual number of admissions to mental illness hospitals increased slowly, except for temporary reductions during the two World Wars, and patients slowly accumulated in hospital under a custodial style of care. However, the introduction of psychotropic drugs in 1945 facilitated the development of short-stay care. This led to a rapid rise in annual admissions from about 30,000 in 1945 to over 170,000 in 1974. These data are reproduced in summary form in Figure 5.10 and, using data from the MHE (DHSS, 1986), extended to 1986, when there were nearly 200,000 admissions to mental illness hospitals and units in England. This estimated number of admissions represents overall rates of 364 and 468 per 100,000 for men and women respectively. Female annual MHE admission rates during 1968–86 were consistently about 30 per cent higher than the corresponding male rates. Foster and Mahadevan (1981) reviewed information sources for planning and evaluating adult psychiatric services.

5.3.2 Oxford Record Linkage Study trends

The Oxford Record Linkage Study (ORLS) dataset is assembled from abstracts of hospital in-patient records (including day cases), cancer registrations and birth and death certificates. The data are collected in such a way that records relating to the same individual can be linked together and analysed to produce time-sequenced information about numbers of people in receipt of care (Acheson, 1967).

Figure 5.10

Admissions to mental illness hospitals and units, 1860–1986

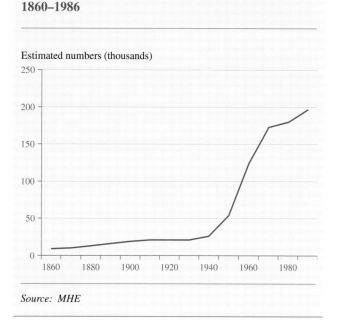

Estimated numbers (thousands)

Source: MHE

Scotland also has such a national dataset, presently covering the years from 1981 to 1994. Data collection for the ORLS began in 1963 and initially covered hospital discharges from the city of Oxford and adjacent parts of the county of Oxfordshire. In 1965, the ORLS expanded to include the present health districts of Oxfordshire and West Berkshire. The area covered increased during the early 1970s until, by 1974, it covered six health districts (Oxfordshire, West Berkshire, East Berkshire, Northampton, Kettering and Wycombe). The linked data have been used extensively to examine time trends in hospital admissions in the ORLS area (see, for example, Goldacre *et al.*, 1988) and numerous studies have examined trends in workload and demographic profiles in various clinical specialties (de Alarcon *et al.*, 1993; Goldacre *et al.*, 1993, 1994; Newton and Goldacre 1993).

The analyses reported here are confined to records of adults (aged 15 and over) who were both resident and treated in the districts of Oxfordshire and West Berkshire (total population about 850,000) at the time of relevant discharge during 1968 to 1985. These two districts were chosen for analysis so that comparisons could be made with trends in the HIPE data described above, during the entire 18-year period. Time trends in both episode-based and person-based rates are analysed for all hospital discharges (including deaths) combined, for ICD chapters, and for some selected diseases where major changes in discharge rates have occurred.

5.3.3 Episode-based discharge rates

As in the HIPE data, the ORLS all-cause 5-year age-specific episode-based discharge rates increased at all ages in both sexes between 1968 and 1985. Again, female rates were higher than male rates in all age-groups under 55 years, but male rates were higher at older ages. Male age-standardised episode

Figure 5.11

Hospital discharges and deaths per 1,000 population, all diagnoses: HIPE compared with ORLS, age-standardised episode-based, 1964–84

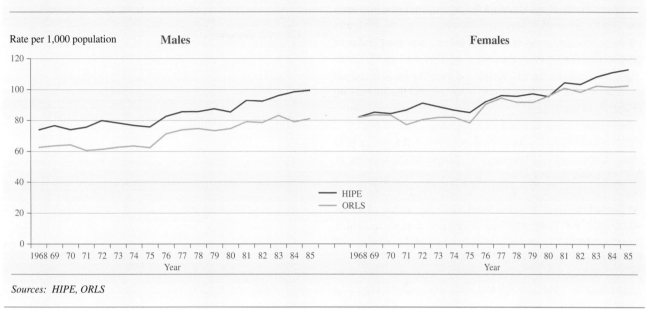

Sources: HIPE, ORLS

rates increased by 30 per cent from 63 per 1,000 in 1968 to 81 per 1,000 in 1985, and female rates increased by 25 per cent from 82 to 103 per 1,000 (see Figure 5.11). The male/female rate ratio remained at about 0.8. In both sexes the ORLS episode rates were lower than the national HIPE discharge rates for the corresponding year. The differences increased with time from 18 to 23 per cent in men, and by 10 per cent in women from initially very similar levels in 1968–70.

Table 5.7

Annual percentage change in episode-based and person-based rates, by ICD chapter, 1968–1985 (ORLS)

	Males			Females		
	Episode rate	Person-based rate	Ratio episode/person	Episode rate	Person-based rate	Ratio episode/person
Symptoms, signs XVI	4.4	4.2	1.05	4.7	4.6	1.02
Musculoskeletal XIII	4.0	3.7	1.08	3.6	3.3	1.09
Skin diseases XII	3.5	3.5	1.00	3.4	3.3	1.03
All malignant IIa,b	1.4	0.9	1.56	2.7	1.7	1.59
Nervous diseases VI	2.5	1.2	2.08	2.5	1.8	1.39
Digestive IX	1.5	1.2	1.25	2.5	2.2	1.14
Pregnancy XI	–	–	–	1.9	1.7	1.12
Respiratory VIII	0.7	0.4	1.75	1.7	1.5	1.13
Mental disorders V	3.3	3.0	1.10	1.7	1.5	1.13
Injury, poison XVII	1.1	1.1	1.00	1.4	1.3	1.08
Blood diseases IV	2.3	0.9	2.56	1.3	0.3	4.33
Genitourinary X	3.6	3.3	1.09	1.2	0.9	1.33
Circulatory VII	1.8	1.4	1.29	0.8	0.8	1.00
Congenital XIV	0.2	0.3	0.67	–0.1	–0.2	0.50
Endocrine III	2.9	2.7	1.07	–0.6	–0.7	0.86
Infective diseases I	–1.9	–1.7	1.12	–1.4	–1.3	1.08
Benign neoplasms IIc	–0.1	–0.1	1.00	–2.6	–2.7	0.96

Source: ORLS

In 1968, men in the ORLS were admitted most frequently for diseases of the digestive system (16 per cent), injury and poisoning (15 per cent), circulatory diseases (14 per cent), malignant neoplasms (11 per cent) and respiratory diseases (10 per cent). Together they comprised over half of all male admissions throughout the study period. Thus, the ORLS percentage distribution was slightly different from that of HIPE, where circulatory diseases comprised 17 per cent of admissions, but by 1976 diseases of the circulatory system had become the commonest cause of hospital admission in the ORLS, too. Female admissions to hospital in the ORLS followed the national pattern. The annual percentage changes in age-standardised episode rates by ICD chapter between 1968 and 1985 are shown in Table 5.6, alongside corresponding HIPE figures.

5.3.4 Person-based discharge rates

The time trends and sex differences in the ORLS all-cause age-specific person-based discharge rates were similar to the episode rates but, not surprisingly, the person-based rates were lower in every age-group. The trends over time in the age-standardised person-based rates are shown in Figure 5.12, alongside the episode rates for the corresponding year. These data illustrate the extent to which the episode rates are inflated by multiple admissions for the same person. In both sexes the episode and person-based rates show significant, but slightly divergent, upward trends, the rate ratios (episodes per person) increasing from about 1.2 to 1.3 during the study period, mainly since 1975. Thus, although there has been an increase in the number of individuals treated in hospital between 1968 and 1985, latterly there has been a greater increase in the average number of admissions per person.

Comparisons between the annual percentage change in episode and person-based rates by ICD chapter (see Table 5.7) show that patients with diseases of the blood and blood-forming organs, nervous system, respiratory system (in men) and all malignant neoplasms have experienced the greatest increases in the average number of episodes per person hospitalised. For malignant neoplasms in women, episodes per person have increased from 1.5 in 1968 to 1.7 in 1985. By contrast, for benign and unspecified neoplasms, there has been a decline in both episode and person-based rates since 1977 but the number of episodes per person has remained constant at about one throughout the study period. It is not possible to deduce from the ORLS data alone the reason(s) for the trends in discharge rates. They may reflect changes in the prevalence or severity of disease, increased detection of disease through screening, a change in referral patterns or a combination of these factors.

For example, for neoplasms of the lymphatic and haematopoietic system , there has been a change of treatment policy towards more frequent admissions of shorter duration, in some cases culminating in increased survival (Stiller, 1994). For patients with Hodgkin's disease, both of these factors have contributed to the marked excess of hospital episodes over people treated. By contrast, data for diabetes mellitus show decreases in both episode and person-based rates since about 1980, following the introduction of a policy of shared care between hospital consultants and general practitioners (Wood, 1990; Sowden et al., 1995). There is now evidence to suggest that general practice can offer the vast majority of diabetic patients a standard of care whose processes and levels of metabolic control are at least equal to those obtained in hospitals (Howitt and Cheales, 1993).

Figure 5.12

Hospital discharge and deaths per 1,000 population, all diagnoses: ORLS age-standardised episode-based rates compared with person-based rates, by age, 1968–85

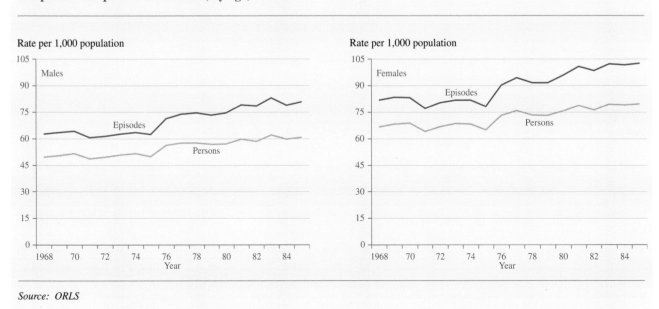

Source: ORLS

5.4 Registers

In addition to the routine collection of hospital morbidity and general practice data from whole populations, there are in existence a number of registers which have been set up for specific purposes, for example, to study specific diseases and the outcome of treatment. Such data are used increasingly in evaluation of services and investigations of equity in health care (Weddell, 1973). Only a few examples of hospital-based registers will be mentioned here.

Regionally and nationally the most important are the cancer registers (see Chapters 2 and 17). Hospital-based cancer registries list and follow up their patients with malignant disease in order to obtain information likely on the efficacy of treatment to be useful in clinical practice and the occurrence of complications, such as late-onset iatrogenic thyroid disease after radiotherapy (Hedley *et al.*, 1970) or leukaemia after multi-agent chemotherapy (Coleman, 1991).

Since 1963, the establishment of kidney registers has made possible the reporting of results based on the pooled experience of centres carrying out renal transplants (Murray and Barnes, 1971).

Diabetes registers are central to running an organised district diabetes service and the local hospital departments have traditionally compiled these registers deriving the information from a variety of sources (Howitt and Cheales, 1993). However, the increasing involvement of general practitioners in the care of their diabetic patients, will require individual practices to maintain their own registers for disease management in future.

For children, malformation and cerebral palsy registers exist, and also genetic registers which record families at high risk of having a child with a serious hereditary disorder and are a valuable source of information both for prevention in high risk and reassurance in low risk families (Weddell, 1973).

Numerous local registers also exist, such as for people with particular psychiatric illnesses, or stroke. Some of these are referred to elsewhere in this book (e.g. arthritis and rheumatism in Chapter 23, and motor neurone disease in Chapter 19). The problems associated with their use relate to migration of subjects into and out of the area, general updating difficulties and worries about completeness. None the less, they represent an important resource.

Chapter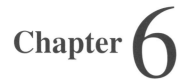

Socioeconomic and demographic trends, 1841-1994

By

Mel Bartley, David Blane and John Charlton

Summary

- Population growth and a falling death rate over the period 1841 to 1991 was accompanied by a falling birth rate. Although the population has aged, the shrinking proportion of children has meant that the total dependency ratio has hardly changed.

- Population health depends not just on the wealth of the nation (typified by the GDP) but on distribution of income, which has changed considerably.

- Increasing urbanisation in the nineteenth century encouraged the rise of infectious epidemics; much of the legislation and social reforms in the 1850s onwards were aimed at combating these.

- Urban epidemics of typhoid, typhus and cholera were effectively eliminated by the building of sewers and a filtered water supply in the second half of the nineteenth century. Changing social attitudes during the second half of the nineteenth century included improved hygiene.

- Medical examination of military volunteers in the Boer War and conscripts in the First World War revealed a high proportion of young men to be physically and medically unfit. Efforts to improve child health among the poorer members of society, at the beginning of the twentieth century, included the School Meals Act and the School Medical Service.

- National Insurance was introduced early in the twentieth century, providing a large part of the population with GP services and sickness benefit.

- Fogs during the years following the Second World War caused several thousand deaths, and the Clean Air Acts resulted.

- Inspired by the Beveridge Report, the National Health Service was established in 1948, alongside other social insurance benefits.

- At the end of the twentieth century we are faced with many further technological and demographic changes – a greater understanding of patterns of the past may help in the attempt to adapt to the changes of the future.

6.1 Introduction

The remainder of volume 1 consists of chapters describing a number of the factors that may be associated with changes in health status. The purpose of this first chapter is to provide a brief introduction, and to sketch in details not included in the other chapters. It is not the intention here to establish a link between health and sociodemographic trends – a separate ONS volume on socio-economic factors and health is in preparation.

The period from 1841 to 1991 has witnessed considerable improvements in survival. The demographic transition from a state of high mortality and high birth rates to low mortality and low birth rates, and the epidemiologic transition from the dominance of infectious to that of chronic disease, have been accompanied by huge changes in the socio-economic and demographic fabric of Britain. Of major interest is the answer to the question: 'What caused these changes?' The data that are available are unfortunately imperfect, and although many have analysed the temporal associations, these types of analyses are fraught with difficulty since most of the variables to be studied are highly intercorrelated, and their separate effects cannot be disentangled from such purely observational data. For example, over time, as real income has risen, sanitation and housing standards have improved, food availability and quality have increased, safety at work has become more regulated and medical advances have taken place. Similarly, at any one time people with lower incomes have tended to live in worse housing conditions, more polluted environments, and to have lower quality diets and more hazardous occupations. Instead of trying to attribute direct effects, in this chapter we largely show trends in factors that are likely to have influenced the health transition. Many factors are likely to be relevant, including: demographic

trends; economic development and standard of living; food availability and nutrition; physical environment; hygiene; lifestyles; the social environment; and the role of health services, medical science and technology. Some of these factors are the subject of separate chapters: diet (Chapter 7), the drugs component of lifestyles (Chapters 8 and 9), housing and households (Chapters 10 and 11), environment (Chapters 12 and 13), and medical advances (Chapter 14). The present chapter concentrates on demographic and economic change and the environment. A chronology of a few selected events is provided as an appendix at the end of this volume. Its purpose is to locate major events that may have influenced health or health statistics in time. A few other dates of well known events have also been added to make this easier.

6.2 Demographic trends 1841–1991

6.2.1 Population growth

The population of England and Wales was growing very rapidly during the nineteenth century: in 1750 it was little more than 6 million, by the first census in 1801 it was nearly 9 million, by 1851 it had doubled to nearly 18 million, and by 1911 it had doubled again to 36 million.

Population growth was brought about initially by increasing birth rates and later by falling death rates. Figure 6.1 shows the trends in crude fertility and death rates for England and Wales.[1] The per capita birth rate rose until the 1870s – the

---

[1] *Historical demographic data are less reliable prior to the introduction of central registration of vital event data in 1838 (see Wrigley and Schofield, 1981)*

Figure 6.1

Fertility and death rates, England and Wales

Rate per 1,000 population

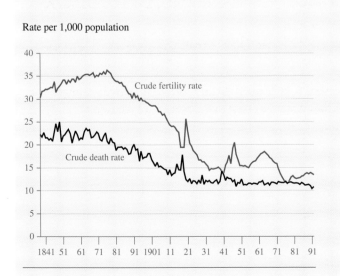

Source: OPCS Birth Statistics, FM1 series No. 13

Figure 6.2

Median age at marriage, England and Wales

Age of bride/groom

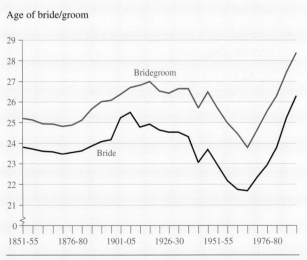

Source: OPCS Marriage and Divorce Statistics, FM2 series

death rate started falling some 10 years previously. After this, the birth rate fell steadily: subsequent population growth was due to the large size of existing cohorts combined with lower death rates.

There is considerable discussion of the causes of the fall in fertility. Much of this centres around the relative importance for national fertility trends of changes in the prevalence and length of marriage versus changes in behaviour within marriage. Notestein (1953) argued that the decline in the death rate changed attitudes, and that this was responsible for the decline in the birth rate:

When death rates are high, the individual's life is relatively insecure and unimportant. The individual's status in life tends to be that to which he is born. There is, therefore, rather little striving for advancement. Education is brief, and the children begin their economic contributions early in life. In such societies, moreover, there is scant opportunity for women to achieve either economic support or personal prestige outside the roles of wife and mother, and women's economic functions are organised in ways that are compatible with continuous childbearing.

Perhaps because of changes in such attitudes, married couples increasingly limited the size of their families: 'Starting in the 1870s, average family size had declined from five or six children to today's two-child family within 60 years' (Coleman and Salt, 1992, 61). Significantly, this reduction in family size was achieved without effective contraceptive aids, with limited lay knowledge of the topic and in the face of opposition from the medical profession. Sexual abstinence, coitus interruptus and, to a lesser extent, abortion were probably the means by which it was effected. Their success illustrates the paramount importance of the 'subjective factor', the desire to limit family size. An increase in the age of

marriage may also have contributed to the decline in births (Burnett, 1989). Women's median age of marriage rose by some two years between 1870 and the early 1900s (Figure 6.2), thereby exposing them to less chance of pregnancy.

Whatever the relative importance of later marriage versus fertility-limiting behaviour, urbanisation and industrialisation place a cost on large family size. In part, this is the opportunity cost to women of child care. As factory jobs with relatively high wages paid year round (unlike seasonal agricultural labour) became available to women, the potential income foregone due to child care increased. Urban working-class families, unlike their peasant forebears, had no access to small plots of land for self-provisioning (which could perhaps be combined with child care), but relied entirely on paid work outside the home. Children were increasingly excluded from paid factory work by legislation, from the time of the 1833 Factory Act. Compulsory education, encouraged by the Education Act of 1870 and enforced to age 14 by the 1880 Act, completed this process. Children ceased to be a potential source of household income and instead became an expense. Lower birth rates and consequent smaller families increased per capita consumption within households and reduced the chronic overcrowding which prevailed in many urban areas.

Population size during the period being considered here was not greatly affected by migration. Emigration exceeded immigration in all years except just before the Second World War and since the 1980s (Figure 6.3). There was little movement during the two World Wars.

6.2.2 Urbanisation

While the British population was undergoing rapid growth the distribution between urban and rural areas completely

---

Figure 6.3

Emigrants and immigrants, United Kingdom, 1855-1992

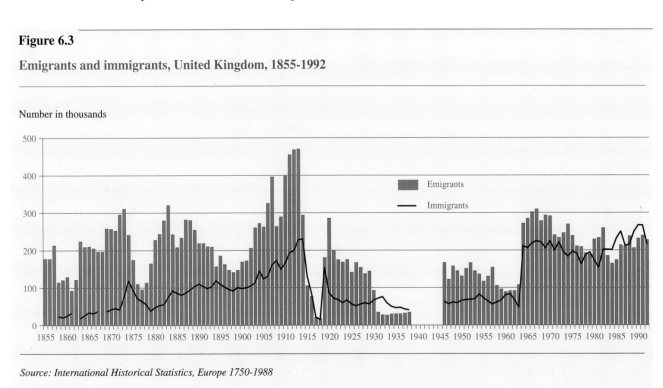

Number in thousands

Source: International Historical Statistics, Europe 1750-1988

reversed: in 1801, 20 per cent of the population were town dwellers, whereas by 1911, 80 per cent were. By 1991, some 90 per cent lived in urban areas. Figure 6.4 shows the growth of population in the major cities of Britain.

Changes in population distribution put pressure on housing, sewage disposal and water supplies in the past, and continue to do so to the present day. Whereas today we see the results in terms of regional 'droughts' and hosepipe bans, early urbanisation had drastic consequences for health. The failure of water provision to keep up with the growth of cities and ignorance of sanitation gave rise to epidemics of infectious disease such as cholera, typhus and typhoid. Overall levels of health in the population were increasingly affected by the ability to control these infectious diseases.

6.2.3 Ratio of 'dependent' to economically active population

Trends in the ratio of economic dependants to people of working age are illustrated in Figure 6.5. The proportion of dependants aged less than 15 years fell dramatically from 1880 to 1940 and again, but more modestly, from 1970 to today. The proportion of dependants aged more than 64 years rose rapidly during the middle half of the twentieth century. The total dependency ratio, which is the outcome of these changes, was highest up to the 1880s; today it is slightly lower than it was in 1900. The remarkably similar total dependency ratios at the start and the end of the twentieth century need to be seen in relation to the prodigious increase in industrial productivity which has occurred between these dates. Taken together, they suggest that the 'problem of the ageing population' concerns not inadequate resources but complex issues of the social division of responsibility for children and infirm elderly people.

Throughout the period since 1840 a proportion of infirm or impoverished elderly people have ended their days in institutions of one type or another. The explicitly punitive workhouse was replaced after the Second World War by long-stay hospitals and nursing homes. Since the 1950s the proportion of all women in such institutions has been higher than that of men, although previously the situation was reversed (Figure 6.6). The currently higher proportion of institutionalised women is partly due to the mean length of widowhood increasing to some 8 years. Although the life expectancy of both men and women has increased during the twentieth century, that of women has increased faster (see Chapter 3). This widening difference has been combined with the unchanging custom of women marrying men who are the older by some 2 years (Figure 6.2). Infirm or terminally ill women are consequently more likely to be institutionalised because they lack a spouse who can nurse them (see Chapter 26).

There remains considerable uncertainty about the processes which underlie these demographic changes. An historical perspective can aid understanding by offering a series of 'natural experiments'. Because the fall in fertility rates *preceded* the introduction of effective contraceptive aids, we can reasonably conclude that effective contraceptive devices are not a *necessary* condition for a falling birth rate and that the 'subjective factor', the choice of fewer children, may be a sufficient condition. McKeown (McKeown and Lowe, 1966; McKeown, 1976, 1979) used a similar 'natural experiment' to examine the fall in infectious disease mortality, which was primarily responsible for the decline in the death rates after 1870. Because most of the fall in infectious mortality preceded the introduction of effective medical interventions (immunisation and antibiotics), we can reasonably conclude that such interventions are not a necessary condition for this transformation in health and that other, probably

---

Table 6.1

Population of five major towns (thousands)

	1801	1831	1861	1891	1911	1931	1961	1991
London	1,117	1,907	3,227	5,638	7,256	8,216	8,183	6,680
Manchester	90	187	358	505	714	766	661	404
Liverpool	80	165	444	518	747	856	748	452
Leeds	53	123	207	367	446	483	510	680
Glasgow	77	202	420	658	784	1,088	1,055	663

Source: Censuses of Population

Figure 6.4

Population of Great Britain living in the major cities, by year

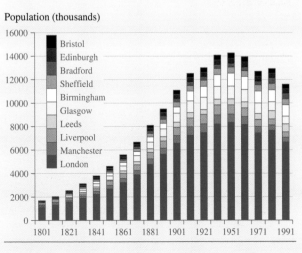

Source: International Historical Statistics, 1750–1988

environmental, factors may be a sufficient condition. Improvements in diet, resulting from both rising real income and technological advances in transport and storage, which made fresh food available for more of the year, may have played an important role. Other plausible factors include personal and public hygiene, housing and local conditions, which were increasingly a focus of attention for reforming municipal and public health officials (Wrigley and Schofield, 1981; Szreter, 1988; Kearns, 1988,1989). Underlying these are more general issues of economic development, income levels and living standards.

6.3 Economic development and standard of living

6.3.1 Income

Figure 6.7 shows how Gross Domestic Product per person, a measure of the United Kingdom's prosperity, has increased over the period. The data have been adjusted to take inflation into account. The first impression is one of cumulative growth. Closer inspection reveals that GDP per person increased during both World Wars and that these wars separated three periods of accelerating sustained growth. The rate prior to the First World War was less than that between the two wars, which was less than that after the Second World War.

Figure 6.5

Dependency ratio (%), 1841-1991
Population aged under 15 and over 64, as a percentage of population aged 15-64

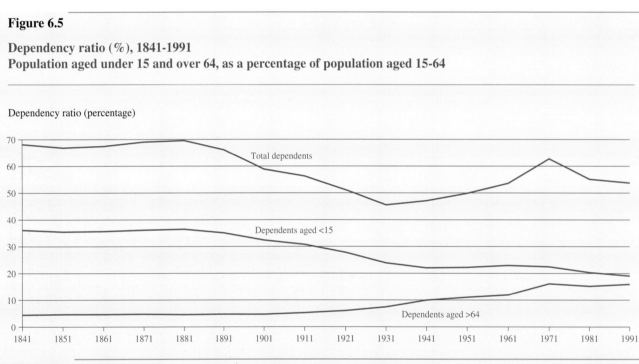

Figure 6.6

Percentage of population in institutions, by sex and type of institution

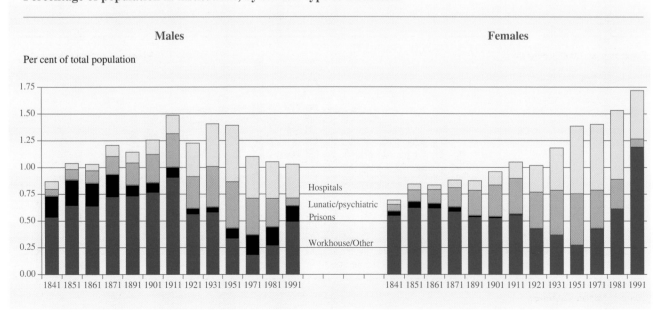

Figure 6.7

Gross domestic product per person, United Kingdom, 1855-1994 at constant prices

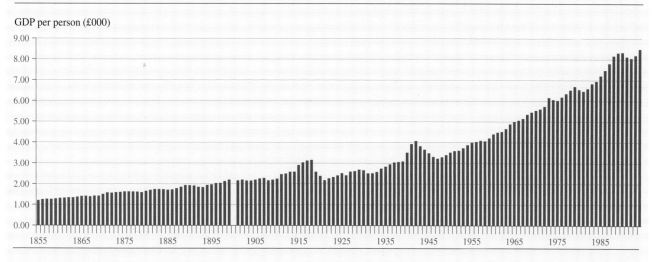

Source: Feinstein; OPCS

Figure 6.8

Car ownership and motor vehicle accidents, 1926-91

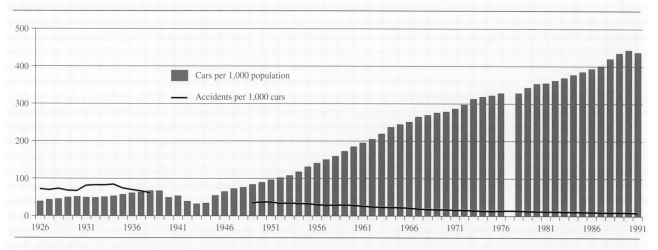

Source: Department of Transport

Figure 6.9

The growth of the railways, 1826-1990

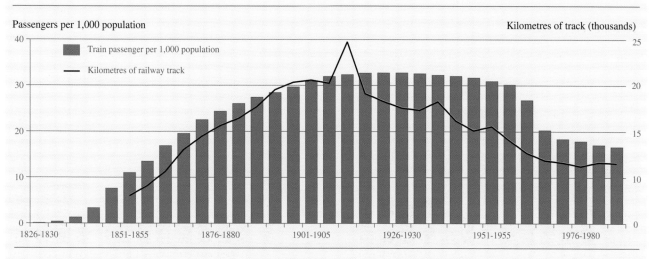

Sources: Statistical Abstract

Car ownership has increased tenfold from its 1926 level to nearly one car for every two persons by 1991 (Figure 6.8), and use of the railways has fallen (Figure 6.9). A motor car widens the options open to, but probably limits the physical exercise of, those who have access to it, its exhaust fumes contribute to atmospheric pollution and its speed makes accidents dangerous. While car ownership currently acts as a powerful predictor of good health (Phillimore and Beattie, 1994; Filakti and Fox, 1995), this is probably because it is a sensitive indicator of income and factors associated with income, rather than a health-enhancing factor in its own right.

The *distribution* of income may be important for population health, since the higher mortality rates of poorer people have a major effect on average mortality rates (Davey Smith, 1996; Kennedy *et al.,*1996; Wilkinson, 1992, 1994). Rodgers (1979) examined international data on income distribution using the Gini coefficient and quintile distribution (two measures of inequality), life expectancy (at birth and at age 5) and infant mortality. He found that mortality was significantly related to income distribution, where the difference in life expectancy at birth between the most and least egalitarian countries was 5 to 10 years. Inequality in income is likely to be associated with inequality in access to education, health care and other social amenities related to health. There are, however, severe limitations in these types of multi-country studies, and there is debate over the relationship between income distribution and health (Judge, 1995; Wilkinson, 1995). In Third World countries mortality decline has stagnated at very high levels, which has been interpreted as demonstrating that health interventions can only reduce mortality up to a point unless poverty, illiteracy, poor nutrition and unsanitary environments and living conditions are ameliorated (Hansluwka, 1975; Gwatkin, 1980; Ruzicka and Hansluwka, 1982).

Income 1841–1914
In Britain, improvement in the social and environmental preconditions of health has been slow. In 1841 the majority of the British population lived in rural areas, where the enclosure of common land was depriving labourers of the option of partial self-sufficiency. William Cobbett gave an account of country conditions in 1830 in his *Rural Rides*. He wrote that the lowest classes of farm labourers were 'the worst used labouring people upon the face of the earth. Dogs and hogs and horses are treated with more civility, and as to food and lodging, how gladly would the labourers change with them!' He was ashamed to see countrymen 'reeling with weakness; their poor faces ... nothing but skin and bone'. The Poor Laws of 1834 made life worse for the agricultural workers (see Section 6.2.1).

The migration from countryside to town was already well under way in Britain by 1841. The conditions of the poorest urban labourers were initially little better than their rural counterparts. Chadwick (1842, 111) quotes Dr Howard's description of Manchester:

Whole streets are unpaved and without drains or main-sewers, are worn into deep ruts and holes, in which water

constantly stagnates, and are so covered with refuse and excrementitious matter as to be almost impassable from depth of mud, and intolerable from stench ... But dwellings perhaps are still more insalubrious ... The doors of these hovels very commonly open upon the uncovered cesspool ...

Conditions in Britain at the start of the period covered by the present volume resemble in important ways those which appear to have stalled improvements in health in the Third World today.

Improvements in living standards in Britain were slow. Separate chapters examine some of the most important components of this change: diet (Chapter 7), housing (Chapter 10) and the environment (Chapter 12). Of particular interest to the present, more general, chapter is the period from the early 1870s to the First World War, when a sustained fall in mortality brought the crude death rate to unprecedently low levels (Figure 6.1). The first two-thirds of this period, from around 1873 to around 1898, was known to contemporaries as 'the great depression' (Webb and Webb, 1920) because of high rates of unemployment. For those who remained employed, however, real wages rose steadily, by 66 per cent, partly because of a sustained fall in prices, rather than a significant improvement in money wages, and partly because of a shift in the distribution of employment (Phelps-Brown and Browne, 1968).

Wood (1909) estimated that some 60 per cent of this rise in real wages had been due to the relative movement of prices and money wages, and some 40 per cent to 'the shifting up of industrial employment', from casual work in small units to more regular work in larger units. Employment contracted in agriculture (and other industries where casual work predominated) and expanded in industries, like mining and

Figure 6.10

Percentage of workforce in various industries in Great Britain, 1841–1981

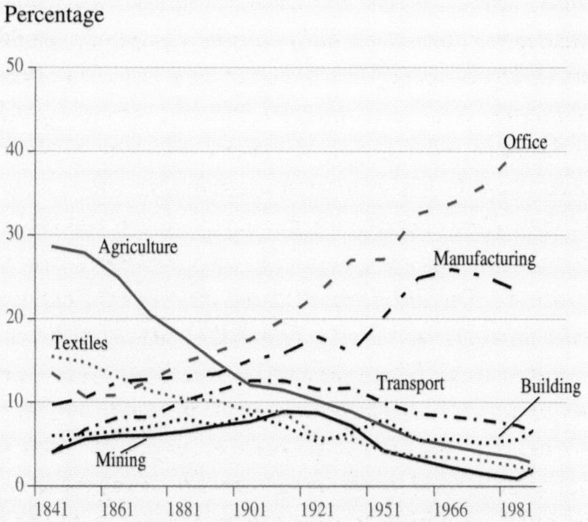

Sources: Censuses of Population, Marks (1996)

railways, which offered regular employment (Figure 6.10). At the same time, production in the established industries moved towards larger units, so that by 1900 the factory had largely replaced home-working and small workshop production.

In contrast to the improving conditions of life of those with paid employment, the situation of the unemployed was one of privation (Webb and Webb, 1920). Able-Bodied Test Workhouses, Stoneyards and Labour Yards were introduced to deter unemployed people from claiming the Poor Law's subsistence safety-net (Webb and Webb, 1929). Figure 6.11 shows the available data on the trends of unemployment during this depression. These were seriously incomplete, a situation which continued to as late as 1922 (Mitchell and Deane, 1962), but contemporaries recognised that unemployment was high, long-term and at 'the centre of popular agitation' (Webb and Webb, 1929).

The rise in pay rates resulted in pressure for a shorter working day: 'the pressure for shorter hours had itself been both permitted and instigated by the rise in real rates of pay, and the same effect was seen in a reduction of effort by piece workers who did not need to produce so much as before in order to obtain a given weekly wage' (Phelps-Brown and Browne, 1968, p.185). The remainder of the increase was spent on commodities, the most costly component of which was food. Unfortunately, the first detailed studies of these issues were not undertaken until around 1900, so there is little information for the period of this depression. Nevertheless, it is possible to extrapolate backwards from the 1900 studies, across 25 years of rising real wages, to suggest the broad outlines of living standards at the start of the depression.

Seebohm Rowntree in his study of poverty in York in 1899 found that the majority of working class people could expect poverty at three points in their lives: as young children; when their own children were growing up; and in old age. He used the following particularly rigorous definition of poverty:

A family living upon a scale allowed for in this estimate must never spend a penny on railway fare or omnibus. They must never go into the country unless they walk. They must never purchase a halfpenny newspaper or spend a penny to buy a ticket for a popular concert. They must write no letters to absent children, for they cannot afford to pay the postage. They must never contribute to their church or chapel, or give help to a neighbour which costs them money. They cannot save, nor can they join sick clubs or trade unions, because they cannot pay the necessary subscriptions. The children must have no pocket money for dolls, marbles or sweets. The father must smoke no tobacco, and must drink no beer. The mother must never buy any pretty clothes for herself or for her children, and the character of the family wardrobe, as for the family diet, being governed by the regulation. Nothing must be bought but that which is absolutely necessary for the maintenance of physical health, and what is bought must be of the plainest and most economical description. Should

a child fall ill, it must be attended by the parish doctor; should it die, it must be buried by the parish. Finally, the wage-earner must never be absent from his work for a single day...If any of these conditions are broken, the extra expenditure involved is met, and can only be met, by limiting the diet, or, in other words, by sacrificing physical efficiency.

Using the above definition Rowntree found that 10 per cent of the population fell below and lived in what he called 'primary poverty', and a further 18 per cent earned higher incomes but lived in poverty because they did not spend their incomes solely on the necessities of life.

Rowntree also estimated the prevalence of malnutrition. Protein and calorie malnutrition were endemic among families earning 26 shillings or less per week, as was borderline protein malnutrition among more affluent working-class families (Rowntree, 1901). These results are broadly consistent with those of the five other similar studies which were undertaken in the final decade of the nineteenth century although, when these results are taken together, 30 shillings per week is a better guide to the level of wages necessary to support adequate family nutrition (Oddy, 1970; Dingle, 1972). At this level, protein and calorie malnutrition and poverty would have been common among all casual workers and all lower grades of unskilled workers, as well as most other unskilled workers in regular employment. Contemporary wage rates reveal the type of occupations involved: agricultural labourers, seamen, wool-spinners, cotton-spinners and weavers, engineering workers and compositors (Bowley, 1900). Medical examination of volunteer recruits to the Army during the Boer War acted as a form of mass screening of the young male population at that time. Forty per cent of army volunteers between 1897 and 1902 were rejected as physically or medically unfit – this figure was as high as 60 per cent in places such as Leeds and Sheffield. Extrapolating back to the start of the depression suggests that in the early 1870s at least half of the working class, which itself comprised some three-quarters of the total population, may have lived in poverty and been protein and calorie malnourished. During the succeeding 25 years the rising real wages of the depression allowed diets to became more varied and adequate, at the same time as employment was becoming more secure and less exhausting, families were having fewer children and all children were going to school. This was the social and economic context in which the crude death rate began the steepest part of its long-term decline.

During the Edwardian years up to the start of the First World War real wages were unchanged, because prices and money wages rose in unison (Phelps-Brown and Browne, 1968). Unemployment fell (see Fig 6.11)[2], so more of the population

2   *Up to the creation of Labour Exchanges after 1911, the unemployment rate was calculated only for workers employed in organised trades which offered some form of out-of-work benefit. As unemployment was more common amongst unorganised, unskilled workers, it is therefore underestimated to an unknown but probably considerable degree.*

benefited from the now established level of real wages. According to the 1911 Census, 29 per cent of the population were skilled workers, 34 per cent semi-skilled, 10 per cent unskilled and 2 per cent self-employed artisans. The skilled worker in regular employment earned around 40s per week – for the semi-skilled and unskilled, on wages of around £1 a week, it was much more difficult to survive financially, especially if they had a family to support. Maud Pember Reeves concluded in 1913 that there were 2 million men, 8 million people in all including dependants, who existed on under 25s a week. 'The great bulk of this enormous mass of people are under-fed, under-housed, and insufficiently clothed. The children among them suffer more than the adults. Their growth is stunted, their mental powers are cramped, their health is undermined.' Even if earnings were above 25s a week, a large family, unemployment, chronic sickness or inability to manage could plunge a family into poverty and debt. The unequal distribution of wealth at this time is illustrated by the fact that in 1914 under 4 per cent of those who died accounted for nearly 90 per cent of the entire capital bequeathed.

> *The upper classes of Edwardian Britain had, generally, been the beneficiaries of a national income which had risen by a fifth between 1900 and 1913... While real wages had remained only constant, if not actually falling, the already wealthy had seen an impressive increase in their accumulated capital ... By 1914 the British upper classes had undergone a significant transformation ... An aristocracy of land was now an aristocracy of wealth*
>
> (Stevenson, 1984).

At the other extreme there was a large supply of cheap domestic labour: 'Even penurious curates and schoolmasters could afford servants when a living-in maid could be employed for £10–12 per year.' In 1901 Seebohm Rowntree rested his distinction between 'middle' and 'working' class on the employment of servants, and one in every three women at some time in their lives worked in domestic service.

Income 1914–94

This way of life was effectively brought to a close by the First World War. Women flocked into munitions factories and other jobs vacated by military conscripts, which offered higher wages and greater freedom than domestic service. Despite wartime disruption to food supplies, civilian health continued to improve (Winter, 1976; Harris, 1993). Gross inequalities in wealth started a slow secular decline: by 1936 the percentage of total personal wealth owned by the richest one per cent of the population had fallen to 54 per cent, from 61 per cent in 1923 (Atkinson and Harrison, 1978).

Economic reorganisation during the inter-war period was as profound as that during the great depression; some industries, like coal mining and textiles, contracted. Others, like motor cars, greatly expanded and were organised around the new production line techniques. New industries, like wireless, aircraft and trucking, emerged. Domestic electrification created a market for household goods such as vacuum cleaners, washing machines and refrigerators which transformed domestic labour. Non-manual occupations grew, particularly clerical and retailing work. Unemployment was high throughout (Figure 6.11). While the average real wages of those in employment rose slowly, poverty and malnutrition were endemic among the unemployed, casual workers and those in receipt of low wages (Boyd Orr, 1936; Le Gros Clark and Titmuss, 1939); such privation affected an estimated 10 per cent of the total population and 25 per cent of all children (Webster, 1985).

Figure 6.11

Unemployment in Great Britain, 1855–1989

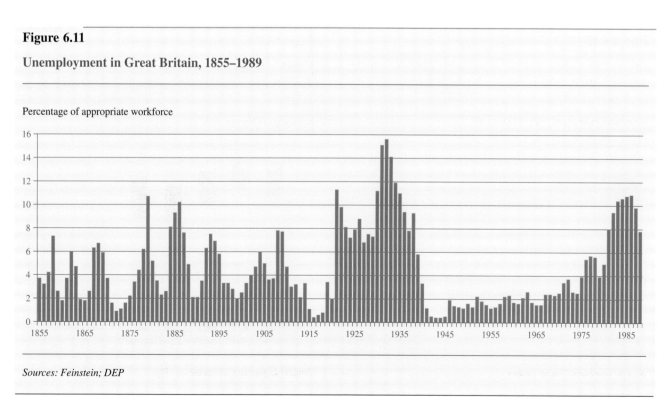

Percentage of appropriate workforce

Sources: Feinstein; DEP

Unemployment started to fall in the late 1930s, owing to rearmament. This accelerated during the Second World War, until even the majority of those previously classified as 'unemployable due to severe disability' had been found suitable work (Calder, 1969). As in the earlier war, millions of women entered paid employment, aided by state nursery provision and workplace canteens (Sheridan, 1990). Civilian morale during this 'total war' was maintained by the idea of 'No Return to The Thirties', which centred on the Beveridge Report (see Section 6.2.3) and its subsequent popularisation (Beveridge, 1943; Clarke, 1943). Popular support for these welfare reforms was indicated by the pattern of voting in the 1945 General Election and gave the incoming government little choice but to implement them.

The legislative introduction of these welfare reforms during the late 1940s coincided with a period of economic austerity. Real incomes did not reach their pre-war level until the early 1950s, although by 1956 they were 16 per cent ahead of the level of real incomes in 1938 (Carr-Saunders, *et al.*, 1958). The subsequent sustained growth in real incomes was, for the first time, combined with full employment, or at least historically low unemployment, and a welfare system which, even if it did not live up to its full promise, offered unprecedented levels of social security. Poverty, it was widely assumed, had been eliminated. The 'rediscovery of poverty' in the late 1960s (Coates and Silburn, 1970; Townsend, 1979) revealed the limits of the welfare state, while the re-emergence of mass

Figure 6.12

Shares of total income received by individuals below various percentiles of the income distribution (after housing costs)

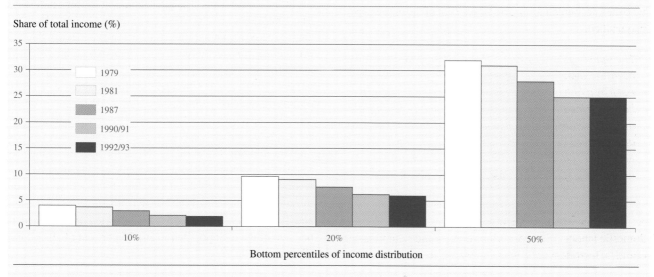

Share of total income (%)

Bottom percentiles of income distribution

Source: Department of Social Security

Figure 6.13

Disposable income per week, persons: 25th percentile and 75th percentile

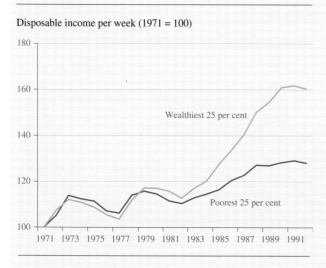

Disposable income per week (1971 = 100)

Source: Institute of Fiscal Studies

Figure 6.14

Composition of bottom 10 per cent of income distribution after housing costs, by household type

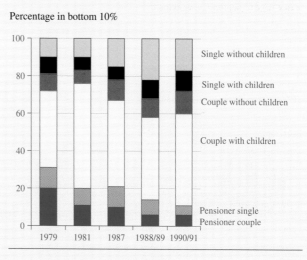

Percentage in bottom 10%

Source: Department of Social Security

unemployment in the late 1970s demonstrated the temporary nature of the post-war settlement.

The subsequent period resembles in important respects the Great Depression and the 1930s. A profound reorganisation of production has led to the contraction, sometimes to near extinction, of industries like coal mining, ship building and steel. A new technology, computers, is working its way through the economy and affecting most types of work. There has been a general 'shifting up' of the occupational structure as non-manual employment has grown and the number of manual jobs fallen. Average real incomes of those with paid employment have increased in most years. Unemployment has been high, access to unemployment benefit has been restricted and a secondary labour market has developed of casual workers, sub-contractors and those employed on short-term contracts.

Recently the gap between the richest and poorest sectors of the population has begun to widen again. Data published by the Department of Social Security show how the proportion of UK disposable income received by the bottom 10, 20 and 50 per cent of income recipients has declined (Figure 6.12). There has been a widening of the gap in disposable income between the richest and poorest quarters of the population (Figure 6.13). Couples with children and single adults with children now form a larger proportion of the poorest 10 per cent, while pensioners now constitute less than 10 per cent of this group (Figure 6.14).

6.4 Food availability and nutrition

Trends in diet and nutrition are described in Chapter 7 in this section, and so are not covered here.

6.5 The physical environment

As discussed above, the 1840s saw the beginnings of major changes in the physical environment for the growing proportion of Britons living in towns and cities.

6.5.1 Sanitation and the urban environment

In his *Report on the Sanitary Condition of the Labouring Population of Great Britain*, published in 1842, the sanitary and social reformer Edwin Chadwick painted a vivid picture of what he regarded as the causes of ill health in industrial cities. For example, in the rapidly growing town of Croydon in 1848 there was only one toilet to every three houses in the poorest courtyards, and the 'town privies' were clustered over an open ditch which ran through the town centre (*Lancet* 13 May 1884: 525, quoted in Smith, 1979). Some of the larger towns had dug closed sewers in the eighteenth century but these were only intended to drain surface water from the streets. They were the wrong shape and did not have sufficient

water flowing through them, allowing stagnant sewage to seep into ground water and pollute drinking supplies. This even affected the houses of the wealthy such as Windsor Castle, which did have piped water, resulting in Prince Albert's death from typhoid in 1861. It was these conditions of life which were widely held to be responsible for the regular epidemics of typhoid and typhus which swept the cities, especially during recessions, as well as a constant burden of tuberculosis and sporadic but alarming outbreaks of cholera. The tendency of life expectancy to rise over the second half of the eighteenth century was threatened by the toll of disease in the new cities. This led to a slow but steady series of measures which eventually brought about improvements in urban conditions.

The Liverpool Sanatory (sic) Act of 1846 established the post of Medical Officer of Health: the first appointment was Dr William Henry Duncan. The Public Health Act of 1848 (much of which was closely based on the earlier Liverpool legislation) gave the Central Board of Health powers to oblige local authorities to set up local health boards in all areas where the mortality rate exceeded 23 per 1,000. The health boards had powers to undertake paving, street cleaning, sewerage and water supply (Flinn, 1965, p.71) and to see that no new houses were built without sewerage. These powers were strengthened by further Acts of Parliament up to 1875. The Metropolitan Water Act of 1852 forbade water companies from taking supplies from tidal sources (the most polluted). In 1865 Bazalgette, the great sanitary engineer, completed his London sewage works, which still exist and can deal with up to 400 million gallons of sewage each day. By 1887 the poorest parish in the London borough of Southwark had filtered water piped to every house, every WC had a water connection and was trapped, as were drains to every house, and all streets and house yards were paved (Smith, 1979, p.228).

The incidence of typhoid in Britain fell dramatically as soon as sewers were built, dropping from 1.2 deaths per 1,000 in 1847–50 to 0.07 in 1906–10 (Parliamentary Papers 1916 vol V, p.60, in Smith, 1979, p.245). The last epidemic of cholera in Britain took place in 1866 and typhus incidence fell rapidly: the last recorded case of typhus in London occurring in 1905 (Smith, 1979, p.244). The Local Government Act of 1888 gave local authorities something like the form which they have at present, and further increased their powers to raise funds for environmental schemes and enforce bye-laws. In 1892 the 'local government debt' of England was about one-sixth of national income (Smith, 1979, p.229; see Millward and Sheard, 1995 for a more detailed account of local authority expenditure on public health).

By the end of the nineteenth century, life expectancy in Britain was at least as great as that in most other Western countries, including ones which had not experienced the same degree of rapid urbanisation: life expectancy at birth being 48 years for British males compared to 45 for those in France and Germany (Coleman and Salt, 1992, pp. 58–61).

6.5.2 The twentieth century urban environment

Although the focus shifted away from sanitation, the beginning of the twentieth century saw a continuing concern with the state of the urban environment and its effects on population health. The Committee on National Deterioration of the Health and Physique of the population was appointed in 1903 in response to the poor health status of Boer War recruits. Its 53 recommendations indicted urban overcrowding, atmospheric pollution, employment conditions, vagrancy, alcohol, venereal disease and, more generally , 'the conditions attending the life of the juvenile population'. Subsequent acts of parliament gave local authorities more powers, for example the Open Spaces Act of 1906. Many of the new measures reflected a shift in concern away from the health of adults to that of children and young people, such as the Education (provision of meals) Act 1906, the Public Health (Amendment) Act of 1907, which established the School Medical Service, and the Maternity and Child Welfare Act of 1918 (Stevenson, 1984).

By 1901 it was estimated that 78 per cent of the population of England and Wales lived in towns or cities. Over half the towns of 50,000 population or above at this time were located on or near to coal fields; more than 80 per cent of the remainder were ports, metal-working towns and textile towns. Areas of dense population, therefore, tended to cluster around sources of pollution. However, transport was already changing the patterns of settlement. Between 1891 and 1911, while the population within six miles of the City of London declined, that of the 'outer ring' (Middlesex and parts of Essex, Surrey, Kent and Hertfordshire) grew from under 1 million to almost 3 million. A similar trend could be seen around other major cities. This was made possible by the growth of suburban railways and electric trams. Railway mileage increased from 8,000 kilometres in 1850 to 21,000 in 1914 (Figure 6.9). The line from Liverpool to Southport was electrified as early as 1904, followed by suburban services on Tyneside. By 1914 all the London underground lines were also electrified, and on some lines cheap fares were available, enabling better off manual workers to move out of the city centre.

Improvement in the physical environment in the period following 1900 was, therefore, less a matter of sanitary reform than of the impact of new technologies of transport and associated changes in patterns of settlement, at least for some sections of society. These changes may have had less impact on working-class than middle-class people. But by 1900 there was a small number of large towns or housing estates which had been 'planned' for the benefit of workers, usually by reforming industrialists such as the Cadbury family who built Bourneville in the East Midlands, and the Lever family who built Port Sunlight in Cheshire. Howard, the initiator of the 'garden city' idea, envisaged towns which combined the advantages of urban living with those of the country, and did not depend upon a single employer. The first 'garden city' was Letchworth, which had grown to a population of 9,000 by 1914 and offered a standard of housing to its working-class inhabitants far superior to anything seen before that time. The underground railway lines allowed the building of the garden city near Hampstead in London between 1905 and 1909: this aimed to be a socially mixed community in which homes of greatly differing sizes would be available, but all of equal quality.

The ideas of Howard influenced a growing tide of opinion amongst those concerned with land use and housing design. During the First World War the government itself built estates designed according to these principles at Gretna in Scotland and Well Hall near London for munitions workers. In 1918 the Tudor Walters Report adopted a standard of 50–60 people per acre and this was widely applied to suburban estates built by municipal authorities in the inter-war period. Second World War bomb damage speeded up the clearance and renewal of older housing around factories, docks and city centres. However, during this period rising concern began to be expressed about the possible social consequences of urban design and re-housing carried out with no consideration of communities and social networks.

Developments in housing policy and household structure and their possible effects on health are further dealt with in Chapters 10 and 11.

6.5.3 Air pollution

Chapter 12 covers this topic in detail.

6.6 The social environment

The major changes in the physical environment which took place during the period 1840–1990 have been accompanied by social change of at least an equal magnitude. Some of these changes can be seen in the sections dealing with fertility and living arrangements – a sharp decrease in the number of children per couple, an increase in both marriage and divorce rates, and the shrinking size of households all indicate great shifts in social relationships. Changes in the workplace can be seen in a similar way. This section will outline some of the other aspects of the social environment which may have had implications for health trends.

6.6.1 Education and attitudes

The very possibility for new ideas to spread themselves depends upon factors such as communication and literacy. When attempting to explain the fall in fertility after 1870, some commentators favour the role of education and the associated spread of new ideas rather than a strictly economic explanation (Coleman and Salt, 1992, p.65; Lesthaeghe, 1983). The 1870 General Education Acts which made education compulsory up to the age of 10 in 1876 and 14 in 1880 will have had a double effect: increasing literacy while at the same time making it impossible for children to work for wages. This will have strengthened the existing tendency of the Factory Acts to increase the economic cost of having children, while improving women's access to new ideas about their role and to contraceptive advice. The spread of education (Figure 6.15) was associated with change in a wide range of attitudes and values; it followed closely upon the 1867 Reform Act which extended the vote to a wider section of the lower middle classes and better off workers who were heads of households. In England church attendance fell markedly (Woods, 1987) while divorce, still a rare event, increased around this time (Figure 6.16), as did suicide (Table 4.2 of Chapter 4) (Coleman and Salt, 1992, p.66).

Attitudes towards the sanitary reforms were at first often hostile: among the middle classes because their rates would have to pay for these, and among the working population because reforms often had greater costs than benefits to them. There was little or no provision for compensation after a home stricken by infectious disease had been fumigated, or for re-housing when slums were cleared. Until the late 1880s, the sanitary department official was regarded in much the same way as the school board officer: someone to be resisted (Smith, 1979). However, as regulation of the activities of the water and food companies made 'healthy behaviour' a possibility and the survival of children more certain for the less privileged, both these attitudes changed. The new enthusiasm for hygiene amongst individuals is reflected in the sales of soap: consumption of soap increased from a total of 10.7 lb per head in 1841 to 14 lb per head of the population per year

Figure 6.15

Children per teacher in primary school, England and Wales

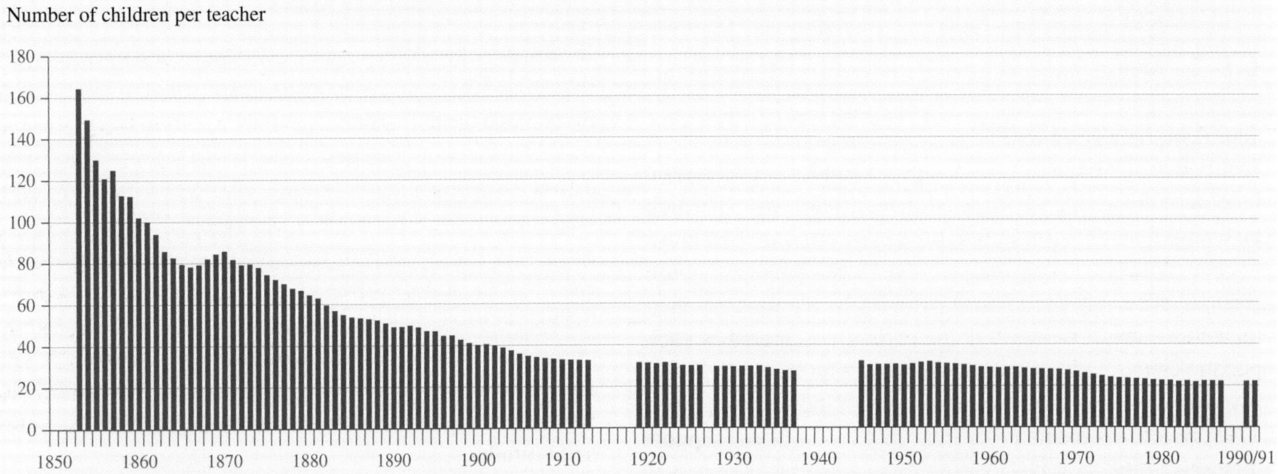

Number of children per teacher

Source: International Historical Statistics, Europe 1750–1988

Figure 6.16

Divorce rate in England and Wales

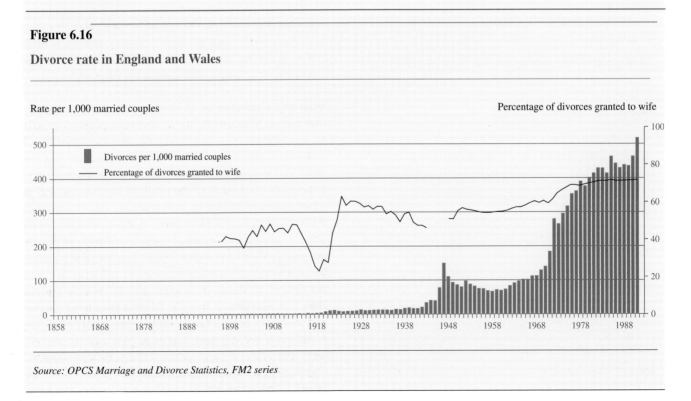

Source: OPCS Marriage and Divorce Statistics, FM2 series

in 1891. The property and business-owning classes increasingly came to accept that public health considerations must sometimes outweigh individual liberty and property rights. By 1870 a wide range of limitations to free market principles had been accepted in the interests of disease control (Porter, 1987), for example, the regulations imposed on private water companies to prevent typhoid and cholera.

Beginning with the extension of the right to vote to all householders and to lodgers paying more than £10 a year in rent in 1885, a wide range of political and social attitudes began to be expressed in a more concrete form, in terms of political pressure for change and in the circumstances of less privileged groups in society. This process was strengthened by the extension of the suffrage to all men and women by 1928. The effects of the ideas and values of citizens from all sections of society are to be seen throughout the history of twentieth century social policy, and in the policies of the present day.

6.6.2   Social policy

The Poor Law 1840–1939
Just before the beginning of the period under consideration here, a major change had taken place in the way in which poverty was dealt with. Before the 1834 Poor Law Act, those unable to earn a living by work (termed 'paupers') were granted 'relief' by each parish, paid for by a poor tax levied on landowners. 'Overseers of the poor' were elected by each parish vestry to administer the system. 'Outdoor relief' was given in cash and kind to those living at home; and, since 1795, relief was extended to those paid too little to support themselves and their families, and was related to the price of bread and the size of family (the price of 12 kg for the man and 6 kg for each other family member per week)

Figure 6.17

People receiving government aid, England and Wales

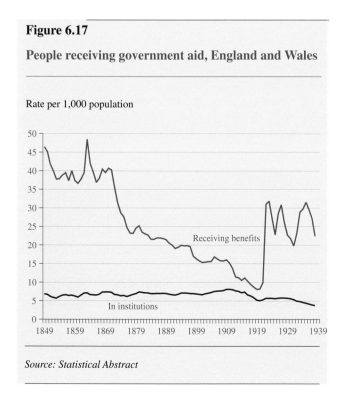

Rate per 1,000 population

Receiving benefits

In institutions

Source: Statistical Abstract

(Speenhamland system). Some healthy men who were judged ineligible for this were placed in a 'workhouse' and made to labour for their keep. The 'able-bodied poor' were obliged to take any work offered to them. Thus, poor relief was supplementing low wages, either because of rises in the price of food or because of large numbers of children in a family. As the population grew this became an increasing economic cost.

Under the 1834 Act (the New Poor Law), workhouses were to be run along more punitive lines, the overseers were re-named 'Guardians', and outdoor relief was severely curtailed. The test of real need was to be the 'workhouse test': anyone refusing to enter the institution was to be judged not poor enough to need support. In addition, conditions within the workhouses were to be more strictly controlled. No-one on relief must be allowed to live at an equal standard of living to that of the poorest labourer. This was the 'principle of less eligibility'.

In practice the effect of the New Poor Law on the cost of relief was not as great as its proponents hoped. It was effective in reducing the proportion of people receiving benefits in their own homes: this dropped from around 5 per cent of the estimated population in 1849 to less than 1 per cent at the beginning of the First World War (Figure 6.17). This fell even further as the coming of old age pensions meant that the elderly were no longer regarded as 'paupers' and a charge on the parish rates. But this was offset by the rising proportion of the poor who were institutionalised, at considerable cost. And as time went on, the deterrent power of the workhouse was drastically curtailed by changes in political institutions and attitudes.

From Poor Law to social insurance

Health: from workhouse to hospital
The impact of health services in Britain will be dealt with in Chapter 14. Here we merely sketch the early changes by which 'hospitals' came to be seen as something separate from 'workhouses': a punitive institution for the poor.

Both before and after the 1834 Act, parish workhouses had a dual role: as places where the healthy unemployed should be set to work, and as a place where the elderly, chronically ill and infants might be housed if there was no other place for them. As urbanisation proceeded, a larger proportion of the population lived far from their village origins, and had no other source of shelter or care when ill, old or orphaned. Between 1870 and 1914, between 6 and 8 per 1,000 of the population were workhouse inmates. However, by the beginning of the twentieth century very few of these could be regarded as able-bodied unemployed. Whereas in 1871 6 per cent of all deaths in England and Wales took place in Poor Law institutions, by 1906 this had risen to 10 per cent and to 21 per cent in London (Crowther, 1981, p.57).[3] As workhouses became more and more places of refuge, they were seen as less and less suitable as a deterrent to 'idleness'. The Poor Law came under increasing criticism (Webb and Webb, 1929). After 1908, a series of policy measures began to break up the 'general mixed workhouse' as the refuge for old, sick, idle, orphaned and unemployed. The coming of old age pensions greatly reduced the demand for 'outdoor' relief but not 'indoor' – the ill elderly still needed institutional care. From 1913, the term 'workhouse' was officially replaced by 'Poor Law institution'; these were separated into infirmaries, children's homes and homes for the elderly, and efforts were made to reduce the degree of stigma associated with institutionalisation. After 1919 Registrars no longer wrote a 'W' on the death certificates of those who died in workhouses, but invented street names and numbers. 1919 was the year in which the first Ministry of Health was set up: the first Health Minister, Addison, regarded the Poor Law as an outdated Victorian institution, but failed to reform it. The granting of the franchise to all men (including the poorest) in 1918 altered attitudes towards workhouses and changes became inevitable.

Since the 1860s 'municipal hospitals' separate from the Poor Law infirmaries had begun to be opened, owing to concerns about infectious disease; by 1911 there were over 1,000 of these. The Local Government Act of 1929 aimed to form a co-ordinated national hospital service with local authorities taking the lead. The coming into reality of the idea of a national health service had to wait, however, until after the Second World War.

Old age and invalidity
From 1908 any citizen over age 70 whose income did not exceed £21 per year could claim a pension of 5s per week (i.e. £13 per annum). Part I of the 1911 National Insurance Act (Part II of which introduced contributory unemployment insurance for some workers) provided 14 million men and women with GP services and income support of 10s a week during the illness of the family breadwinner. After 26 weeks the 10s was reduced to 5s; it then became a long-term invalidity benefit and was paid indefinitely. Like unemployment benefit, National Health Insurance was a contributory benefit, financed by a contribution of 4d from working men, or 3d from women, in addition to 3d from the employer. Soon after the end of the First World War the Adkins Committee concluded that there should be a comprehensive system of non-contributory public assistance for all those in need, whether from old age, illness or unemployment. These proposals were dismissed as far too expensive in a time of recession, but in early 1924, William Beveridge first put forward his plans for contributory insurance against the full range of possible misfortunes (Beveridge, 1924). Once again, the full impact of these ideas had to wait until after the Second World War.

Poverty, nutrition and physical efficiency
As we have seen, by 1900 the major health problems for population health were no longer seen as those related to

infectious disease spread by unhygienic conditions. However, the Royal Commission on Physical Training (Scotland) Report of 1903 and the Committee on Physical Deterioration Report of 1904 found plenty to be concerned about in the health of recruits to the armed forces. Some 40 per cent had been found unfit for service, and the reasons they pin-pointed were related to poverty and poor nutrition amongst the families of urban labourers, and policy measures were focused on child health. In 1906 the School Meals Act was passed and in 1908 the School Medical Service was established. The examinations carried out under this legislation gave rise to increased concern with nutrition. Rickets was found to be widespread, and provision of milk and meals to schoolchildren was encouraged. This period saw the beginnings of the 'open air school' movement, which provided residential schooling for children who were debilitated and 'pre-tubercular' (much of this will have been due to malnutrition). However, all these measures were either undertaken by voluntary effort or under enabling legislation: there were no compulsory standards of provision, so that by 1936 fewer children were receiving school meals than in 1911 (Hewetson, 1946, p.40). In many areas this was under 10 per cent. However these 'new' health problems associated with poverty rather than with dirt could not be solved without a change in attitudes towards the wider issues of poverty. Parents who were receiving poor relief or unemployment benefit had the cost of meals deducted from their benefits. School meals had to be financed by local rates, but the poorest areas with the most children in need and bearing the greatest cost were the ones which received least in local rates.

The failure of social policies of the early twentieth century to deal with the health effects of poverty came alarmingly to light during recruitment for the First and Second World Wars. Between November 1917 and October 1918 the Ministry of National Service examined some 2.5 million young men of military age. It concluded that 'of every 9 men of military age ... on average three were perfectly fit and healthy; two were upon a definitely infirm plane of health and strength ... three ... could almost be described ... as physical wrecks; and the remaining man was a chronic invalid with a precarious hold on life,' (quoted in Le Gros Clark and Titmuss, 1939, p.125). Between 1934 and 1936 over 30 per cent of recruits were being rejected on health grounds, excluding those rejected due to poor sight (Le Gros Clark and Titmuss, 1939, pp.127–8).

Unemployment
The development of unemployment benefit shows the way in which social policies undergo violent shifts according to changes in political attitudes. Although up to 1900 those without work received an income, the term 'pauper' was intended to stigmatise, as were the rules for entering and living in the workhouses. Before 1885, those entitled to vote on both national and local methods for dealing with the poor and unemployed were the upper- and middle-classes who were unlikely to experience such contingencies themselves. However, after the introduction of votes for all householders, policies began to change. After 1905, policy emphasis turned

---

3   *These figures should be interpreted with some caution, as by the late nineteenth century many local authorities were sending non-pauper infectious disease patients to the workhouse infirmaries.*

towards the provision of training and of better access to information on work availability through Labour Exchanges, and the development of 'social insurance' schemes. The National Insurance Act of 1911 introduced the world's first compulsory state unemployment insurance scheme into Britain. The idea of 'social insurance' was that while earning, not only the worker but also the employer and central government would contribute a small proportion of salary towards old age, illness and unemployment. The benefits thus accrued belonged to the insured person as of right, and were not subject to the 'workhouse test' or to means testing (that is, benefits were received regardless of the income of the person at the time they became eligible). The 1911 and 1916 Unemployment Insurance Acts applied only to occupations such as building and engineering, where unemployment was relatively frequent. Workers and employers paid $2^1/_2$d per week and the government added $1^2/_3$d. In return workers received as of right 7s per week for up to 15 weeks of unemployment in any single year. At that time, this represented around one-third of the average weekly wage for low paid urban workers (Gilbert, 1970, p.52). However, those with insufficient contributions were still dependent on the Poor Law.

Between 1920 and 1921 the numbers reliant on poor relief grew from 664,000 to 1,498,000 (almost 4 per cent of the population) (Gilbert, 1970, p. 211). As the inter-war recession went on it became impossible to maintain the Poor Law principles of deterrence and punishment of the poor. Wages in the lowest paid jobs fell so low that even the most draconian workhouse manager was providing more food and warmth than a low-paid worker could afford. In 1922 the so-called 'Mond Scale' was published, setting a semi-official going rate for poor relief (i.e. the benefits available to people not eligible for unemployment insurance benefits). This went up to a maximum of 54s a week for a family of eight: much higher than the available unemployment insurance benefit of 23s 4d for an equivalent household. Under the pressure of political change, the local Guardians of the Poor were now providing a better standard of living than that available either to low-paid workers or under social insurance. Under these same pressures, the degree of stigma associated with being 'on relief' had also reduced. Attitudinal changes allowed local expenditure on the relief of poverty to rise rapidly at a time of economic crisis, and led to the abolition of the Poor Law and the advent of a modern Welfare State.

The end of the War saw large numbers of men thrown back into the open labour market after years either in the armed forces or the munitions industries, and the 1911 and 1916 measures were inadequate to meet the ensuing recession. Many women drafted into the workforce during the war now saw employment as a right. Political ideas which had inspired the Russian revolution had wide currency among British workers, and political anxieties were great. As an emergency measure the government made an allowance to all unemployed (whether insured or not) based on the cost of living and including a dependants' allowance. This allowance was known as 'the dole'; it was paid at a much higher level

of 29s for men and 25 for women for the first 13 weeks, with additions for dependents (Gilbert, 1970, p.62). The 1920 Unemployment Insurance Act increased the rate of contributions and reduced the rate of benefit paid. However, the attempt to establish an actuarially sound system of contributory unemployment insurance was doomed by the onset of mass unemployment, and extra benefits were paid in various forms throughout the period. Despite this, studies in the 1930s showed that the allowances available to the unemployed were not sufficient to provide the diet judged by the British Medical Association necessary to maintain health (Vernon, 1936; cited in Hewetson, 1946, p.43). An aspect of British unemployment which has continued to the present is that the labour market is 'segmented' into more and less discrete groups of people. What happens during recession is that those losing work find it harder to regain employment, and those whose work is normally insecure become long-term unemployed rather than intermittently employed. Thus in the 1930s those at risk of unemployment were also most likely to have been only intermittently employed in the past, and therefore to have been unable to pay full insurance contributions. A large number of the unemployed during the 1930s were not insured, or had run out of benefit, and were therefore reliant on the Poor Law.

Social policy after 1940

A unified scheme: the Beveridge Plan
By 1939 nearly 21 million people were covered by the state old age insurance schemes, 15.5 million by unemployment insurance and 20 million by national health insurance (Calder, 1969, p.607). The aim of the benefits received under each of these schemes was the same: to reduce dependency on the Poor Law and restore dignity to those unable to earn as a consequence of illness, unemployment or old age by giving benefit as of right. However, national health insurance did not include any supplement for dependants, and wives and children were not insurable under it, and was undermined by low levels of benefit as well as relatively high levels available under the Poor Law. The aim of the Beveridge Report was to design ways to make social insurance live up to its intended aims.

The Report was based on the simple principle that all needs would be covered by a single contribution. Anyone unable to contribute, and those who 'fell through the net', would be given a non-contributory benefit (a residual Poor Law) called 'National Assistance'. In either of these ways, all citizens were to be assured a national minimum income sufficient for a decent level of subsistence. However, for the great majority of people, this income was to be paid for by their own, as well as their employers', contributions – it was neither 'relief' nor a 'dole'. All citizens would pay contributions and receive benefits: there was no income limit. This was thought to be a vital socially unifying element in the Beveridge Plan. It was not a system for the poor only, but for the whole of society. Beveridge identified Five Great Evils: Want, Disease, Ignorance, Squalor and Idleness. Future social welfare depended on keeping all of these at bay. For example, if Want and Squalor were to be abolished, something like full employment must be ensured to avoid the problem of labour market segmentation and the attending poverty. Providing free health care would prevent loss of work due to chronic illness, and improvements in education would have a similarly benign effect on employability.

Contributions to the new scheme were to be far higher than the old rates, but no-one would be obliged to carry private insurance. Benefits were also to be far higher. In the original Report it was envisaged that a man with a wife and two children would, under the Plan, receive 56s per week for an unlimited time when out of work, as compared to the 1942 level of 38s a week for 26 weeks. The same man, if disabled, would receive 56s a week as compared to the 1942 benefit of 18s for the first 26 weeks followed by 10s 6d.

Although the Beveridge Plan and the associated scheme for a national health service set out the framework for the welfare state we have today, there were from the beginning visible signs of future difficulties. One of the most important of these was the level at which benefits were actually paid. The rate of subsistence was calculated on the basis of research by Rowntree, who had tried to establish scientifically the amount of money necessary to prevent malnutrition. Rowntree had included a number of 'social sundries' in his calculations, all of which were cut out. By the time the first benefits began to be paid in 1948 the cost of living had also risen. The net result of this was that benefits only represented 75 per cent of Rowntree's minimum. The scheme also failed to deal with variations in housing costs. As a result, people had to resort to National Assistance from the very beginning of the scheme: the ideal of comprehensive social insurance was never realised at all (Wilson, 1977, p.149).

Beyond the post-war settlement
The level of benefits was not an overwhelming problem while something near to full employment existed up to the 'oil shocks' of the mid-1970s. However, once unemployment began to rise (see Figure 6.11), the cracks in the post-war welfare system widened rapidly. The increasing power of technology made many forms of routine and unskilled labour unnecessary. As the demand for labour fell (Nickell and Bell, 1995), wages for unskilled work also decreased in relative value. Those with lower levels of skill fell behind the rising trend in income of the more prosperous (Goodman and Webb, 1995; Central Statistical Office, 1995). Means-tested benefits always raise the problem of people becoming 'trapped in benefit': taking a low-paid job may increase income by so little (if at all) that any increase is swallowed up in the cost of fares to work and wear on clothing. In addition, although the relative value of low wages was falling, the money wage at which individuals began to pay tax had changed little during the high-inflation years of the mid-1970s, meaning that by the end of that decade very large numbers of low paid workers lost over 30 per cent in taxation. The cost of the welfare state had also been rising faster than GDP (Figure 6.18). The failure of successive post-war governments to overcome these problems was in part responsible for a disenchantment with

re-distributive policies, and led the voting public to elect governments promising lower taxes and a return to 'free market' economics. By the mid-1990s top rates of taxation had fallen from over 80 per cent to 40 per cent, and the rate for the low-paid had fallen to 20 per cent. Inflation of under 3 per cent protected those on fixed incomes. However, the problems surrounding the collapse in demand for manual and less skilled non-manual labour persisted in the United Kingdom, as in most other advanced industrial nations. Combined with improving life expectancy, this was, by the end of the Millennium, creating the problem of an increasingly large non-employed and retired population, supported by a diminishing number of employed tax-payers determined to maintain control of their incomes.

The 1980s saw a large number of changes in the rules relating to unemployment, disability, housing and other benefits. Many of the underlying problems were little different from those faced during the recession of the 1930s, but because of the difference in political attitudes, some solutions resembled a move towards to the policies of the nineteenth century. Tests of eligibility for unemployment benefit were tightened in a series of measures. The right to unemployment benefit was withdrawn altogether from young people aged 16–18. Funding of care of the elderly shifted away from collective and towards personal responsibility, including the requirement that old people who owned their homes should sell them to pay for institutional care, effectively re-introducing a 'means test'. The value of the old age pension itself, as well as that of other benefits, was detached from the average wage and linked instead to the level of inflation. In this way, those on benefit, while protected from the effects of inflation, were excluded from any general rise in the standard of living of the rest of the population. In at least one respect, however, there were radical differences between the 1980s and 1930s. Legal and attitudinal changes over the 1960s and 1970s radically changed the situation of women. The assumption of the Beveridge Plan was that married women would be predominantly concerned with the care of the home and children, and that divorce and single parenthood not due to widowhood would be relatively rare. By the 1980s these assumptions were completely overtaken by events (Figures 6.19 and 6.20), and these changes continue to represent a challenge to policy makers.

At the same time as these changes in the economy and in public attitudes and values have taken place, there have been continuing increases in the income of those in well-paid jobs, falling living standards amongst the low paid and those not in paid work, and rising levels of uneasiness about the state of society at large (Davey Smith, 1996; Hutton, 1995; Watt, 1996) (Figures 6.12 and 6.13). It is also reflected in increasing levels of variation in health between different social groups (McCarron, *et al.*, 1994; McLoone and Boddy, 1994; Phillimore *et al.*, 1994). Whereas in 1955 Morris and Heady could write, in the face of the Beveridge reforms, that future differences in health must be tackled by changing individual behaviour, in 1995 the Chief Medical Officer for England and Wales' sub-group on social variation in health was less

Figure 6.18

General government expenditure as a percentage of the GDP, United Kingdom

Per cent of total GDP

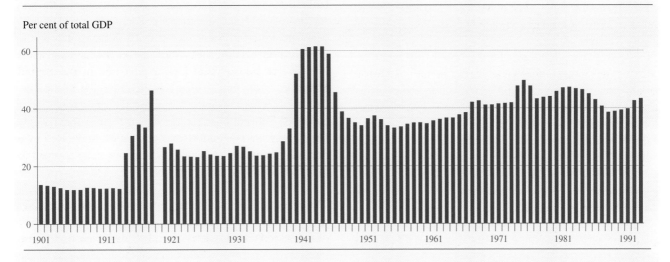

Source: CSO

Figure 6.19

Changing composition of the workforce, 1959-93

Workforce (millions)

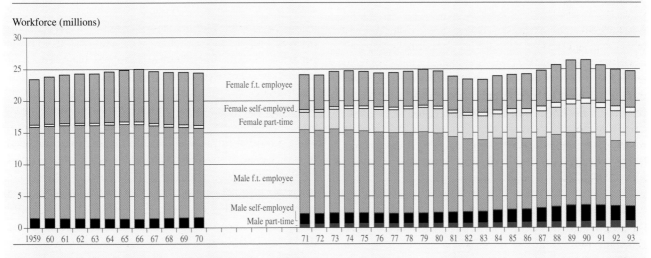

Note:Data on part-time workers only available from 1971 onwards
Source: Department of Transport

Figure 6.20

Families headed by lone parents as a percentage of all families with dependents

Percentage

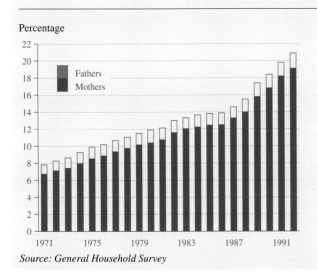

Source: General Household Survey

certain of this (Variations Sub-group, 1995). Research evidence shows that differences in lifestyle such as smoking, diet and exercise can only account for around a third of the differences in heart disease between better and worse off sections of the community (Rose and Marmot, 1981; Woodward *et al.*, 1990). Furthermore, social inequality in health is not just a matter of illness and early death amongst the very poor. Life expectancy is finely graded throughout the social scale – 'higher' professionals and managers live longer than 'intermediate' ones – and is probably influenced by differences in the risk of adverse experiences throughout the course of life. Insecurity of employment is no longer the prerogative of lower-skilled manual workers: large numbers of managers, scientists and civil servants are becoming familiar with threats of redundancy. Like the changing attitudes to the family among women, changing attitudes to, and experiences of, work among middle-class men may be one of the moving forces for the future of social policy.

6.7 Conclusion

The period from 1841 to 1994 might be characterised as one in which very great changes in the technology of production were accompanied by equally major changes in attitudes and values. The coming of the factory production system led to the growth of cities, the concentration of production in large workplaces, the separation of paid labour from domestic work and child care, and the availability of non-seasonal work for the majority of the population. Industrial production was far more powerful than agricultural and craft methods, although it involved the subjection of workers to mass production methods and crowded urban life. Populations responded to these massive changes in many ways: by limiting their fertility in ways which are still not understood, by organising Friendly Societies to tide over the boom and bust rhythms of the new economic regime, by combining into trade unions and eventually creating new political parties. The policies which evolved from these processes aimed to spread the wealth created by the new industrial technologies to create a more general prosperity, one which was more evenly spread both over time (straddling the economic cycles) and between richer and poorer regions and social groups. Parallel with these economic, political and demographic changes, there have been great improvements in population health. These improvements have been somewhat uneven in their distribution, however. At the end of the twentieth century, industrialised countries are faced with yet another major set of technological and demographic changes: from mass heavy industry dominated by iron, steel and coal to highly automated, flexible production dominated by advances in electronics and information science; from a younger to an older age profile; from lives taken up by work and child rearing to lives in which adaptation to rapid change through re-education may take a central part. A greater understanding of the patterns of the past may help in the attempt to adapt to the changes of the future.

Acknowledgements

The authors would like to thank Anita Brock and Karen Quaife for their help in collating much of the tabular and graphical material.

Chapter 7

Trends in diet 1841–1994

By
John Charlton and Karen Quaife

Summary

- Nutritional status can be influenced by illness and other factors, and is thus not solely determined by diet. In turn, it can influence resistance to infection, health and growth, particularly in children.

- For women obesity is the next best predictor of cardiovascular disease after age and blood pressure, and is a risk factor for men and women without other major risk factors.

- By 1900, food regulation and better transport offered an improved choice of food for the burgeoning urban population, although there remained a large undernourished underclass – 31 per cent of the population of London lived below the poverty line.

- During the Second World War rationing and other factors affecting redistribution raised nutritional standards for the poor and may also have provided health gains for the wealthy.

- Energy intakes have decreased steadily since the 1960s in adults and children, which may reflect a more sedentary lifestyle. In spite of these dietary changes the proportion of adults who are obese or overweight has increased.

- In the 1950s affluent households were the greatest consumers of sugars, fats and eggs, but by 1993 their consumption was the lowest.

- A recent survey showed that parents who suffered the most severe financial pressures spent least on food and had the lowest nutrient intakes.

7.1 Introduction

This chapter presents trends over the period 1841 to 1993 because of the important bearing that nutritional status has on health. Although McKeown (1976) attributed most of the mortality decline in the eighteenth and nineteenth centuries to improved nutrition, other factors such as public health, sanitation, housing, living standards, social organisation and scientific advance are also important, and it is difficult to disentangle the contributions of each using the available data. Nutritional status, which is dependent upon the body's absorption of nutrients, can be influenced by illness and other factors (see section 7.2), and is thus not solely determined by diet. The data in the chapter cover two distinct periods, up to the First World War, and afterwards. Data for more recent times are more reliable, since survey methodology has advanced. In the earlier period, concern had been focused on under-nutrition amongst the poorest individuals, and only working-class diets tended to be studied. Since 1950 nationally representative data have become available. As the country has become more affluent, British dietary concerns have shifted from the problems of under-nutrition towards the problems of over-nutrition (and hence obesity), and the health- related properties of particular foods (Buss, 1993).

7.2 The role of nutritional status in maintaining health

Food is the body's source of energy and means of material growth, and problems arise when the balance and adequacy of nutrients in the diet exceed or are less than what is required. Energy is required to drive the metabolic process and the

Table 7.1

Daily dietary reference values for men aged 19–50 years

| | Quantity | | |
	Truswell (1983)	DoH (1991a)	Units
Total energy (EARs)*	10.31 (2,480)	10.60 (2,550)	*MJ (kcal)*
Total fat	-	33 (35)	
Saturated fatty acids	-	10 (11)	
Cis-polyunsaturated fatty acids	-	6 (6.5)	*% of Daily total energy*
Cis-monosaturated fatty acids	-	12 (13)	*(% of food energy)*
Trans fatty acids	-	2 (2)	
Total carbohydrate	-	47 (50)	
Non starch polysaccharide	-	18	
Protein	66.1	55.5	*g*
Vitamin A	910	700	*µg*
Thiamin	1.26	1	*mg*
Riboflavin	-	1.3	*mg*
Niacin	18.3	17	*mg*
Vitamin B6	2.0	1.4	*µg*
Vitamin B12	2.52	1.5	*µg*
Folate	194	200	*µg*
Vitamin C	47.4	-	*mg*
Vitamin D	4.4	-	*mg*
Vitamin E	12.0	-	*mg*
Calcium	610	700	*mg*
Phosphorus	960	550	*mg*
Magnesium	345	300	*mg*
Sodium	-	1,600	*mg*
Potassium	-	3,500	*mg*
Chloride	-	2,500	*mg*
Iron	20.0	8.7	*mg*
Zinc	13.2	9.5	*mg*
Copper	-	1.2	*mg*
Selenium	-	75	*µg*
Iodine	145.7	140	*µg*

* Estimated Average Requirements
Sources: Truswell (1983); Department of Health, (1991a)

body's stores of nutrients must be maintained, with at least 30 g of protein required per day to maintain equilibrium. Vitamins are essential co-factors for many metabolic processes. The first United Kingdom recommendations, by the British Medical Association, followed a review of diets during and after the Second World War. These have since been updated at regular intervals. There is uncertainty about the levels of nutrients sufficient to prevent signs of deficiency, and experts differ in their assessment of the evidence. Table 7.1 shows the energy, protein and other major nutrients considered necessary for the health of normal adult men, based on the average recommendations of nutritional committees in 40 countries (Truswell, 1983), and recent United Kingdom standards (DoH, 1991a). Dietary reference values (DRVs) are estimated averages intended as a guide to nutritional assessment of large groups or populations. Typically, they are levels necessary to prevent clinical deficiency, allowing also for the possibility of periods of high demand. Nutrient requirements differ widely between similar individuals, as well as being dependent upon age, sex, size, physical activity and physiological state (Wenlock, 1992). The difference between total energy and food energy is due to alcohol consumption. Ninety five per cent of ingested alcohol is converted to energy – it provides almost as much energy as pure fat (29 kilojoules per gram).

One problem in assessing needs is that when the body is undernourished it adapts by lowering the resting metabolic rate, achieving a new steady state with lower body weight and energy requirements. Other adaptations also occur. For example, in West Holland during the hungry winter of 1944–45, when the average energy intake fell below 1,000 kcal per person per day, virtually all women of child-bearing age ceased to menstruate (Stein *et al.*, 1975). In spite of the uncertainties, evidence is accumulating that a diet meeting certain criteria is predictive of survival to old age. In a recent study among elderly people, Trichopoulou *et al.* (1995) established that a one unit increase in a dietary score, that had been devised on the basis of eight component characteristics of the traditional Mediterranean region, was associated with a significant 17 per cent reduction in overall mortality.

Estimated energy requirements have decreased over time – the 1950 recommendations of the BMA for a moderately active man were 3,000 kcals per day (BMA, 1950), which decreased to 2,900 kcals/d in 1979 (DHSS, 1979). The most recent recommendations in 1991 (DoH, 1991a) now assume that a man will be occupied in light activity and is relatively sedentary during leisure time, requiring 2,550 kcals. This contrasts with Joseph Rowntree's calculations in 1901 that 3,500 kcals was the lowest possible threshold for a working man without damaging his physical health (Rowntree, 1901). Children and lactating women have different nutritional requirements from men – for children the process of growth requires relatively higher intakes, with a 1-year-old requiring about half the protein and energy of a sedentary adult, who might weigh six to seven times as much. If a growing child does not get enough to eat it adapts by growing less – the velocity of height growth in children is an extremely sensitive

index of nutritional status, with the usual provisos that other factors (genetic and infective) may also affect height growth. This measure is most useful in populations where marginal malnutrition is common, and less so in more affluent societies (Garrow, 1991).

7.2.1 Low nutritional status, immunity and infection

Studies of the developing countries have improved our understanding of the role of nutrition in our susceptibility to infectious and parasitic diseases. Poor nutritional status has a definite influence on the incidence, severity, duration and outcome of tuberculosis, bacterial diarrhoea, cholera, leprosy, pertussis, respiratory infections, measles, rotavirus diarrhoea, herpes and a number of parasitic and fungal diseases, and a variable influence on others such as diphtheria, staphylococcus, streptococcus, influenza, etc. – see Table 7.2 (Chandra, 1983). The mechanisms include depression of the immune system's response to infection, and thus increasing susceptibility to infections, discussed in detail by Lunn (1991). Improvements in food intake in poorly nourished communities lead to better resistance to infection and lowered mortality,

Table 7.2

Infectious diseases influenced by low nutritional status

Disease category	Influence		
	Definite	**Variable**	**Slight**
Bacterial	Tuberculosis	Diphtheria	Typhoid
	Bacterial	Straphylococcus	Plague
	diarrhoea	Streptococcus	Tetanus
	Cholera		Bacterial
	Leprosy		toxins
	Pertussis		
	Respiratory		
	infections		
Viral	Measles	Influenza	Smallpox
	Rotavirus		Yellow
	diarrhoea		fever
	Respiratory		Arthropod-
	infections		borne virus
	Herpes		
Parasitic	Pneumocystis	Giardia	
	carinii	Filiariasis	
	Intestinal		
	parasites		
	Trypanosomiasis		
	Leishmaniasis		
	Schistosomiasis		
Fungal	Candida	Mould toxins	
	Aspergillus		
Other		Syphilis	
		Typhus	

Source: Lunn (1991)

especially in infancy and childhood. Infection and nutritional status interact, however, since virtually all infections are associated with loss of appetite, particularly marked in children. Even when food is consumed it may not be absorbed effectively. For example, diarrhoea is associated with decreased absorption of carbohydrate, fat and protein, together with a number of trace elements and vitamins (Scrimshaw, 1981). Inflammation occurring in response to infection mobilises body tissues and reserves to provide energy to fuel the immune response. Powander (1977) has calculated an average loss of 0.6 g of protein/kg/day during most illnesses, rising to 0.9 g/kg/day with diarrhoea.

7.2.2 Height, growth and nutritional status

Floud (1991) has reviewed the evidence linking height with nutritional status. Heights have been increasing. Based on statistically adjusted army recruitment data, Floud et al., (1990) showed that a working class boy of 14 in the 1990s is almost as tall as a working class adult of the mid-eighteenth century. However, there have been periods when height has decreased. During the middle of the nineteenth century, particularly for men born between 1830 and 1860, there was a moderately sustained decline in height in Britain. Floud concludes that '... broadly, these different levels and patterns

Figure 7.1

The heights of boys at Christchurch School, by age

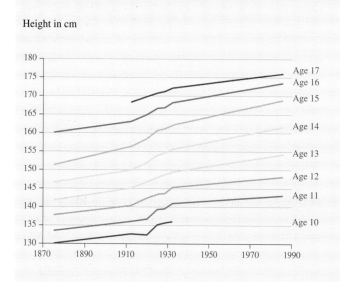

Figure 7.2

Trends in height distribution of men and women aged 25–34

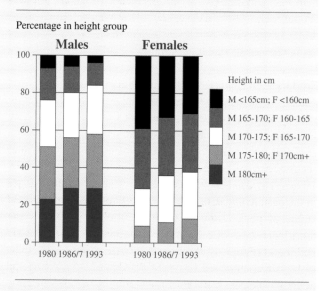

Source: ONS

Table 7.3

Height and weight of toddlers

Mean weight (kg) of children aged 1½–4½ years, 1967/8 and 1992/3

Age (years)	Boys		Girls	
	1967/8	1992/3	1967/8	1992/3
1½–2½	12.9	12.6	12.2	11.9
2½–3½	14.7	14.9	13.9	14.3
3½–4½	16.5	16.6	16.0	16.4

Mean height (cm) of children aged 1½–4½ years, 1967/8 and 1992/3

Age (years)	Boys		Girls	
	1967/8	1992/3	1967/8	1992/3
1½–2½	85.9	86.9	84.9	85.3
2½–3½	94.3	95.6	92.8	94.7
3½–4½	101.7	102.1	100.4	101.3

Source: Gregory et al., (1995)

Table 7.4

Incidence and prevalence of breast feeding 1975–1990

Percentage breast feeding at each age

	England and Wales				Scotland		
	1975	1980	1985	1990	1980	1985	1990
Birth	51	67	65	64	50	48	50
1 week	-	58	56	54	44	41	41
2 weeks	-	54	53	51	41	38	39
6 weeks	-	42	40	39	32	29	30
4 months	-	27	26	25	21	22	20
6 months	-	23	21	21	18	18	16
9 months	-	12	11	12	9	9	9
Base	1,544	3,755	4,671	4,942	1,718	1,895	1,981

Source: White et al., (1990)

appear to be associated with levels of income and of mortality, although many features remain unexplained'. There were large differences between different population subgroups. For example, in the early nineteenth century boys from the Marine Society, which took boys from the London slums, were below the first centile of modern height distributions, whereas boys at the Royal Military College at Sandhurst (upper classes) were some 25 cm (10 inches) taller, at the fiftieth centile of modern height distributions. It is suggested that the Sandhurst children (who are likely to have been well nourished) would have been even taller had their exposure to disease been less (Rea, 1971). Data from army recruitment records have shown that white-collar workers were taller than skilled and semi-skilled industrial workers, who were taller than most labourers, who were taller than domestic servants. Analysis of recruitment data which provided measures of both height and health showed that the two were inversely related, a short man being more likely to be rejected on medical grounds (Fogel *et al.*, 1986). Marmot *et al.*, (1984) have found similar relationships between height and the probability of early death, using recent data on civil servants.

Studies in the developing world have shown that food deprivation between weaning and the age of 3 can permanently stunt growth (Falkner and Tanner, 1986). Other environmental influences such as disease, socio-economic level, urbanisation, seasonal and climatic variation, psycho-social stress and secular trend are, however, also important (Eveleth and Tanner, 1990). Provided that we can reliably estimate height changes in the past, height data may accurately reflect the nutritional status of populations in the past, and in particular the nutritional status of cohorts of populations during their early childhood (Floud, 1991). Figure 7.1 shows how the heights of boys has increased since the 1870s in Christ's Hospital School, which has had a policy of admitting boys of moderate means throughout the period (Rosenbaum, 1988). The heights of 15-year-old boys, for example, increased by 10.9 cm (4.3 inches) from 1870 to 1933, and by 17.6 cm to 1986. However, improvement in nutritional status also results in earlier maturation, and the boys in the 1870s may have caught up some of the height differential later – for 16-year-olds the difference between the 1870s and 1986 was less – 13.4cm. Figure 7.1 shows, also, that the biggest increase in average height occurred between 1910 and the 1940s.

Comparison of anthropometric measurements from the 1993 dietary and nutritional survey of toddlers with the earlier 1967–68 survey (Gregory, 1995), shows an increase in both mean height and weight for toddlers (see Table 7.3), which has resulted in little change in body mass index (see 7.2.3 below). In addition, the different methods used to measure height in the two surveys may mean that increase in height may be even more pronounced. Anthropometric comparisons from three surveys conducted between 1980 and 1993 show that the heights of men and women are still increasing (Figure 7.2 shows ages 25–34), with mean height increasing by 0.8 cm for men and 1 cm for women. Most notable is the reduction in the proportion of people in the shortest categories.

Barker (1994) has gone further in hypothesising that a baby's nourishment before birth and during infancy 'programmes' the development of risk factors in adult life such as raised blood pressure, fibrinogen concentration, factor VIII concentration and glucose intolerance, and hence alters the risk of coronary heart disease. In the studies undertaken by him and his colleagues, early nutrition is inferred indirectly from foetal and infant growth. However, foetal growth may be a doubtful surrogate measure (Paneth and Susser, 1995). Paneth and Susser found the evidence to be mixed, and in need of more rigorous testing.

Breast feeding is a major factor in influencing infant survival, being nutritionally ideal and rich in antibodies that provide immunity against a number of common childhood infections. Early weaning carries the dangers of exposure to, among others, protein-energy malnutrition and deficiencies of iron, iodine and vitamin A (Lopez, 1986). A longitudinal study from birth to age 17 has demonstrated that, in addition, breast feeding is protective throughout childhood and adolescence against atopy, specifically eczema, food allergy and respiratory allergy (Saarinen and Kajosaari, 1995). Data on the prevalence of breast feeding has only been collected since 1965, and Table 7.4 shows the proportions breast feeding at birth and at subsequent intervals (White *et al.*, 1990).

7.2.3 Obesity and health

In affluent societies, over-nutrition is more likely to be a problem, when some nutrients are taken in excess. The most important problem is excess energy intake, leading to increases in body fat. A lesser problem is an excess of fat-soluble vitamins resulting in poisoning. The body can compensate for excesses in other nutrients by increasing excretion or diminishing absorption.

People above a certain weight-for-height tend to die young, a fact that has been used by insurance companies for many years. Quetelet (1869) established that for adults of normal build the ratio of weight (kg) to the square of height (m²) is constant. Quetelet's index, renamed the Body Mass Index (BMI) by Keys (1972) is the standard measure of obesity in adults: 20–24.9 is 'desirable'; 25–29.9 is 'overweight'; and more than 30 is 'obese'. Ninety per cent of the variation in BMI is explained by variations in body fat (Garrow and Webster, 1985).

A consensus conference in the USA in 1985 (NIHCDP, 1985) concluded that obesity is undoubtedly associated with hypertension, hypercholesterolaemia, non-insulin-dependent diabetes mellitus, certain cancers, and has adverse effects on health and longevity. The medical importance of obesity has been concealed in the past by the fact that several life-threatening chronic diseases cause weight loss; smokers tend to have lower BMIs than non-smokers, but die younger. For women, obesity is the next best predictor of cardiovascular disease after age and blood pressure, and is a risk factor for men and women without other major risk factors (Hubert, 1984). Excess weight is also associated with gallbladder disease (Bray, 1985), menstrual irregularity (Friedman and Kim, 1985) and cancers of the colon, rectum and prostate in men, and gallbladder, endometrium, cervix, ovary and breast in women (Garfinkel, 1985). Substances such as alcohol and sugar, which contain energy but virtually no other nutrient, contribute to excess energy intakes.

Burkitt and Trowell (1975) have compared consumption per capita of various foodstuffs in the United Kingdom over the past three centuries, as shown in Table 7.5. Most striking is the increase in consumption of sugar and fat, resulting in an increase in total energy intake. Associated with this trend is the growth of processed foods, which tend to contain saturated fats, as unsaturated fats are more likely to go rancid (Garrow 1991). High consumption of saturated fatty acids, derived mainly from animal fats, increases the risk of cardiovascular disease by increasing serum cholesterol (DoH, 1991a).

Later in this chapter we discuss the increasing problem of obesity, in response to which the following Health of the Nation targets were set (DoH, 1995):

A7 To reduce the percentage of men and women aged 16–64 who are obese by at least 33 per cent for women by the year 2005 (from 7 per cent for men and 12 per cent for women in 1986/87 to no more than 6 per cent and 8 per cent, respectively);

A8 To reduce the average percentage of food energy derived by the population from saturated fatty acids by at least 35 per cent by 2005 (from 17 per cent in 1990 to no more than 11 per cent);

A9 To reduce the average percentage of food energy derived by the population from total fat by at least 12 per cent by 2005 (from about 40 per cent in 1990 to no more than 35 per cent);

A10 To reduce the proportion of men drinking more than 21 units of alcohol per week from 28 per cent in 1990 to 18 per cent by 2005, and the proportion of women drinking more than 14 units of alcohol per week from 11 per cent in 1990 to 7 per cent by 2005.

7.2.4 Methodological issues in monitoring trends in nutritional status

The most direct way to assess nutritional status in a population is to survey the diet of a sample of the population and compare the intake with the recommended allowances, which needs to be for a reasonable period since there are large variations in an individual's diet from day to day (Garrow, 1991). Recall of diet can be unreliable when used to assess individual consumption patterns. Acheson et al., (1980) showed, with data from a British Antarctic Expedition, that when dietary recall was compared with careful measurements, the recalled energy intake ranged from 32 to 132 per cent of the true intake. Prospective recording of diet yields better data, but introduces new errors since the process of weighing and recording food intake may inhibit normal eating behaviour – subjects required to record their intake usually lose weight over the study period – especially true for obese subjects (Prentice et al., 1986). It can also be misleading to use mean intake to represent the nutrition of a group, since the distribution of particular nutrients can be very skewed by a few atypical individuals (Garrow, 1991). The available data from the nineteenth century consist primarily of very small surveys, where the main aim was often to describe what sort of diets were 'typically' achieved on various low levels of income. They will not be truly representative of the whole population. The modern surveys during and after the First World War involve much larger, representative samples, based on diaries of food eaten (see Chapter 2).

7.3 The British diet 1841–1914

The first half of the nineteenth century witnessed a rapid rise in the population of England that was becoming concentrated mainly in towns and had to be fed. Fortuitously, the railways arrived in the 1830s and brought about a revolution in the supply of food to towns, providing rapid and cheap distribution. They also created a national market, levelling out regional variations in prices, and played a role in lowering costs. The period from 1830 to 1850 was a period of recession. At the end of the Napoleonic wars in 1815 the price of wheat had fallen, but so too had the wages of the agricultural workers, while at the same time their rents had increased. Many labourers became desperately poor (Chadwick, 1842). Before the Poor Laws of 1834 the earnings of the poorest had been supported by an allowance based on the price of wheat and the size of the family. A new law replaced this relief with workhouses where the destitute had to work unpaid in return

Table 7.5

Per capita consumption in the UK of various foodstuffs over the last three centuries

G/day per head	1770	1870	1970
Fat	25	75	145
Sugar	10	80	150
Potatoes	120	400	240
Wheat flour	500	375	200
Cereal crude fibre	5	1	0.2

Source: Burkitt and Trowell (1975)

for food and shelter. Many would rather starve than enter the workhouses, which separated families, men from women, and children from parents. The loss of the allowance meant that, to a greater extent than before, the labourer's wife and children needed to work in order to make ends meet. In the countryside, too, living standards were falling. The enclosure of land meant that labourers who previously had kept a cow could no longer do so. With the agricultural slump many small farms closed down, putting labourers out of work. William Cobbett gave an account of country conditions in 1830 in his *Rural Rides*. He wrote that the lowest classes of farm labourers were 'the worst used labouring people upon the face of the earth. Dogs and hogs and horses are treated with more civility, and as to food and lodging, how gladly would the labourers change with them!' He was ashamed to see countrymen 'reeling with weakness; their poor faces ... nothing but skin and bone.' Burnett (1989) wrote: 'Within one generation, high prices had first transformed the farm servant into a day labourer; low prices and the Poor Law turned the day labourer into a pauper.'

Oddy (1981) evaluated the recorded diets of farm labourers in present day nutritional terms. These represented inadequate nutritional levels for manual workers – 1,900 kilocalories of energy per person per day, 49 g of protein, 31 of fat, and 0.25 of calcium. There was at this time a growing public concern for the labourer's plight. Both Houses of Parliament debated the situation at length, and an official report published in 1843 quoted a physician from Wiltshire who said that four out of every five of his female patients suffered from a diet 'insufficient in quantity and not good enough in quality ... I am always more and more astonished how the labourers continue to live at all.' It also gave the example shown in Table 7.6 of a weekly family budget and stated: 'But there are numbers of families who, although in the possession of the same amount of wages ... do not dispose of it with such frugality, but appear in the greatest state of destitution; many others, with the same number of children, do not get the wages this man's family have.' The table describes the budget of

Robert Crick, his wife and five children aged 12, 11, 8, 6 and 4. All children worked, barring the two youngest, bringing in 4s of the family's 13s 9d income between them. The wife earned 9d per week.

In the towns there were large swings in the purchasing power of industrial workers between good years and bad – the depression of the 1840s was the worst of the whole century, with about 10 per cent of the population officially classified as paupers (Hobsbawm, 1975). In Bolton in 1842, 60 per cent of millworkers, 87 per cent of bricklayers, 84 per cent of carpenters and 36 per cent of ironworkers were unemployed. Between 15 and 20 per cent of Leeds inhabitants had an income of less than 1s per head per week. Food prices fluctuated widely – the price of four 6 lb loaves, which represent the weekly ration for a family of two adults and three children, rose from 3s 6d in 1835 to 5s in 1840, falling to 3s 9d in 1845 and 3s 5d in 1850. The early 1840s were called the 'hungry forties'.

In the first half of the nineteenth century white bread constituted virtually the total diet of the poorest. Oddy (1977) calculated that at least 70 per cent of the total energy value of the national diet was derived from carbohydrate, and only 20 per cent from fat. Wheat availability fell continuously from 1.6 lb/head per day in 1825 to 1.25 lb in 1846, the year of the repeal of the Corn Laws, increasing to 1.6 lb in 1851 and 2.0 lb in 1879 (Salaman, 1949). Per capita consumption was 0.6 lb/head per day by 1838 (Salaman, 1949). Tea was important for the poor, because it converted a cold meal into the semblance of a hot one. It was the national beverage of all classes by 1850, and was included alongside white bread in the poverty-line dietaries of the time. Potatoes were seen as a substitute for grain, but generally regarded as inferior. David Davies (1795) wrote 'Wheaten bread may be eaten alone with pleasure; but potatoes require either meat or milk to make

Table 7.6

A family budget of a poor rural family of 7 in 1841 (Robert Crick)

Total earnings   13s 9d

Weekly expenditure

Bread	9s 0d	Potatoes	1s 0d
Rent	1s 2d	Tea	2d
Sugar	3¹/₂d	Soap	3d
Blue	¹/₂d	Thread	2d
Candles	3d	Salt	¹/₂d
Coal and wood	9d	Butter	4¹/₂d
Cheese	3d		

Total expenditure   13s 9d

Table 7.7

The daily nutritional intake and weekly earnings of skilled cotton workers in Manchester and Dukinfield, 1841

	Protein (g)	Calories	Iron (mg)	Vit C (mg)	Earnings
Averages					
All families	65	2300	15	50	
Manchester	71	2600	16	57	
Dukinfield	51	1900	12	36	
Selected families					
No. occupation (family size)					
4 storeman (8)	79	2600	17	75	£2 0s 1d
6 overlooker (6)	65	2100	13	58	£1 7s 10d
14 dresser (6)	44	1700	11	33	£1 1s 1¹/₂d
19 mechanic's asst	45	1600	11	25	£1 0s 4¹/₂d

Source: Nield (1841); McKenzie (1962).

them go down; you cannot make many hearty meals of them with salt and water only. Poor people indeed give them to their children in the greasy water in which they have boiled their greens and their morsel of bacon.' Meat was produced at the equivalent of 72 lb per head a year in 1850 (Williams, 1976), but this was not evenly distributed among the population. Alexander Somerville (1843), son of a farm labourer, wrote 'we never had butcher's meat', and Caird (1880) commented that 'thirty years ago not more than one third of the people of this country consumed animal produce more than once a week'. Fish became more readily available as a result of the railways – by the middle of the nineteenth century around 90 lb per head per year was sold. Herrings were commonly eaten by the poorer population, and accounted for half the weight of fish sold. Fuel was scarce – before the enclosure of land it could be collected freely. Now it had to be bought. This limited the capacity of poor people to cook food. Thus bread was generally bought, in both town and country, and not home baked.

There were marked variations in earnings between different types of worker, which influenced the food they could buy. The Statistical Society carried out a survey of 19 skilled cotton workers in employment, 12 in Manchester and 7 in Dukenfield (Nield, 1841). The Dukenfield workers are more typical of the Lancashire cotton workers at that time (Burnett, 1989). McKenzie (1962) has evaluated these budgets in modern nutritional terms. The results are given in Table 7.7. Only the best-paid workers achieved a diet that we would regard as adequate in calorific and protein intake today. Since men tended to eat the lion's share of the food this would still have meant undernourishment in women and children, which could lead to restricted physical growth and rickets in children, and susceptibility to infectious diseases such as tuberculosis and typhus.

The Statistical Society's survey was of skilled workers – Somerville (1843) collected budgets for less skilled workers in northern industrial towns, and presented average budgets for four levels of wealth. The lowest two are given in Table 7.8 – the higher two overlap with the Manchester and Dukenfield budgets.

It is not known what proportion of families were in each of the income categories given above, and this would in any case have varied from time to time with people's changing fortunes and the economic cycles. Somerville said that

When trade was in a thriving condition, by far the greatest proportion of families belonged to this fourth class (26s 6d per week), a smaller proportion to the third (15s 6d) and comparatively few to the second (10s) or first (5s). Now in 1842 when trade is prostrate, the greatest proportion of families belong to the first and second classes, and comparatively few to the third and fourth.

The year 1848 marks the end of the 'hungry half century', when about half the children born died before they reached the age of 5, and a high proportion of those who survived grew up rickety, deformed and undernourished. By 1850, for the better-off worker, the towns offered a greater choice of food than the country, and the average consumption of meat, fats, sugar and milk was higher in towns than in the country (Oddy, 1982).

During the first half of the nineteenth century food adulteration became increasingly common as suppliers tried to keep down costs to compete with each other for trade. Fredrick Accum (1820) published a 'Treatise on adulterations of Food and culinary poisons', drawing attention to the widespread adulteration of food that was taking place in order to offer more competitive prices. London bakers frequently added alum and inferior flour and sometimes beans and peas or potatoes to bread. Ale could contain cocculus indicus, a dangerous poison containing picrotoxin, multum, capiscum, copperas, quassia, mixed drugs, harts-horn shavings, orange powder, caraway seeds, ginger and coriander as cheap substitutes for malt and hops, allowing the beer to be diluted and appear strong. Green tea was sometimes manufactured from local leaves – ash, sloe and elder – which had been coloured and curled on copper plates to give it a green verdigris colour. Black tea was made using iron plates and adding logwood or black lead. These 'teas' were mixed in with genuine tea. Cheeses were sometimes coloured with red lead. While the book was a great success, Accum had to leave the country and take up a professorial post in Berlin, ostensibly because of charges of mutilating books in the Royal Institution's library, but possibly because there was a conspiracy of vested interests to discredit him (Burnett, 1989). In the 1840s there were at least eight factories in London for drying used tea leaves and making them appear to be genuine tea. George Phillips, head of the Chemical Department of the Inland Revenue wrote:

Persons were employed to buy up exhausted leaves at hotels, coffee-houses and other places at 2¹/₂d and 3d per

Table 7.8

Alexander Somerville's budgets of northern industrial workers' families, 1842

	Weekly earnings per family			
	5s	6d	10s	0d
Bread and flour	1	9	2	6
Oatmeal	1	0	1	10
Potatoes		10	1	8
Milk		11		6
Bacon		2		8
Soap and candles		4		6
Coals		6		9
Sugar and treacle		-		5
Tobacco and snuff		-		2
Clothing		-		6
Rent		-		6
Total	5s	6d	10s	0d

pound. These were taken to the factories, mixed with a solution of gum, and re-dried. After this the dried leaves, if for black tea, were mixed with rose-pink and black lead to 'face' them as it is termed by the trade. (Hassall, 1855)

Hassall drew attention to such problems through a series of articles in the *Lancet*, which precipitated a Parliamentary inquiry, and eventually, legislation (the Adulteration of Foods Act of 1860). However, the Act was merely permissive and not very effective. It was replaced in 1872 by the more enforceable Adulteration of Food, Drink and Drugs Act, and the Sale of Food and Drugs Act of 1875. Statutory standards for spirits were established in 1879, for milk in 1901 and for butter in 1902. The Co-operative Movement also played a part in improving the standard of food for the working classes by providing quality food, although the purchasers had to pay in cash, which was not possible for all.

After 1850, wealth began to be shared more equally between different sections of society as factory acts were introduced and trade unionism grew. During the second half of the nineteenth century co-operative retail societies sprang up to ensure that the workers got a fair deal for their money and received unadulterated food. They bought wholesale, sold for cash and divided up profits as dividends at the end of each year. A Quaker, John Horniman, had the idea of selling tea in sealed packets to prevent adulteration, and by 1884 packed tea was mass produced. Tax on tea, sugar, coffee and wheat was reduced from £15.8 million to £4.8 million between 1841 and 1882. Before income tax was reintroduced in 1842 customs and excise duties on basic foods made up almost half of total national revenue. In 1834 a working man earning £22 annually paid a total of £9 12s 7d in tax on malt, sugar, tea, coffee and other foods (Thompson, 1980).

The reduction in customs and excise duties made it easier for poorer people to obtain an adequate diet, helped, too, by the large-scale import of cheap wheat and meat. Tea consumption increased from 1.6 lb per person per year to 5.7 lb by 1891–1900. Alcohol consumption rose, too, to reach a peak in 1875–76 at 34 gallons of beer and almost 1.5 gallons of spirit per head per year (Burkitt, 1989). Rowntree and Sherwell (1900) estimated that the average adult male consumed 73 gallons of beer and 2.4 gallons of spirit per year in 1900. By 1878 some employers provided subsidised canteens for their workers, including Coleman's, Cadbury's, Fry's and Lever Bros. Bowley (1895) made a study for the Statistical Society which showed that real wages had risen by 92 per cent between 1860 and 1891, mainly owing to falling prices. At the same time the supply and distribution of quality food improved due to better transport and stricter food regulations, especially the pasteurisation of milk (Burnett, 1989).

But there was still evidence of poverty, ill health, overcrowded and insanitary housing, and poor nutrition among large sections of the population. Throughout the period 1850–1914 the rural labourer lived a life of poverty, and Canon Girdlestone remarked that labourers 'did not live in the proper sense of the word, they merely didn't die' (Burnett, 1989). The penalty for poaching was transportation, even in 1857.

In 1867 women, and children from the age of 6 upwards, still had to work in organised gangs on farms (Burnett, 1989). The better-off labourers kept a pig as a food luxury. In the towns, those who had employment were better off, but periods of unemployment created hardships. For 3 years the American Civil War interrupted cotton imports and resulted in half-time work for thousands in the cotton industry. In 1863 Edward Smith (1864) collected weekly budgets from 370 agricultural labourers and poorly-paid industrial workers for an official report, and found the diets, especially those of infants, were wanting. Gin and narcotics were given to babies 'to allay the fretfulness which the want of proper food causes'. He concluded that 'The average quantity of food supplied is too little for health and strength.' The diets of farm labourers were generally superior to those of indoor workers, and were on average above the minimum subsistence level – 2,190 kilocalories, 55g of protein, 53 g of fat, 12.5 mg of iron and 0.36 g of calcium, with the poorest receiving only 1,950 kcal and 49 g of protein on average. Since the men took the lion's share of meals, women and children would have fared worse. The nutritional levels would have been low enough to retard children's growth and the protein was insufficient for pregnant or lactating women. The average working class household spent between £15 and £20 a year on drink, and when allowance is made for the growing number of teetotallers this meant that some families spent between a third and a half of their income on alcohol (Levi, 1885).

Even at the beginning of the twentieth century there was widespread poverty. A survey by Charles Booth (1902) found that 31 per cent of the population of London lived below his poverty line, with daily diets yielding on average 2,620 kilocalories, 61g protein, 57 g of fat, 10.6 mg of iron and 0.3 g of calcium (Oddy, 1970). Most of these levels are higher than the modern average levels for men aged 19–50 years given in Table 7.1, but Booth's subjects were manual workers, without the benefits of central heating, and thus would have had higher energy and protein requirements than today's sedentary workers. In 1901, 3,500 kilocalories were deemed necessary for a man in moderate work (Rowntree, 1901). Rowntree did a similar survey in York and concluded that 10 per cent of the whole population were in 'primary poverty', defined as earnings insufficient to maintain physical health, and 18 per cent in 'secondary poverty', where expenditure depleted income that would otherwise have been just sufficient (see also Chapter 6). The poorest families in his survey received only 1,578 kilocalories a day, 42 g of protein and 40 g of fat, while the middle class families had 3,526 kilocalories, 96 g protein and 139 g of fat. Three government enquiries at that time confirmed that there was a large underclass with malnourished children, and one third of the population died in the workhouse (Report, 1899; Report, 1904; Reports, 1905–9). General Booth started the Salvation Army in 1878 in response to the thousands of unemployed and casual labourers who lived and slept on the streets of London and provincial cities. In 1885 James Cantlie described the poor condition of town dwellers, where the average male was 'height 5 ft 1 in; chest measurement 28 in. His aspect is pale, waxy: he is very narrow between the eyes, and with a decided squint' (Jones, 1976). The Inspector-General of army recruiting for the Boer

War (1899–1902) reported that 38 per cent of volunteers had been found unfit for service or had been invalided out subsequently. Heart afflictions, poor sight and hearing, height less than 5 feet, and bad teeth were cited. The Committee on Physical Deterioration found evidence of a generally low standard of health, particularly among children of the working classes. In 1911, infant mortality was 77 deaths per 1,000 among the middle and upper classes, but 152 per 1,000 among unskilled labourers, where 13-year-old boys were 4 inches shorter than sons of middle-class parents (Oddy, 1982).

In 1906, the Education (Provision of Meals) Act allowed local authorities to levy a rate of a halfpenny in the pound to provide meals for 'children unable by reason of lack of food to take full advantage of the education provided to them'. However, by 1914, meals were provided for only 200,000 children out of a school population of 6,000,000. In 1908, a means-tested old-age pension of 5s a week was granted to people over the age of 70. Rowntree and Kendall, investigating the diets and budgets of 42 labourers in 1913, found that only in five northern counties was 'the wage paid by farmers sufficient to maintain a family of average size in a state of merely physical efficiency'. In many households fresh meat was for the man only, and milk consumption was only 5½ pints per family per week. One in six working-class babies died in their first year of life, and in 1913 the President of the Board of Education stated on the basis of a recently introduced inspection of elementary school children, that 10 per cent suffered from defective nutrition (Oddy, 1982). Orr (1936) calculated the average food consumption up until immediately prior to the First World War, and this is summarised in Table 7.9. In 1902 a 4-week diary survey of 220 households was undertaken for the Statistical Society into food consumption, which showed that there were steep economic gradients, with higher income groups consuming the largest quantities of meat, milk and butter (see Table 7.10).

7.4 Diet during the First World War

In 1917, with the German U-boat threatening British supplies, the Ministry of Food took control of essential food supplies which were centrally requisitioned and distributed at fixed prices by the government. Bread was subsidised, saving an estimated 2s a week on the working-class budget. The price of milk was fixed. Civilian rationing began on 1 January 1918 starting with sugar, later extended to 8 oz sugar, 5 oz butter and margarine combined, 4 oz jam, 2 oz tea, 8 oz bacon, rising to 16 after July 1918. Fresh meat was rationed by price. Bread was not rationed at all, nor were potatoes, and many people grew vegetables. Factory canteens were provided which benefited many workers – by the end of the war, 1,000 industrial canteens supplied a million meals a day. Drummond and Wilbraham (1957) claim that the restricted diet caused a decline in health, exacerbating the effect of the influenza epidemic in 1918. There was, however, a negligible fall in the average number of calories consumed per head compared with the pre-war period average of 3,442 (Burnett, 1989). For the poorer sectors of the community the diet was actually improved, according to the Sumner Committee of 1918: '... families of unskilled workmen were slightly better fed at the later date, in spite of the rise in the price of food ... From London it is officially reported, after inspection of all the

Table 7.9

Estimated average annual consumption per head of certain foods in the UK, 1903-1934

	1903–13	1924–28	1934
Fruit	61 lb	91 lb	115 lb
Vegetables (not potatoes)	60 lb	78 lb	98 lb
Potatoes	208 lb	194 lb	210 lb
Butter	16 lb	16 lb	25 lb
Eggs	104 no	120 no.	152 no.
Cheese	7 lb	9 lb	10 lb
Margarine	6 lb	12 lb	8 lb
Sugar	79 lb	87 lb	94 lb
Meat	135 lb	134 lb	143 lb
Wheat flour	211 lb	198 lb	197 lb

Source: Orr, 1936.

Table 7.10

Food consumption per head per annum in 1902: survey carried out by the Statistical Society

Group	No. of h\holds	Meat lb	Milk gals	Cheese lb	Butter lb
Wage earners	82	107	8.5	10	15
Lower middle class	60	122	25	10	23
Professional classes	46	182	39	8.5	29
Upper classes	32	300	31	10.5	41

Source: Jnl.S.S. (1904)

Table 7.11

Some results from Crawford's household survey of 1936–1937: comparison by class

N = 5,000 households

Class	% of population in group	Est weekly income per capita	Food expenditure as % of income	Interest in dietary subjects	Families with food expend. below BMA minimum
	%	d	%	%	%
AA	1	159s 6d	12	34	0.0
A	4	88s 4d	18	34	0.0
B	20	43s 0d	29	27	0.4
C	60	20s 3d	39	17	17.0
D	15	12s 6d	47	8	48.2

Source: Crawford (1938)

children entering school, that "the percentage of children found in poorly nourished condition is considerably less than half the percentage in 1913 ... borne out by the information we have received as to the number of meals provided to 'necessitous' children'". One factor in improving living standards during the war was the virtual disappearance of unemployment, coupled with women earning comparatively good wages. Winter (1977) claimed that mortality rates among working-class children fell during the war, partly due to higher standards of maternal and child care, but especially to 'a major improvement in nutrition after 1914'.

7.5 Diet from 1919 to 1939

Between 1924 and 1936 real wages rose considerably (Oddy, 1982), and this resulted in increasing consumption of meat, butter, eggs, fruit and vegetables (Table 7.9). Refrigeration, canning and an increase in the international food trade extended the eating season for fruit and other perishable produce. British farmers increased production of 'health protective foods' with the aid of government subsidies. The proportion of the very poor fell between the wars – for example, in 1936 Rowntree found that in York the number living in poverty (using the same definition of primary poverty as in 1901) had fallen to 6.8 per cent (Rowntree, 1941). The workers benefited from council housing, medical services and insurance benefits that had not existed before. A 'Milk in Schools' scheme was started in 1934, supplying a third of a pint of milk daily to 50 per cent of elementary school children, at half cost or free. School meals were introduced for those in need, with 5 per cent of children benefiting (HMSO, 1946).

By 1939, health departments were providing milk, cod liver oil, iron and vitamin products at low cost or free to mothers and children who were 'clear cases of malnutrition', and there were 3,000 infant welfare centres (Burnett, 1989). An experiment sponsored by the Milk Nutrition Committee in 1938–39 showed that supplementary milk benefited not only the children's health but also their educational achievements (National Diary Council, 1939). When soldiers were conscripted for the Second World War, 70 per cent were graded as 'fully fit' – twice the proportion in 1917-18. The number of schoolchildren showing signs of malnutrition fell from 15–20 per cent before 1914 to 1 per cent in 1925–32 (Burnett, 1989).

During the same period there were also hunger marches and dole queues. Oddy calculated that some women's diets yielded as little as 1,305 kilocalories and 36 g of protein per day (Oddy, 1982). Maternal mortality rates peaked in 1933 and 1934, suggesting this may have been related to the economic depression. Orr (1936) found that his 'standard of perfect nutrition' ('a state of well-being such that no improvement can be effected by a change in the diet') was realised only in the wealthiest 50 per cent of the population – the poorest 10 per cent lacked calories, protein, fat, calcium, phosphorous, iron, and vitamins A and C. The diets of the next 20 per cent only satisfied protein and fat requirements. By the minimum dietary standards established by Orr in the 1930s, some 30 per cent of the country's population could be considered undernourished in 1933. McGonigle (1936) found in Stockton-on-Tees that even with new, more sanitary, houses there was no improvement in health since higher rents and travelling expenses reduced the income available for food –

Table 7.12

Working-class diet – 1932–93: consumption per person per week (1952=100)

(Category C in MAFF surveys)

	Milk and cream pts	Cheese oz	Meat oz	Fish oz	Eggs no.	Fats oz	Sugar and preserves oz	Vege-tables oz	Fruit oz	Cereals oz	Beverages fl oz
1952 consumption	4.88	2.21	28.86	7.10	2.93	9.75	17.08	101.26	22.16	89.90	2.93
1932-35*	47	113	-	52	119	-	102	-	-	-	-
1938-39**	37	77	-	80	89	-	91	-	-	-	-
1941	68	86	-	66	48	-	50	-	-	-	-
1945	90	113	94	128	96	89	87	-	-	-	-
1952	100	100	100	100	100	100	100	100	100	100	100
1955	100	129	118	79	139	122	126	93	108	93	120
1960	101	140	125	80	155	122	124	91	119	82	121
1965	101	138	130	81	160	123	116	91	115	77	120
1970	100	157	134	73	177	124	109	90	117	74	120
1975	103	161	128	60	140	114	74	86	90	66	102
1980	91	162	138	67	125	115	66	88	109	64	101
1985	84	175	131	63	104	104	48	85	104	61	89
1990	77	170	120	64	77	90	36	81	119	58	79
1994	78	171	121	69	62	84	36	74	129	57	71

*Source: Orr (1936)
**Source: Carnegie (1951)

the death rate on a new housing estate rose, while the rates in the slum areas from which the inhabitants had moved, and death rates in the town itself, fell. Crawford (1938) undertook a dietary survey in 1936–37 involving 5,000 family budgets in seven principal cities, covering all social classes, and involving house-to-house interviews in seven principal cities (see Table 7. 11).

7.6 Diet from 1939 to 1950

Government food control planning for wartime was more advanced in 1939 than it had been at the outbreak of the first world war (Burnett, 1989). The rationing schemes devised were concerned mainly with protein foods, milk and fats. Fresh vegetables, fruit and fish were allowed unrestricted supply, although availability (other than potatoes) was variable. The extraction rate of flour was raised to 85 per cent to increase the intake of iron, riboflavin and nicotinic acid. Calcium carbonate was added to flour, making up for the loss of calcium. Margarine was fortified with vitamins A and D. Additional proteins, mainly in the form of milk, were supplied to children and nursing or pregnant mothers, as were orange juice, cod-liver oil and vitamin tablets, although the take-up was not complete (orange juice 46 per cent; vitamin A and D tablets 34 per cent; cod-liver oil 21 per cent). A National Milk Scheme allowed free or cheap milk to all children under 5 years and expectant mothers. Eggs too were made available to pregnant women and mothers. The school milk system was expanded (Ministry of Food, 1951). Changes in the war time diet, estimated through food supplies moving into civilian consumption, showed a decrease in the consumption of fish, meat, fats, eggs, sugar and fruit, and an increase of dairy products, potatoes and cereals (Ministry of Food, 1951). Over 11,000 work-site canteens were set up by 1943 and school canteens fulfilled a similar role. Before the war, 4 per cent of children took school dinners, by 1945 the figure had risen to 36 per cent, and milk was received by three quarters of all schoolchildren (HMSO, 1946). Throughout the war period the Ministry of Food undertook surveys of working-class diets to monitor the situation (MAFF, 1951). The results, including those of subsequent surveys, are shown in Table 7.12. During the war the consumption of milk and cheese increased relative to 1938–39 levels. Egg consumption was reduced during the war, but rose dramatically afterwards until around 1970, since when it has fallen equally dramatically. Fat consumption increased after the war until around 1970, and has been declining thereafter. Sugar consumption reduced during the war, but rose to pre-1932 levels by 1955, since when it has fallen below 1932 levels. Meat consumption increased after the war until around 1980, but has declined since. Fruit consumption has increased, particularly since 1980. The consumption of cereals (including bread) and vegetables (including potatoes) has been declining ever since the MAFF surveys began.

The *State of the Public Health* (HMSO, 1946) declared of the war period that 'the average diet of all classes was better balanced than ever before. Luxury items soon disappeared... but it was, nevertheless, always physiologically a better diet

and more evenly distributed'. Demands for the war production meant that wages increased more sharply than prices, and unemployment largely disappeared. Wages increased particularly for the growing numbers of women in the workforce, and also for working teenagers. Price control measures on staple food and other minor articles curbed inflationary pressures which, together with special distribution schemes, probably had a levelling effect on dietary variation between rich and poor; raising nutritional standards for the poor and possibly also providing health gains for the wealthy. Food was rationed for 14 years – 1939–53, and in some respects the post-1945 diet was more frugal than the wartime one, especially for fat, whose shortage was felt particularly during the icy winter of 1946–47 (Burnett, 1989). In 1946–48 rations were cut, and fat consumption was 84 per cent of its 1939 value and, energy was 97 per cent.

7.7 Diet from 1950 to 1993

7.7.1 General changes in food consumption and current patterns

By 1954, foods that had been so scarce during the austerity of rationing were widely available and eagerly consumed by the population, particularly butter, eggs, meat, sugar and white bread. Post-war British society continued to increase in affluence, associated with higher levels of consumption, until the oil crisis in the mid-1970s. Since then, lower paid workers have done less well (Halsey, 1987). Other social changes have probably influenced our diet, including the participation of women in the workforce, together with car ownership, growth of supermarkets and widespread use of freezers and microwaves. Holidays abroad and a multicultural restaurant boom have coincided with the availability of out-of-season vegetables and 'exotic' foods in the supermarkets. Nevertheless, the constituents of the British diet have not changed greatly post-war. Breakfast is now more likely to consist of breakfast cereal and fruit juice than the traditional bacon and eggs (Buss, 1988). There are fewer formal multi-course family meals and snacks have become more frequent but less filling (MAFF, 1990). Consumption has shifted from canned foods to frozen and other convenience food, including take-away meals eaten at home. Consumption of potato products, such as crisps and potato snack foods, has risen by 50% since 1983 (MAFF, 1994).

In a recent study, Gregory *et al.* (1990) found that women currently were more likely than men to prefer foods with a healthier profile, such as wholemeal and other non-white breads, cottage cheese, yogurts, salad vegetables and fresh fruit. They are also more partial to chocolates and other sweets. Men prefer chips and roast potatoes, are more likely to add sugar to drinks and cereals and also to eat meat. Among beverages, women tend to drink more fresh fruit juice, wine and fortified wine, and men to drink beer as an alcoholic drink. Gregory *et al.* (1995) found that, among toddlers, biscuits were the food most often eaten, followed by white bread, non-diet soft drinks, whole milk, savoury snacks, boiled or baked potatoes, and chocolates. More than half the sample had not eaten any leafy green vegetables or drunk fruit juice during the 4-day study period. Similarly, more than half had not eaten coated or fried white fish, and only 16 per cent had eaten oily fish. Raw vegetables and salads appeared to be fairly unpopular with toddlers, with only 10 per cent having eaten raw carrots and 17 per cent raw tomatoes. Over half had added sugar with cereals or drinks. The majority consumed whole milk, although semi-skimmed milk was most likely to be used for cooking or for breakfast cereal, and the likelihood of drinking whole milk decreased with age. A third of toddlers drank tea.

It was generally found that toddlers from manual households were more likely to eat white bread and non-wholegrain cereals, non-polyunsaturated soft margarine and reduced fat

spreads. They were also more likely to use table sugar, drink tea and coffee, and eat confectionery. Those from non-manual households were more likely to eat buns and pastries, ice cream, fromage frais and cheese (other than cottage cheese). They also were more likely to eat salads, raw vegetables, fruit and fruit juice. Recent qualitative research undertaken by Dobson *et al.,* (1994) of 48 low-income families living in the Midlands looked at the social, cultural and nutritional aspects of food consumption. The food bill was perceived as being the most flexible item that could be cut to pay for any unexpected bills. Shopping and managing the household budget were normally handled by women, who also tended to protect the other members of the household where possible and do without themselves. Children were given crisps and chocolate for school breaks to prevent peer ridicule – expensive waste was avoided by giving their favourite food,

Figure 7.3

Fats consumption per person per week by income group

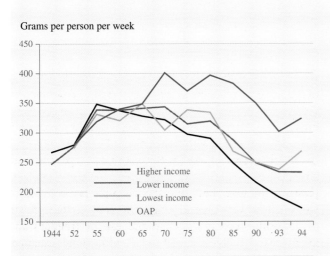

Source: MAFF

Figure 7.4

Eggs consumption per person per week by income group

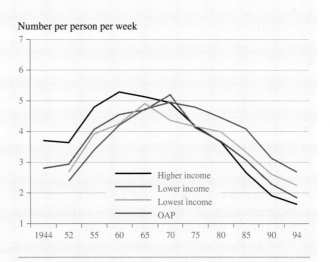

Source: MAFF

Figure 7.5

Fruit consumed by income group

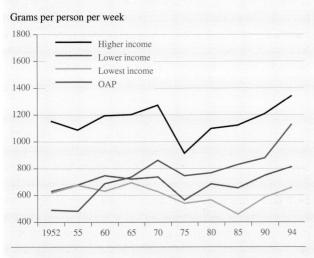

Note: This does not include fruit juice but does include tomatoes after 1975.

Source: MAFF

Figure 7.6

Sugars and preserves consumption per person per week by income group

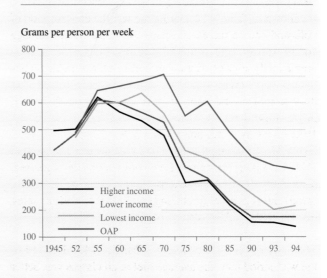

Figure 7.7

Average consumption of fats per person per week

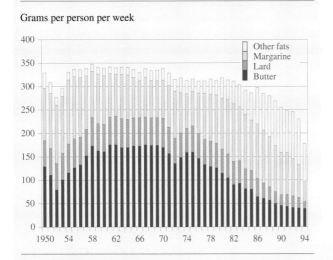

Grams per person per week

Source: MAFF.

Figure 7.8

Changing patterns in consumption of food at home

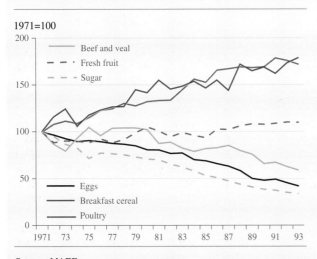

Source: MAFF.

Figure 7.10

Consumption of fresh vegetables per person per week

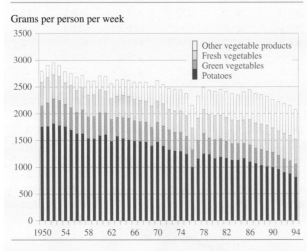

Grams per person per week

Source: MAFF.

although this was not always the healthiest choice. Modifying the diet to promote healthier eating was difficult, either because it was more expensive or because other members of the family did not like it. Dowler (1995) conducted a nutrition survey among 189 lone parent family households using a 3 day food intake diary. Nearly 30 per cent of the sample admitted to missing meals when money was scarce but nearly all managed to find food for their children. This was reflected in the nutrient intake of adults, which was invariably lower as a percentage of dietary reference intake than the childrens'. Parents who suffered the most severe financial pressures spent least on food and had the lowest nutrient intakes. Black British or Afro-Caribbean households tended to have a higher nutrient intake and were more likely to eat brown bread, rice, beans, tropical root vegetables, fish and fruit.

Figure 7.9

Consumption of fresh fruit and fruit juices per person per week

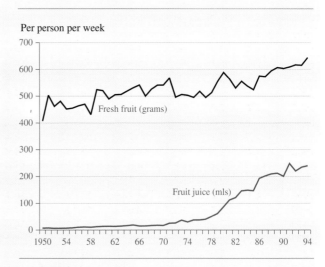

Per person per week

Source: MAFF.

Figure 7.11

Consumption of total meat and meat products per person per week

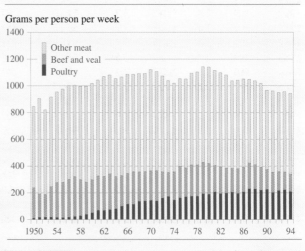

Grams per person per week

Source: MAFF

7.7.2 Evidence from the NFS and other surveys, 1950–94

The dietary surveys commissioned by the Ministry of Food (MAFF) became nationally representative since 1950. Previously they related to working class diets. Figures 7.3 to 7.6 provide some examples of different trends by income group, where the 'lower-income' group corresponds approximately to the 'working-class' figures previously published. The early data show affluent households as the greatest consumers of sugars, fats and eggs, but by 1993 their consumption was the lowest. Old-age pensioners had the lowest egg consumption, but now have the highest. Egg and total fat consumption in all groups has, however, declined since the 1970s, but the decline began first in the higher income group. Fruit consumption has always been highest in

Table 7.13

Consumption of foods per person per week: 1950–1994, Great Britain

Year	Bread (kilo)	Milk (ltrs)	Cheese (g)	Eggs (no.)	Fresh fruit (g)	Fruit juice (ml)	Potatoes (g)	Fresh veg (g)	Fresh green veg (g)	Other fresh veg (g)	Other veg products (g)	Sugar (g)
1950	1.6	2.7	72.0	3.5	408.6	7.1	1,759.0	824.8	391.6	433.2	214.1	287.2
1951	1.7	2.8	78.3	2.8	504.7	7.6	1,763.8	914.4	441.2	473.2	226.0	324.4
1952	1.7	2.7	61.5	3.0	463.3	6.2	1,816.6	911.3	462.4	448.8	228.2	311.9
1953	1.6	2.7	70.9	4.0	482.6	6.5	1,779.7	918.9	469.0	450.0	200.7	384.7
1954	1.6	2.7	82.2	4.3	453.4	7.1	1,761.3	815.7	419.3	396.4	207.5	480.9
1955	1.6	2.7	80.2	4.2	456.8	8.2	1,698.3	829.9	414.8	415.1	223.7	500.1
1956	1.4	2.7	80.8	4.4	465.6	10.4	1,624.6	808.1	400.9	407.1	250.9	510.3
1957	1.4	2.7	81.9	4.4	471.5	11.3	1,626.9	858.5	446.0	412.5	229.4	501.8
1958	1.3	2.7	84.5	4.4	432.7	10.4	1,535.3	812.6	408.0	404.6	264.2	525.9
1959	1.3	2.7	82.8	4.5	525.7	12.4	1,530.8	822.5	416.8	405.7	256.6	524.5
1960	1.3	2.7	86.2	4.6	522.0	13.6	1,588.6	857.1	430.4	426.7	260.3	503.5
1961	1.3	2.8	87.0	4.7	491.1	14.1	1,607.3	812.6	409.4	403.2	281.5	513.2
1962	1.2	2.8	88.5	4.7	506.7	13.6	1,484.5	799.8	407.4	392.4	274.7	521.7
1963	1.2	2.8	89.6	4.6	507.8	14.7	1,575.6	753.9	353.8	400.1	300.5	524.2
1964	1.2	2.7	89.9	4.7	520.3	16.4	1,534.2	808.9	393.0	415.9	300.3	492.5
1965	1.2	2.7	90.7	4.8	532.7	18.9	1,509.5	812.9	406.6	406.3	303.7	497.9
1966	1.1	2.8	88.2	4.8	543.0	15.0	1,488.2	777.4	382.8	394.7	324.9	483.4
1967	1.1	2.8	95.0	4.7	501.3	15.2	1,481.1	767.2	373.4	393.8	340.8	487.9
1968	1.1	2.7	96.7	4.7	527.1	16.7	1,472.1	765.0	370.0	395.0	351.9	463.6
1969	1.1	2.8	99.2	4.6	542.1	17.5	1,398.1	747.4	347.3	400.1	368.9	458.7
1970	1.1	2.6	101.8	4.7	542.7	16.9	1,469.8	766.1	372.0	394.1	381.6	480.3
1971	1.0	2.7	102.9	4.6	569.0	25.4	1,394.4	792.5	379.6	412.8	359.2	448.0
1972	1.0	2.6	100.1	4.4	497.3	26.3	1,324.1	760.1	376.8	383.3	388.4	425.9
1973	0.9	2.7	106.3	4.2	507.5	36.7	1,302.2	748.8	353.8	395.0	405.4	388.1
1974	0.9	2.7	106.0	4.1	504.4	30.2	1,294.6	755.6	360.1	395.5	394.4	369.6
1975	1.0	2.7	107.5	4.1	496.5	37.6	1,244.7	719.0	328.3	390.7	417.4	320.1
1976	0.9	2.7	107.5	4.1	519.1	37.6	1,000.9	734.6	323.2	411.4	421.3	345.9
1977	0.9	2.6	107.7	4.0	496.2	40.4	1,156.5	761.6	344.5	417.1	412.5	342.8
1978	0.9	2.6	105.5	4.0	514.6	50.8	1,248.9	829.3	381.3	448.0	416.8	337.1
1979	0.9	2.5	108.9	3.9	556.3	62.1	1,235.9	747.4	308.5	438.9	454.8	327.5
1980	0.9	2.4	110.3	3.7	590.0	87.0	1,161.0	801.0	352.1	448.8	458.5	316.7
1981	0.9	2.4	110.3	3.7	565.6	112.7	1,187.1	785.9	339.7	446.3	482.3	314.1
1982	0.9	2.3	107.7	3.5	531.6	121.4	1,165.6	762.7	318.7	444.0	489.7	292.3
1983	0.9	2.3	113.7	3.5	556.8	146.8	1,130.7	751.1	305.6	445.4	492.5	279.0
1984	0.9	2.3	108.9	3.2	538.4	149.1	1,129.0	739.7	307.1	432.7	480.0	259.4
1985	0.9	2.2	110.9	3.2	525.1	147.1	1,161.3	722.4	277.3	445.1	524.0	238.4
1986	0.9	2.2	117.9	3.0	576.4	193.1	1,099.0	791.9	315.0	476.9	555.1	228.0
1987	0.9	2.1	116.0	2.9	574.1	202.4	1,068.3	755.3	282.7	472.6	552.0	212.1
1988	0.9	2.1	117.1	2.7	596.0	209.8	1,032.9	772.0	295.4	476.6	550.9	196.8
1989	0.8	2.1	115.4	2.3	608.2	212.3	1,009.1	775.7	290.0	485.7	540.4	183.2
1990	0.8	2.0	113.4	2.2	604.8	200.8	997.2	736.6	277.6	459.0	528.5	171.3
1991	0.8	2.0	116.5	2.3	610.4	248.5	958.6	719.9	258.9	461.0	545.2	166.7
1992	0.8	2.1	113.7	2.1	618.1	220.5	901.0	724.4	249.8	474.6	567.9	156.2
1993	0.8	2.0	109.2	1.9	616.7	234.6	875.5	717.0	239.9	477.2	561.7	151.1
1994	0.8	2.2	106.0	1.9	645.0	240.0	812.0		245.0	464.0	561.0	187.0

Source: Household food consumption and expenditure, 1990, MAFF, HMSO:1991.

Table 7.13 (continued)

Consumption of foods per person per week: 1950–1994, Great Britain

Year	Butter (g)	Lard (g)	Margarine (g)	Other fats (g)	Total Fats (g)	Fish & products (g)	Meat & products (g)	liquid wholemilk	skimmed milk	yoghurt	Poultry (g)	Beef & veal (g)	Other meat (g)
1950	129.3	55.6	111.7	32.6	329.2	187.7	846.3	4.8			9.9	228.5	607.9
1951	110.9	57.6	117.1	23.2	308.8	217.2	906.2	4.9			16.2	176.6	713.4
1952	79.1	57.0	124.5	16.7	277.3	213.2	821.1	4.8			17.0	170.1	634.0
1953	100.9	56.7	121.3	18.1	297.1	178.6	916.9	4.8			17.0	229.1	670.8
1954	116.0	61.8	136.4	16.7	330.9	161.0	954.6	4.8			14.7	261.7	678.2
1955	126.7	61.8	132.7	15.6	336.8	168.7	975.9	4.8			13.6	265.4	696.9
1956	133.3	59.0	127.0	16.4	335.7	173.8	1,002.3	4.8			16.7	283.5	702.0
1957	152.3	56.1	114.0	16.7	339.1	168.4	1,004.8	4.8			22.7	298.8	683.3
1958	173.0	61.0	98.1	15.0	347.0	161.6	997.2	4.8			27.5	271.3	698.3
1959	162.7	57.8	106.0	14.5	341.1	168.1	997.4	4.8			38.3	242.4	716.8
1960	161.0	58.4	103.8	16.2	339.4	166.1	1,017.6	4.8			50.2	247.8	719.6
1961	175.8	58.7	93.6	13.9	341.9	161.3	1,043.1	4.9			68.6	258.0	716.5
1962	175.8	60.7	89.3	14.2	339.9	164.2	1,069.5	5.0			67.5	255.5	746.5
1963	169.5	62.1	94.1	15.6	341.4	164.7	1,080.2	5.0			73.4	268.5	738.3
1964	169.5	60.1	95.0	16.4	341.1	168.4	1,054.4	4.9			80.0	241.8	732.6
1965	173.0	60.1	86.2	17.0	336.3	163.9	1,066.1	4.9			99.5	229.1	737.5
1966	172.7	60.4	79.1	17.6	329.7	164.2	1,085.6	4.9			115.1	230.5	740.0
1967	175.5	59.3	85.1	18.1	338.0	164.2	1,085.6	4.9			113.7	244.1	727.8
1968	174.1	59.0	79.7	21.0	333.7	161.3	1,090.7	4.8			136.4	220.0	734.3
1969	174.4	59.0	78.8	22.4	334.6	154.8	1,091.6	4.9			139.8	218.3	733.5
1970	169.8	62.7	81.1	25.2	338.8	151.7	1,120.8	4.6			143.5	221.2	756.2
1971	156.8	56.1	89.0	26.9	328.9	146.0	1,106.0	4.7			139.5	225.7	740.9
1972	135.8	53.6	99.8	26.1	315.3	143.2	1,072.9	4.6	0.0	0.0	161.3	195.6	715.9
1973	148.6	51.9	85.9	31.8	318.1	133.5	1,038.6	4.8	0.0	0.0	172.7	178.9	687.0
1974	159.1	51.6	73.7	28.6	313.0	122.8	1,019.3	4.7	0.0	0.1	146.9	210.1	662.3
1975	159.6	55.9	73.7	26.7	315.8	126.5	1,052.5	4.8	0.0	0.0	162.5	235.9	654.1
1976	146.3	52.7	86.8	25.5	311.3	129.9	1,050.8	4.7	0.0	0.1	170.1	216.0	664.6
1977	133.3	53.3	98.7	26.4	311.6	117.1	1,093.8	4.5	0.0	0.1	174.9	233.9	685.0
1978	129.0	54.2	100.4	32.3	315.8	120.5	1,103.5	4.4	0.0	0.1	174.4	234.5	694.6
1979	126.2	52.7	102.9	31.2	313.0	127.9	1,141.8	4.3	0.0	0.1	193.4	234.5	713.9
1980	114.8	51.3	108.6	43.4	318.1	136.1	1,139.5	4.2	0.0	0.1	189.1	230.5	719.9
1981	104.6	51.0	116.5	41.4	313.6	139.5	1,115.4	4.0	0.1	0.1	207.0	197.3	711.1
1982	89.9	49.9	122.8	48.8	311.3	142.9	1,097.5	4.0	0.1	0.1	194.2	200.2	703.1
1983	92.7	48.2	115.7	46.5	303.1	145.7	1,081.1	3.8	0.1	0.1	198.2	186.3	696.6
1984	81.4	42.8	115.7	51.9	291.7	138.6	1,037.7	3.6	0.3	0.1	205.3	177.8	654.7
1985	80.2	40.8	106.6	57.8	285.5	138.9	1,042.5	3.3	0.4	0.1	195.6	184.6	662.3
1986	64.4	38.6	116.2	78.3	297.4	146.3	1,051.3	3.0	0.7	0.1	207.0	186.6	657.8
1987	60.7	32.6	112.8	78.5	284.7	144.3	1,048.2	2.9	0.8	0.1	230.8	191.9	625.5
1988	56.7	28.4	107.2	87.3	279.6	143.5	1,037.4	2.7	0.9	0.2	229.4	180.0	628.0
1989	49.6	25.2	98.4	95.5	268.8	147.4	1,019.0	2.4	1.1	0.2	220.0	171.0	628.0
1990	45.6	22.7	90.4	96.4	255.2	144.0	967.1	2.2	1.3	0.2	225.4	148.6	593.1
1991	43.7	25.2	89.0	90.4	248.4	138.9	962.0	1.9	1.4	0.2	202.4	151.7	607.9
1992	40.8	25.0	79.1	100.7	245.5	141.5	950.4	1.8	1.7	0.2	216.6	141.2	592.6
1993	40.0	22.4	70.3	97.2	229.9	144.6	955.8	1.6	1.8	0.2	222.3	132.7	600.8
1994	39.0	15.0	43.0	81.0	226.0	145.0	943.0	1.5	1.9	0.2	208.0	131.0	604.5

Source: Household food consumption and expenditure, 1990, MAFF, HMSO:1991.

the higher income group, and it has increased markedly in recent times. Old-age pensioners have doubled their fruit consumption since 1952, but consumption in the lowest income group has remained relatively low. In all groups fruit consumption has increased since 1985. Changing patterns of consumption now also mean that pensioner households consume 82 per cent more table sugar and preserves than the average, and 'higher-income' households consume 30 per cent less. This category, however, does not include other sugars such as those found in confectionery and soft drinks.

Table 7.13 shows trends for the British population between 1950, when the NFS became representative of the British population, and 1994. Consumption of fats (see Figure 7.7) increased in the immediate post-war period, but has declined since 1970. Within this group there has been a move away from butter and lard, and an increase in consumption of 'other fats', which includes polyunsaturates and monounsaturates. Figure 7.8 and Table 7.13 show that egg and sugar consumption have fallen sharply. The temporal pattern in consumption of high cholesterol foods mirrors the epidemic in heart disease (see Chapter 18). The consumption of bread has more than halved since 1953, and that of milk has fallen by a quarter since 1970. Cheese consumption has increased over the period, but consumption of whole milk has decreased steadily, with low-fat milks increasing since the 1980s (not shown in table), probably associated with a wish to reduce saturated fat and cholesterol intake. Figure 7.9 shows the trends for fresh fruit and fruit juices – per capita consumption of fruit has risen some 40 per cent since 1950, but on top of this there has been a dramatic increase in fruit juice consumption. Nevertheless, consumption of fresh fruit and vegetables remains among the lowest in the developed world (Buss, 1988). Figure 7.10 shows that the consumption of potatoes, while still important, has more than halved. Fresh green vegetables, including brussels sprouts and cabbage, have declined steadily in popularity since 1950. Other vegetable products (including frozen and canned vegetables) have become more popular. Meat consumption is now higher than it was in 1950 but lower than it was in the 1970s (Figure 7.11), with poultry replacing more traditional meats.

7.7.3 Protein and energy intake

Largely as a result of the decreased consumption of high carbohydrate foods such as potatoes, bread, fats and sugars, there has been a reduction in total energy intake in the population since the mid-1960s (Figure 7.12). The National Food Surveys do not account for the energy intake of soft and alcoholic drinks and confectionery or food eaten outside the home, although the monitoring of the numbers and types of meals eaten away from home by the National Food Survey do not show a marked increase over the previous decade (NFS, 1990). The rising prevalence of obesity and those of above desirable weight (see later in this chapter) indicates that there is, on average, more than adequate energy intake. Energy intake in the Dietary and Nutritional Survey of British Adults also showed a 'low' energy intake, particularly among women.

The low figures could reflect under-reporting or the diary keeper unconsciously eating less than normal, or they could indicate that energy requirements are falling (Gregory et al., 1990). The average total energy intake for men was 2,450 kcals and for women 1,680 kcals, around 46 per cent lower than men. The National Diet and Nutrition Survey of toddlers (Gregory et al., 1995) found that toddlers' mean energy intake was 1,172 kcal for boys and 1,108 kcal for girls, about 82 to 90 per cent of the estimated average intake requirement. The results are likely to reflect an over-estimate of energy requirement since the survey results show an average increase in height and weight compared to a previous (1967/8) survey.

To some extent the reduction in energy intake of adults can be explained by less strenuous work – according to census results, the proportion of the male workforce which is non-manual has increased from 28 per cent in 1951 to 48 per cent in 1991. For females the corresponding figures are 36 and 69 per cent. Non-manual workers have much lower energy requirements than manual workers. There has also been an increase in unemployment, which is associated with lower energy intake – unemployed men consume on average 2,060 kcal, and working men 2,520 kcal (Gregory et al., 1990). Among women, variations in energy intake occurred according to household composition: lone mothers had the lowest average energy intake (1,580 kcal), compared with other women with dependent children (1,720 kcal). Within the same survey, unemployed men similarly had a lower mean body mass index (BMI) compared with other employment categories, and lone mothers had a lower BMI than other women with dependent children. Other reasons for lower energy requirement, which also apply to children, are central heating (less need for the body to burn food to keep warm), the use of motor cars instead of walking, and a generally more sedentary lifestyle, with watching television as the main form of recreation (Foster et al., 1995).

Figure 7.12

Average protein and energy intake

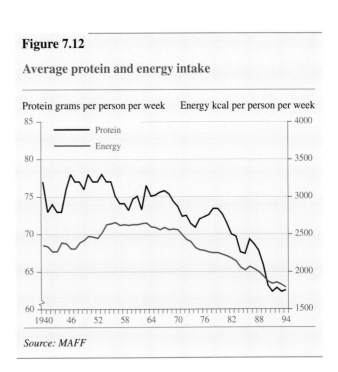

Source: MAFF

Protein consumption has also fallen since the 1960s, but intake is still greater than the recommended daily intake (DH, 1991a). Among women, lone mothers had the lowest average daily intakes of protein, carbohydrate, sugars and fibre. Unemployed men had lowest absolute intakes of protein and carbohydrate.

7.7.4 Fat intake

High consumption of saturated fatty acids, derived mainly from animal fats, is linked to increased serum cholesterol (DH, 1994a) and this is a major risk factor for cardiovascular disease. The 1984 Committee on Medical Aspects of food policy (COMA) recommended a reduction in the consumption of saturated fatty acids plus *trans* fatty acids to 15 per cent of total energy intake, and total fat to 35 per cent as a proportion of energy intake (DHSS, 1984). This was later incorporated within the government health targets set out in the 'Health of the Nation' (DH, 1991). In 1991 COMA recommended further that saturated fatty acids should be reduced to 10 per cent of total dietary energy, and fat intake to 33 per cent of total energy, which includes alcohol (DH, 1991a). A recent meta-analysis of fat intake from 1900 to 1985 by Stephen and Sieber (1994) indicated that among British adults, total fat intake as a percentage of dietary energy increased from 25 per cent during the early part of the century to 33 per cent by the late 1930s. It continued to increase after the war to peak at 40 per cent of dietary energy by the late 1970s before falling again (see Table 18.6 of Chapter 18). The NFS figures, on which the 'Health of the Nation' targets are based, are slightly higher, but show that this measure is currently falling slowly, from a high of 42.6 per cent in 1980 to 40.5 per cent in 1994. Only 12 per cent of men and 15 per cent of women achieved the 35 per cent limit of fat as a percentage of total food energy in the 1987 OPCS Nutritional and Dietary Survey (Gregory *et al.*, 1990). Thus, although total fat consumption has been substantially reduced, reduced energy intakes as a whole have

meant that the percentage energy from fat has fallen more slowly.

The COMA panel also recommended that the ratio of polyunsaturated fatty acids to saturated fatty acids (the P/S ratio) should be increased to approximately 0.45, which would mean eating less saturated fat compared to the amounts of polyunsaturated fats. Saturated fat as a percentage of total energy intake has steadily declined, with a related increase in polyunsaturated fat (Figure 7.13). The 1987 OPCS Nutritional and Dietary Survey (Gregory *et al.*, 1990) revealed that saturated fats contributed on average 15.4 per cent of total food energy for men and 16.5 per cent for women, compared with the target of 10 per cent. For men, the proportion of energy derived from saturated fats is lower because they consume more alcohol rather than because they consume less saturated fat. The P/S ratios for men and women were respectively 0.40 and 0.38, which decreased for both men and women with age. The P/S ratio was found to be significantly lower for men and women in social classes IV and V, but there was no difference in the level of total fat as a percentage of total energy intake.

7.7.5 Calcium, vitamin C and iron intake

The decline in bread consumption has contributed to the decrease in the nutritional intake of calcium and iron – flour has continued since 1943 to be fortified with calcium, as well as iron, thiamin and niacin (see Figure 7.14). The problem has been exacerbated by the decreased consumption of milk. The association between dietary calcium intake and healthy bones and teeth has long been recognised. COMA recommends higher intakes of dietary calcium where there is a higher risk of osteoporosis (DH, 1991a). Although the national consumption of calcium has decreased, intakes among adults and children are still within the levels needed for health.

Figure 7.13

Per cent of energy derived from fat per day

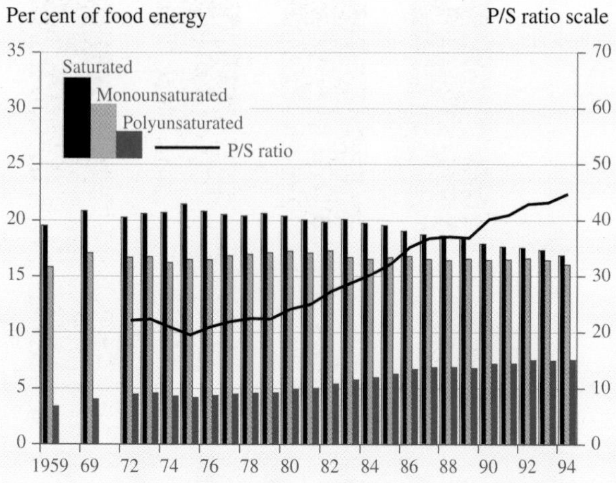

Source: MAFF

Figure 7.14

Calcium, vitamin C and iron intake per person

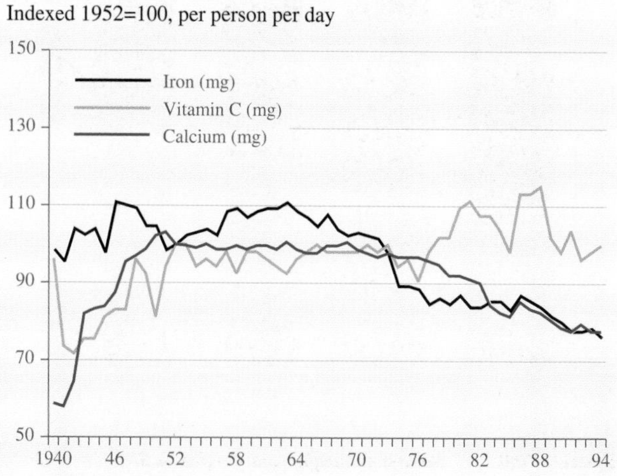

Source: MAFF

Children and adults generally now have vitamin intakes within the range of the reference nutrient intake (RNI), although family type and socio-economic factors are associated with variations. Intake of vitamin C increased between the war period and 1952, and again between the mid-1970s and the present, although in recent years consumption appears to have reduced. It has remained markedly higher in the 'higher income' group since the 1950s (and presumably before then). Intake of vitamin A has fallen since the mid-1960s, and vitamin D intake has been falling since 1950 (not shown). Intakes of vitamin C and total carotene are lower in lone mothers and their children, particularly where there is more than one child (Gregory *et al.*, 1990). Similarly, vitamin C, niacin and total carotene intakes were significantly lower for toddlers whose parents were receiving benefits, where the head of household was not working and where the toddler's mother had no formal qualification (Gregory *et al.*, 1995). The low popularity of fruit and vegetables meant that potatoes, particularly chips and savoury snacks were an important source of vitamin C, carotene and iron. Vitamin A is needed for growth in children and is found in many fruits and vegetables, and there is evidence suggesting protective properties of carotene and Vitamins C and E against certain cancers (Austoker, 1994). Similarly, research has found an association between a diet rich in Vitamin C and decreased risk of death from cardiovascular disease (Gale *et al.*, 1995). It is hypothesised that there may be a link between increased winter infections, increased plasma fibrinogen, factor VIII and vitamin C (Khaw and Woodhouse, 1995). Increased fruit and vegetable consumption may have beneficial effects against colorectal cancer, possibly through vegetable fibre (Austoker, 1994). Strachan (1991) found in an analysis of lung function that even after adjusting for sex, age, height, cigarette consumption, region of residence and household socio-economic group, lung function (FEV_1) was significantly worse (by 78 ml) in those who never drank fresh fruit juice and ate fresh fruit less than once a week during the winter.

There has been a decline in the intake of iron since the mid-1960s, with the average iron intake now at 10.2 mg (Gregory *et al.*, 1990). The higher recommended levels of total iron intake for women under 50 years of 12 mg daily were not met, particularly the average intakes of women aged 16–34 years, with median values of 10.0 mg and a mean value of 12.3 mg. The toddler's survey similarly found a low intake of iron among young children. For 84 per cent of toddlers under 4 years of age, total iron intake was below the recommended nutrient intake (RNI) of 6.9 mg/d (Gregory *et al.*, 1990). This level is considered sufficient for 97 per cent of a group for healthy growth and development. The lower recommended nutrient intake (LRNI) constitutes the lowest range sufficient for those with low needs (DH, 1991a). Of the toddlers, 16 per cent had intakes below the LRNI, with the likelihood that they were receiving insufficient for their needs. Total iron intake tended to increase with age. Nevertheless, 57 per cent of toddlers in the sample had intakes below the RNI of 6.1 mg/day. Meat and meat products were the main source of haem iron for 89 per cent of toddlers, the most readily absorbed source of dietary iron. Non-haem iron contributed 96 per cent of total iron intake for the toddlers, of which half was provided by fortified cereal and cereal products. The absorption of non-haem iron may be inhibited by some foods, including tannin from tea, which was drunk by 37 per cent of the children. Ascorbic acid (vitamin C), fish, meat and poultry enhance absorption. The intake of iron, calcium, phosphorus and potassium were lower among children from manual class backgrounds.

Figure 7.15

Trends in distribution of Body Mass Index in population aged 16–64

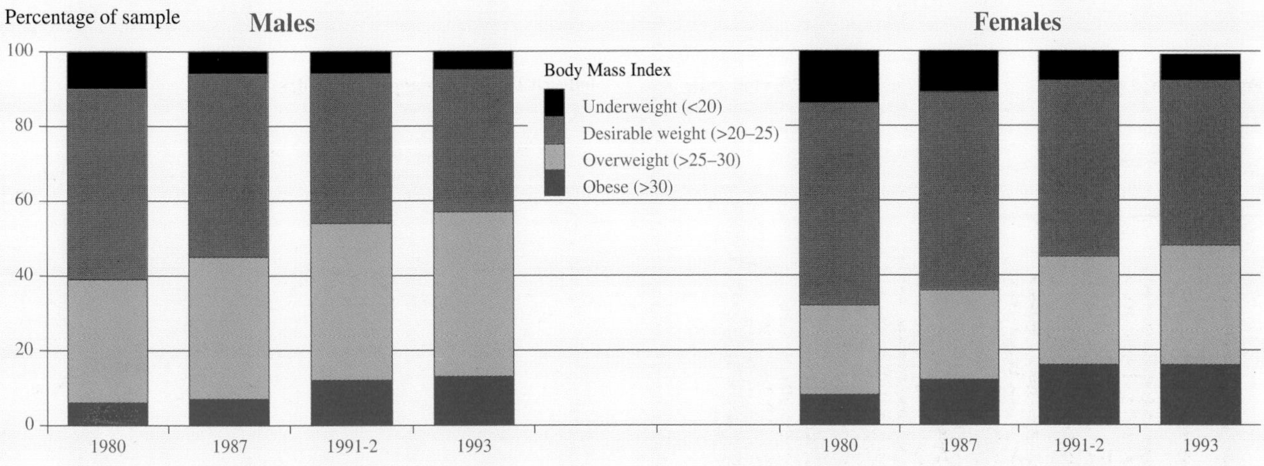

Percentage of sample — Males — Females

Body Mass Index
- Underweight (<20)
- Desirable weight (>20–25)
- Overweight (>25–30)
- Obese (>30)

Source: 1980: Surveys of Heights and Weights in GB
1987: Dietry and Nutritional Survey, GB
1991–93: Health Survey of England

7.7.6 Other dietary constituents

Average sodium intake has remained relatively constant over the period that MAFF have analysed the data (1991–94): sodium is 70 per cent above reference nutrient intake, and potassium is 20 per cent below RNI (MAFF, 1995). Among toddlers, the levels of sodium chloride consumed were also above the RNI, even when table salt and additions during cooking were excluded (Gregory *et al.*, 1995). The mean value of sodium intake among toddlers was 233 per cent of the RNI and 280 per cent of the RNI of chloride. In addition, over half of parents in the sample used salt in cooking their toddlers' food. Intakes of sodium per 1,000 kcal of energy were higher among toddlers from manual class backgrounds, and those living with a lone parent.

The COMA report on dietary reference values (DH, 1991a) reports some detrimental effects from a diet high in wheat bran and instead recommends an increased intake in foods naturally rich in non-starch polysaccharides, found in cereals and vegetables. Fibre consumption did tend to increase with age for women but did not tend to vary with age in men (Gregory *et al.*, 1990).

7.8 Weight changes since 1980

Obesity and excess weight are associated with a higher risk of hypertension, high serum lipids and diabetes mellitis, indirectly contributing to increased risk of coronary heart disease (DH, 1994a). The 1993 Health Survey (Bennett, 1995) found a strong positive relationship between body mass index (BMI – see section 7.2.3) and mean blood pressure, indicating that blood pressure rises incrementally with BMI. Those classified as at or below the desirable weight for height were less likely to have a raised blood pressure for their age, whereas those who were classified as overweight or obese were more likely to have a high blood pressure. One of the 'Health of the Nation' targets aims to reduce the percentage of those aged 16–64 years who are obese from the 8 per cent of men and 12 per cent of women in 1986/87 to no more than 6 per cent and 8 per cent, respectively, by 2005.

Bennett *et al.,* (1995) have shown that the proportions of men and women with a BMI of over 30 have increased steadily since 1980 to 13 per cent of men and 16 per cent of women (see Figure 7.15). For men, this meant an increase in the mean BMI from 24.3 in 1980 to 25.9 in 1993 (23.9 to 25.7 for women). The proportions overweight but not obese have also increased. The proportion of the population who are obese increases with age (see Figure 7.16). The increases in the proportion obese or overweight have been greatest in those aged 35 and over, but the younger age-groups, 16–24 and 25–34 years, also showed substantial increases. The National Study of Health and Growth (NSHG) has similarly noted the marked increase in obesity among children of primary school age (Rona, in press).

This increase in mean BMI and the prevalence of obesity, observed also in Europe and the US (Kuskowska-Wolk and Bergstrom, 1993), suggests that calorific intake is exceeding our requirements, in spite of the steadily declining energy intake. The reasons for this are not fully understood (Prentice and Jebb, 1995). The prevalence of a sedentary lifestyle is considered the most likely cause of excess weight gain. Other factors include the move from manual work to non-manual occupations, number of hours watching television and a net decrease in the number of periods of exercise, and increasing

---

Figure 7.16

Percentage of people who were obese (Body Mass Index > 30)

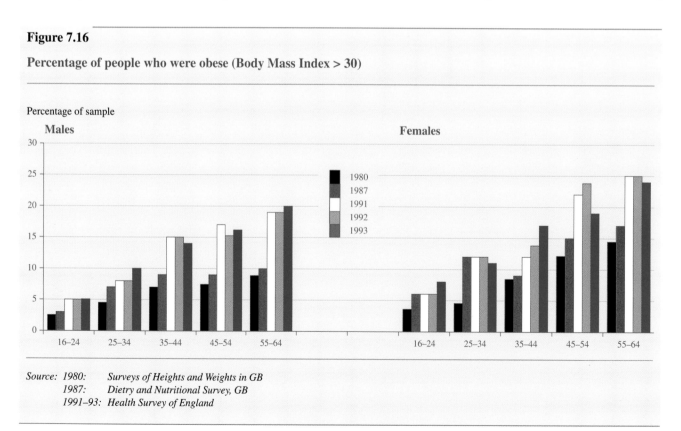

Source: 1980: *Surveys of Heights and Weights in GB*
1987: *Dietry and Nutritional Survey, GB*
1991–93: *Health Survey of England*

unemployment. The Health Survey of England (Bennett, 1995) has found a significantly higher proportion of 16–24-year-old women (12 per cent compared to 8 per cent of men) who have no occasions of moderate activity and are classified as 'inactive'; a proportion similar to women who are 10–20 years older. Men and women in the manual classes are generally more likely to be overweight or obese than the non-manual classes. Ex-regular smokers were significantly more likely to be either overweight or obese for both men and women. Those men and women who did not undertake any physical activity were more likely to be obese than those who engaged in 12 or more periods of moderate or vigorous activity in the 4 weeks prior to interview. This occurred across all age-groups but was particularly noticeable in the 45–64 year age band.

7.9 Conclusions

The period from 1841 to 1994 has witnessed large changes in British society, with much greater protection now provided by the welfare state. While the earlier data showed evidence of under-nutrition, this is not so much evident now. In the modern, affluent, consuming Britain attention is now being focused on the problems of over-consumption, particularly of energy. We are getting taller and heavier, even though we are eating less, and the increase in obesity, which carries with it increased risk of heart disease and stroke, is worrying. Despite this, there are still vulnerable groups in the population, particularly those in receipt of benefits and their children, who eat less, or less well. They also weigh less and have poorer nutritional status.

There are, nevertheless, encouraging signs. As a nation we eat more fruit than hitherto, and are cutting down on saturated fatty acids, although overall fat consumption as a proportion of total energy intake has fallen only slightly over the past two decades. In theory, these improvements in eating habits may pay dividends in terms of reduced risk of cardiovascular disease mortality later on in life, although other risk factors also play a part. Mortality from cardiovascular disease is indeed falling (see Chapter 18). But although the British diet is improving, it still has some way to go.

Chapter 8

Trends in alcohol and illicit drug-related diseases

By
Martin A Plant

Summary

- An increase in the consumption of alcohol in the nineteenth century was reversed by the introduction of a number of licensing controls in 1872. The decline continued until after the Second World War, when per capita consumption doubled between 1945 and 1979.

- Rates of alcohol morbidity and mortality are associated with trends in per capita alcohol consumption. However, certain measures of alcohol problems, for example drunkenness offences, have shown opposing trends.

- Although the numbers of drivers and two-wheeled vehicle riders killed in road accidents who were found to be over the legal blood alcohol level has fallen, there has been an increase in fatalities involving intoxicated pedestrians.

- Reported trends in mortality rates resulting from alcohol dependence in England, Scotland and Wales show considerable variation. This may be due partly to the different ways in which alcohol dependence is defined in these regions.

- Death rates from alcohol-related diseases, including liver disease and alcohol- and tobacco-related cancers, show different trends for men and women. Trends also vary between age-groups.

- Mortality associated with the recreational use of drugs other than alcohol and tobacco has been reduced over the last 150 years by control legislation.

- Recent surveys of self-reported drug use, focusing on groups of adolescents and young people, suggest that a large and growing minority have at least limited experience of illicit drug use.

- There has been a steady increase since 1965 in the number of notified drug addicts in England and Wales. However, the pattern of deaths is changing.

- The number of deaths involving people previously notified as drug addicts has risen.

- Drug-related deaths, including those with an underlying cause of death recorded as drug dependency or non-dependent abuse of drugs, are increasing.

8.1 Introduction

This chapter reviews evidence related to alcohol, the most widely used legal drug in Britain, and to 'illicit drugs'. For the purposes of this review an 'illicit' drug is defined as a substance the use of which is controlled under the Misuse of Drugs Act 1971 or by related legislation. This encompasses substances such as cannabis, LSD, cocaine, the opiates and ecstasy. Glues and volatile solvents, although not controlled in this way, are also cited if used for recreational purposes.

Alcohol has been used since prehistoric times, whereas concerns about illicit drugs are of much more recent origin. It has been noted that virtually all societies have adopted and valued some form of 'psychoactive' drug use. A 'psychoactive' drug is a substance the use of which causes some form of change of consciousness. Alcohol, tobacco, cannabis, heroin and LSD are examples of such drugs. The legal status of psychoactive drugs has varied at different times and in different places. Alcohol use is legal in most countries, albeit subject to a variety of regulations. Cannabis, heroin and a wide range of other substances are proscribed under both international and national laws.

Drug use has long been a cause for concern, provoked by moral disapproval and the fact that the use of both legal and illicit drugs is invariably accompanied by heavy or problematic use. One of the key features of drug use throughout history has been the fact that, although many people enjoy or value the use of such substances, their use is also associated with a range of adverse consequences that are frequently identified as being among the major health and social problems of the age. Recent concern about illicit drug use, especially by young people, parallels public and political alarm about problems associated with alcohol and with the use of opium in Britain in the eighteenth and nineteenth centuries.

Available evidence supports the conclusions that, although most adults in Britain drink in moderation, a minority experience serious adverse consequences. Similarly, although most illicit drug use is extremely limited, such behaviour is increasing, as is associated morbidity and premature mortality.

This chapter reviews evidence of morbidity and mortality associated with alcohol and illicit drugs. This is related to evidence on the patterns of use of these substances in Britain since 1841. It is emphasised that there is an obvious link between the use of alcohol and illicit drugs and levels of adverse consequences related to these substances. History demonstrates that the greatest levels of alcohol- and drug-related problems have been evident when the use of these has been at its greatest. The link between use and 'abuse', mortality and morbidity is well established, even though different problem indicators are related in different ways to overall trends in alcohol and drug use (Royal College of Psychiatrists, 1986; Sales *et al.*, 1989; Edwards *et al.*, 1994).

8.2 Alcohol

8.2.1 Drinking patterns

Alcohol has been described as 'our favourite drug' (Royal College of Psychiatrists, 1986). Certainly, alcohol consumption has been an integral part of the social life of Britain since early times. Indeed, the simple invitation to 'have a drink' is widely assumed to refer to alcohol. The earliest inhabitants of Britain consumed alcohol. By Roman times a network of Tabernae was established along the road system. By the Middle Ages, taverns or ale houses were widespread. Spring and Buss (1979) commented that ale had been consumed in England since Celtic times, while hopped beer had been in use since the fifteenth century. Alcohol consumption in mediaeval Britain was, by modern standards, very high. Warner (1992), for example, has reported that in northern Europe alcohol consumption was particularly great. In the fourteenth century the daily consumption of one or two gallons of beer by men was not uncommon. The 'Gin Epidemic' of the eighteenth century was linked with the rise of an increasingly urban and industrial society, together with the widespread availability of cheap alcohol. During the nineteenth century consumption of spirits rose, reaching a peak in around 1880. Wine consumption also increased between 1860 and the 1870s. Increasing alcohol consumption was accompanied by rising problems such as drunkenness, which prompted widespread concern, including the rise of an active prohibitionist movement. A number of licensing controls were introduced in 1872. The precise impact of these, together with the vigorous campaign against alcohol, or its heavy use, is unclear. Even so, as reported by Harrison (1971), the number of licensed premises fell after 1870 and the level of alcohol consumption declined after the mid-1870s (Wilson, 1940). Between 1880 and 1899 annual per capita alcohol consumption ranged from 9.7 to 11.2 litres (Witheridge, 1994, personal communication).

During the First World War it was feared that heavy drinking was undermining the war effort. The Defence of the Realm Act of 1916 reduced the availability of alcohol through licensing restrictions. Per capita alcohol consumption in the United Kingdom continued to fall until the 1930s. This trend was, however, reversed after the Second World War, per capita consumption virtually doubling between 1945 and 1979. As during earlier periods of increasing alcohol consumption, this rise was accompanied by the proliferation of alcohol-related problems and by a rise in concern. The pattern of per capita alcohol consumption levels in the twentieth century is shown in Figure 8.1.

The twentieth century consumption of alcohol has been regulated and influenced by a number of events. These have been reviewed elsewhere. Consumption levels reached their nadir during the First World War and the Depression of the

1930s. The rise in alcohol consumption after 1945 was part of an international trend. Recent levels of per capita alcohol consumption in the United Kingdom are not, however, high by international standards. For example, the United Kingdom level in 1993 was 7.0 litres of absolute alcohol. The corresponding levels in France, Portugal and Spain were 12.3, 11.4 and 9.7 litres respectively. Countries in which per capita consumption levels were similar to those of the United Kingdom included Ireland, Canada, the USA and New Zealand (Brewers' Society, 1995).

The post-war increase of alcohol consumption and alcohol-related problems has prompted a considerable number of social and behavioural studies of drinking habits and their associated consequences. The number of such studies reached a peak in the 1980s (May, 1992). Several surveys have been carried out into the drinking habits of adolescents and adults. These support a number of main conclusions. For example, people in Northern Ireland are more likely than those in England, Wales and Scotland to be non-drinkers. In Britain only 12 per cent of women and 7 per cent of men are abstainers, compared with over 50 per cent of women and nearly a third of men in Northern Ireland (Wilson, 1980; Foster et al., 1990). It is evident that there are regional variations in levels of alcohol consumption and rates of alcohol-related problems in Britain. Contrary to some popular beliefs, recent studies have indicated that the areas with the highest proportions of heavy drinkers are the north and north-west of England and not Scotland (Foster et al., 1990). Even so there is some evidence to indicate that Scottish teenagers are more likely to be heavy and infrequent drinkers than are their counterparts in England (Marsh et al., 1986; Plant and Foster, 1991; Anderson et al., 1995).

Survey data from Britain and from other countries clearly indicate that women are more likely than men to be abstainers.

Figure 8.1

Per capita alcohol consumption in United Kingdom, 1900 – 93

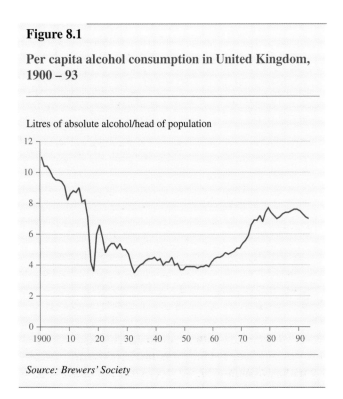

Litres of absolute alcohol/head of population

Source: Brewers' Society

They also drink smaller quantities than men. There is some evidence that drinking habits of women are 'converging' slightly with those of men (Breeze, 1989; Plant, 1996). Most people start to drink regularly after or around adolescence, although even young children form a clear, if rather eccentric, view of drinking as a popular adult form of behaviour (Fossey, 1994). Most British teenagers consume alcohol and many experience minor adverse consequences such as hangovers and intoxication. Individuals who drink heavily are especially likely to smoke tobacco, to use illicit drugs and to engage in other forms of potentially high-risk behaviour (Plant and Plant, 1992). British men typically drink on 3 or 4 days each week. Women typically do so on 2 or 3 days. However, there is evidence of a more concentrated pattern of drinking in Scotland and in Northern Ireland (Loretto, 1994; Anderson et al., 1995). It is far more common for British drinkers to drink to intoxication periodically than to imbibe large amounts habitually. This fact is reflected in the general pattern of alcohol-related morbidity and mortality.

The connection between general levels of alcohol consumption and the pattern of associated harm has long been controversial. It is, however, evident that overall levels of adverse consequences do fluctuate with per capita alcohol consumption. There are also some exceptions to this (Sales et al., 1989; Plant and Plant, 1992).

8.2.2   Alcohol-related diseases

Although most drinkers consume alcohol in relatively small quantities, it is well established that heavy drinking is associated with morbidity and premature mortality (Royal College of Psychiatrists, 1986; Royal College of Physicians, 1987; Faculty of Public Health, 1991; Verschuren, 1993; Edwards et al., 1994). Ulpian, in Roman times, wrote that 'inebriety' was a disease. Trotter (1813) wrote one of the most detailed British nineteenth century accounts of the medical problems associated with alcohol. Carpenter (1850) described three types of 'oenomania' or problematic drinking.

Space does not permit a detailed review of this evidence. Even so a useful recent review of some of the available medical evidence has been provided by Verschuren (1993). This concluded that alcohol consumption was associated with hypertension. Indeed, it was noted that chronic consumption above 4–8 units of alcohol per day might be the second most important factor for this condition. A unit is equivalent to a single glass of wine, a bar room measure of spirits or half a pint of normal strength beer/lager/stout/cider. It was further concluded that alcohol was a significant factor in haemorrhagic stroke, but not in ischaemic stroke. The latter currently account for 85 per cent of all strokes in Britain. Studies further indicate that heavier drinking is a factor in coronary heart disease. Alcohol is causally related to cancers of the larynx, pharynx, liver, oesophagus and the mouth (International Agency for Research on Cancers, 1988; Duffy and Sharples, 1992). In some cases this link is increased by smoking. Evidence on the possible role of alcohol in relation to cancers of the breast, stomach and pancreas is unclear. Alcohol is a major factor in liver cirrhosis and liver disease. This connection is so clear that rates of liver cirrhosis and chronic liver disease are frequently used as key epidemiological markers for rates of 'problem' or heavy drinking in a population (Williams *et al.*, 1994). Even so, it has been concluded that even among heavily alcohol-dependent people, only a minority, around 12 per cent, die from liver cirrhosis or allied conditions. Most 'alcohol problems' involve other factors.

Alcohol consumption has also been linked with a number of other conditions, including oesophageal disorders, peptic ulcers (gastric and duodenal), gastritis, coeliac disease, Crohn's disease, ulcerative colitis and pancreatic disease. In spite of this, a recent review concluded that there is 'no evidence' to support the conclusion that drinking is causally connected with oesophageal disorders, coeliac disease, Crohn's disease or ulcerative colitis. It was further concluded:

The position is less clear for ulcers and gastritis. There is evidence that alcohol consumption is greater in patients with peptic ulcers. However, it is associated with other risk factors for ulcer such as smoking and emotional stress, and does not emerge as an independent risk factor in multivariate analysis.

Raab (1992, p. 136)

As noted by Plant (1992), it is sometimes difficult to demonstrate or to refute the existence of a clear causal link between drinking and some diseases as a result of the limitations of available studies. Concern about women's drinking has included interest in the possibility that maternal alcohol consumption during pregnancy might damage the developing foetus. In 1973 the term 'foetal alcohol syndrome' was introduced to describe features noted in the babies of a small group of women who were believed to have drunk heavily while pregnant. A considerable amount of research has been conducted into the topic. Recent reviews have concluded that the foetal alcohol syndrome is rare and that it appears to be attributable to a constellation of factors including smoking, illicit drug use, poor health and diet, low socio-economic status and heavy drinking. Most pregnant women do not drink heavily enough to put their offspring at risk and the foetal alcohol syndrome is unusual in most populations (Plant, 1985; Plant *et al.*, 1993; Plant, 1996).

Acute heavy drinking and its associated intoxication are important factors in accidental injuries and deaths. These include industrial, domestic and traffic accidents. Moreover, heavy drinking is also associated with public disorder and with crimes, especially crimes of violence (Collins, 1982; Giesbrecht *et al.*, 1989). Continued heavy drinking may lead, not only to conditions such as liver cirrhosis, but also to alcohol dependence (sometimes referred to as 'alcoholism'). Available statistics on the prevalence of alcohol dependence are strongly influenced by the policies and availability of treatment agencies, especially in-patient facilities within or attached to psychiatric institutions. In fact many 'problem drinkers' do not contact such agencies, and some of those will contact the fellowship of Alcoholics Anonymous, local councils on alcohol, family doctors or social workers. Others,

particularly women, will contact agencies with no specialist alcohol remit. The first alcohol treatment clinics in Britain opened in the early 1960s.

Recorded patterns of alcohol-related morbidity and mortality are influenced and distorted by a variety of factors. These have made it hard even to compare such rates in different areas of Britain (Crawford and Plant, 1986). Studies of alcohol-related mortality have universally found that 'heavy drinking' is a factor in a wide range of conditions. A growing body of evidence supports the conclusion that moderate levels of alcohol consumption are protective in relation to coronary heart disease. Higher rates of premature mortality have been found among abstainers and heavy drinkers than amongst those who consume moderate/intermediate quantities of alcohol. This conclusion has been described as the 'U'- or 'J'-shaped mortality curve. The evidence has been reviewed elsewhere (see Doll *et al.*, 1994; Gronbaek *et al.*, 1994). The first of these groups of authors found that the lowest mortality rates were among men and women who consumed 1–6 UK alcohol units per week. Doll *et al.*, describing the results of a study of male doctors, concluded that (p. 911):

Above three units . . . of alcohol a day, progressively greater levels of alcohol consumption are associated with progressively higher all cause mortality.

Gronbaek *et al.* (1995) have further reported that the low-to-moderate consumption of wine is associated with lower mortality as a result of cardiovascular and cerebrovascular disease and other causes. These authors concluded that a similar level of spirits consumption was associated with an increased risk, whereas beer consumption did not influence mortality. The 'J'-shaped curve has survived analysis designed to examine whether 'abstainers' are former drinkers or heavy drinkers and the possible confounding influence of smoking. More research is needed to examine what mechanisms may explain this effect. The work of Gronbaek *et al.* suggests that the 'J'-shaped curve may reflect a combination of different risks associated with different types of alcoholic drink. In addition, it is emphasised that the existence of an apparent protective effect from moderate drinking should not be interpreted as a reason for abstainers to start to drink, or for drinkers to increase their consumption. Overall, such a step would be likely to elevate levels of alcohol-related problems.

People who drink to acute intoxication or who chronically drink heavily may place themselves and sometimes others at risk from illness or death. To provide clear practical advice the royal medical colleges have suggested that adult male drinkers should limit themselves to 21 units per week and that the corresponding 'low-risk' level for women is 14 units (Royal College of Psychiatrists, 1986). It should, however, be emphasised that the consequences of drinking vary with the individual, their pattern of drinking and their circumstances. Pregnant women, for example, are recommended either to abstain or to restrict their alcohol consumption to one or two units once or twice a week. Drinking and driving are mutually incompatible.

As noted above, rates of alcohol-related ill health are associated with trends in per capita alcohol consumption. In spite of this some measures of 'alcohol problems' have moved in a different direction from alcohol consumption. For example, drunkenness offences in Scotland fell to a fifth of their original level between 1964 and 1991. In England and Wales the decline has been much smaller – 18 per cent. Over the same period per capita alcohol consumption rose from 4.8 litres to 7.3 litres. During the period 1979–89 the numbers of drivers and riders killed in road accidents who were found to be over the legal blood alcohol level dropped dramatically (Department of Transport, 1990a). This is shown in Table 8.1. During the same period the level of per capita alcohol consumption in the United Kingdom remained little changed.

As shown in Table 8.1, the decline in alcohol involvement in driver/rider deaths has been evident among all age-groups. The greatest improvements have been among the youngest individuals, those aged 16–19. Among the latter the proportion over the legal blood alcohol level fell by 50 per cent among two-wheeled vehicle riders and by 66 per cent among young drivers. Fatalities among two-wheeled vehicle riders in the 30–39 age-group have also exhibited a marked fall in alcohol involvement, dropping from 46 per cent to 17 per cent. It should, however, be noted that these improvements in alcohol-impaired driver/rider deaths have been accompanied by recent evidence suggesting that there has been a rise in fatalities involving intoxicated pedestrians (Christie, 1993). Although, there has been a reduction in driver/rider fatalities involving alcohol, the Department of Transport (1990b) has reported that 840 people were still being killed annually in accidents involving alcohol-impaired drivers or riders.

Recent trends in British rates of alcohol-related morbidity and mortality have been reviewed by Noble (1994), Pinot de Moira and Duffy (1994) and Duffy and Plant (1986). The first of these studies examined the period from 1970 until the early 1980s. This showed that hospital admissions for alcohol dependence in England rose over this period, but those in Scotland fell from 1976 for men and 1977 for women. Rates of first admissions for alcohol dependence among Scottish men rose until 1974–5, then declined. Rates among Scottish women reached a peak in 1980. In England such rates for men and women rose steadily until 1980–81. In spite of this, the Scottish risk of being recorded as a 'first admission' for alcohol dependence was more than three times higher for men and nearly as high for women.

The information considered by Duffy and Plant related to a diagnosis of 'alcoholism' between 1970 and 1978 in England. Thereafter they related to alcohol dependence and non-dependent abuse of alcohol. Scottish figures before 1975 related to 'alcoholism' in general. It was noted that these data only referred to psychiatric in-patients, other alcohol agencies not being included. In addition, such figures are influenced by hospital admission policies. Duffy and Plant also examined mortality resulting from alcohol dependence. Before 1978 such deaths were recorded under the International Classification of Diseases (ICD 8) as being attributable to 'alcoholism' (ICD 303) and 'alcoholic psychosis' (ICD 290). Since 1979 the first of these categories has been replaced by 'alcohol dependence'. A comparison between England and Wales and Scotland is complicated because, before June 1984, the certification of a death caused by alcohol dependence (in England and Wales) led to referral to a coroner. This may

Table 8.1

Drivers and riders killed: percentages over the legal blood alcohol limit in Great Britain, 1979–89

Year	Two-wheeled motor vehicle riders age-groups				Driver of cars and other motor vehicles age-groups			
	16–19 %	20–29 %	30–39 %	40+ %	16–19 %	20–29 %	30–39 %	40+ %
1979	26	40	46	19	34	42	47	20
1980	22	39	38	24	33	43	35	22
1981	16	39	38	29	20	45	39	20
1982	17	43	34	17	31	50	52	20
1983	17	29	30	8	34	42	43	14
1984	24	30	28	22	18	39	33	15
1985	15	27	39	11	25	40	38	14
1986	15	28	33	14	19	36	33	13
1987	16	31	24	16	16	32	27	13
1988	10	33	33	9	12	30	27	9
1989	13	25	17	17	11	24	31	9

Source: Department of Transport (1990a, p.25)

have discouraged the use of such a diagnosis. Such rates had, for some time, been markedly higher in Scotland than they were south of the border. In spite of this, trends in mortality resulting from alcohol dependence in Scotland were similar to those in England and Wales. Such deaths rose throughout Britain in the early 1970s, but declined during the later part of that decade. A more inclusive measure of alcohol-related mortality was also examined. This combined deaths from liver cirrhosis, 'alcoholism', and alcoholic psychosis and alcohol poisoning (ICD E860). This composite rate rose slightly and fairly uniformly throughout Britain between 1970 and the early 1980s. Scottish rates were higher than those in England and Wales.

A second review has examined a broader group of mortality indicators in Britain over the period 1980–91 (Pinot de Moira and Duffy, 1994). This related to chronic liver disease and cirrhosis (ICD 571), pancreatitis (ICD 577), alcohol dependence or psychosis (ICD 303 and 291), and alcohol poisoning (ICD E860). This review showed that liver cirrhosis deaths rose slightly over this period and that these were recorded as having a markedly higher rate in Scotland than in England. The rate of deaths attributed to alcoholic psychosis and alcohol dependence was also much higher in Scotland than in England and Wales. Between 1980 and 1991 the Scottish rates declined whereas those in England rose, albeit at a very low level. In 1991 the rates per 100,000 population for men and women in Scotland were 3.4 and 1.7 respectively. The corresponding rates in England and Wales were 0.6 and 0.3.

Throughout Britain during this period the death rates from pancreatitis changed very little. The death rates from alcoholic poisoning fell markedly in Scotland but rose slightly in England and Wales. A review by Noble (1994) has also provided a clear account of trends in alcohol-related deaths in England and Wales since 1979. It should be noted that this was the peak year for post-war per capita alcohol consumption in the United Kingdom (see Figure 8.1).

Figure 8.2 shows that rates of deaths from liver disease in which alcohol was mentioned have risen fairly steadily since 1979. The rate among women has been similar. In addition, the rate of increase in women has been less marked. It is emphasised that data related to liver cancer may be misleading. Some deaths attributed to this cause relate to secondary liver cancer, rather than to primary cancer as the cause of death. The rates in Figure 8.2 are standardised for age.

Figure 8.3 shows that although rates of alcohol- and tobacco-related cancers have been increasing among men, they have changed very little among women. Such rates are also much lower in women than in men. The increase is mainly due to increases in oesophageal cancer.

Rates of four categories of alcohol-related death are shown in Figure 8.4. This relates to alcoholic psychosis, the toxic effect of alcohol, alcoholic cardiomyopathy, the non-dependent abuse of alcohol and the alcohol dependence syndrome. As this figure indicates, there has been little change

in these rates among women, although those among men have increased. Older people are most at risk from deaths caused by liver disease and the alcohol dependence syndrome. Younger people are most at risk from non-dependent abuse and the toxic effects of alcohol. This is shown in Figure 8.5. It should be noted that in Figures 8.3–8.5 the rates for the disease groups shown vary considerably.

Overall trends in alcohol-related mortality for those aged 25 and above rose between 1979 and around 1990 (see Figure 8.6).

8.3 Illicit drugs

8.3.1 Drug use

The use of illicit drugs has grown steadily since the 1960s. The recreational use of drugs other than alcohol and tobacco has a long history. Opium was extensively used in Britain, both as a medicine and for the pleasure of its effects. As noted by Edwards (1971), the use of substances such as peyote, coca, opium and cannabis has long been a feature of most societies. The use of some drugs has been linked with religion in some contexts, although it is purely hedonistic or illegal in others. The use of opium was legal and widespread in eighteenth and nineteenth century Britain, both as a medicine and as a recreational substance. Its use was especially commonplace in the Fens. Laudanum, a tincture of opium, was a standard drug (Berridge and Edwards, 1979). The ill-effects associated with opiates are described below. The Pharmacy Acts of 1868 and 1908 restricted the availability of opium. In spite of the former legislation, associated mortality only began to decline at the end of the nineteenth century. Even so, the 1868 law did appear to reduce the level of infant deaths associated with opium. In spite of this, as Berridge (1979) notes, accidental deaths were little influenced and there was an increase in poisonings involving adult men.

In 1916 the Commissioner of Police for London reported trafficking in cocaine, mainly by prostitutes and service personnel. It has been noted that opium and cocaine use continued to be evident during the 1920s. This was reflected by a small number of convictions under the Defence of the Realm Act 1916 and the Dangerous Drugs Act 1920. Between the two World Wars, drug use in Britain apparently declined, though some opium use was evident (Phillipson, 1970). In 1924 the Rolleston Committee was set up to consider the United Kingdom approach to drug dependence. In 1926 this body reported and laid the foundations of what has been described as the 'British System', which involved providing drug-dependent people with controlled drug supplies if this facilitated the leading of a fairly 'normal' life. During the following two decades, this system had to handle a few hundred 'therapeutic' patients, mainly middle-aged people.

During the Second World War, returning troops and immigrants introduced some cannabis smoking to Britain. There was also some evidence of a rise in heroin use. In 1958 the Brain Committee reviewed the situation. They reported in 1961,

Figure 8.2

Deaths from alcohol-related liver disease, rate per 100,000, England and Wales

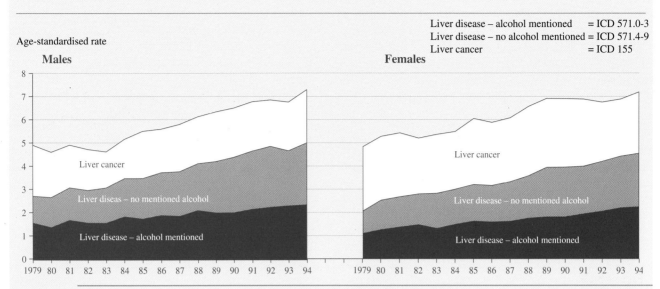

Liver disease – alcohol mentioned	= ICD 571.0-3
Liver disease – no alcohol mentioned	= ICD 571.4-9
Liver cancer	= ICD 155

Age-standardised rate

Figure 8.3

Deaths from cancers associated with smoking and alcohol, rate per 100,000, England and Wales

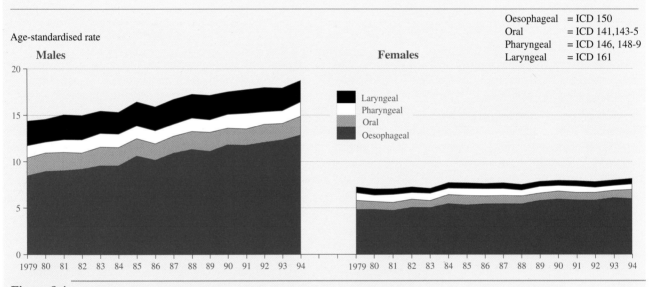

Oesophageal	= ICD 150
Oral	= ICD 141,143-5
Pharyngeal	= ICD 146, 148-9
Laryngeal	= ICD 161

Age-standardised rate

Figure 8.4

Deaths from causes linked to alcohol*, rate per 100,000, England and Wales

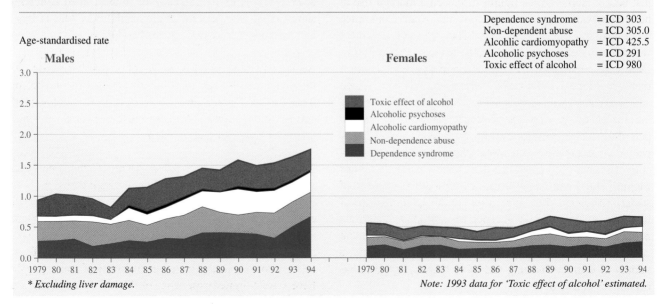

Dependence syndrome	= ICD 303
Non-dependent abuse	= ICD 305.0
Alcoholic cardiomyopathy	= ICD 425.5
Alcoholic psychoses	= ICD 291
Toxic effect of alcohol	= ICD 980

Age-standardised rate

Excluding liver damage.

Note: 1993 data for 'Toxic effect of alcohol' estimated.

Figure 8.5a

Liver disease: average rates, England and Wales, by age and sex, 1990–94

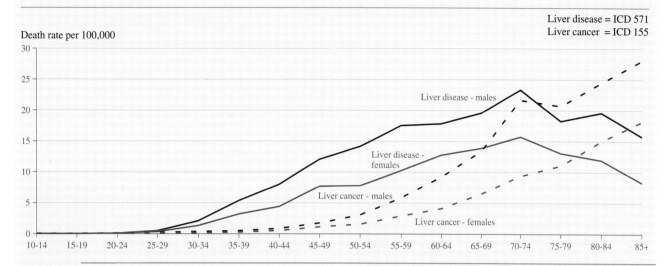

Liver disease = ICD 571
Liver cancer = ICD 155

Figure 8.5b

Abuse of alcohol: average rates, England and Wales, by age and sex, 1990-94

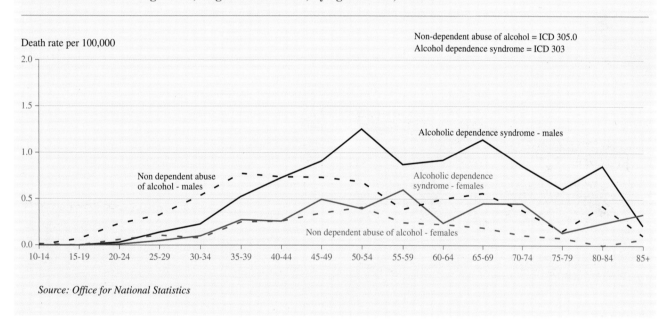

Source: Office for National Statistics

just before Home Office figures disclosed a marked rise in heroin dependence. In 1965 a reconvened Brain Committee reported that, since they had first reviewed the situation, there was a considerable increase in illicit drug use (Plant, 1975). During the 1960s, both in Britain and in many other countries, there developed a distinctive subculture. This embraced adolescents and young, even not so young adults. Illicit drug use, mainly convivial and recreational, gained acceptance as part of a more general set of values, music and fashion. Many people were attracted, at least peripherally, to this 'counter-culture'. It has been noted that this had particular attractions for individuals who had little status within the mainstream of society (Young, 1971). In response to the spreading use of illicit drugs, new control legislation was introduced, both at a national and an international level. In addition, drug treatment centres were introduced in the late 1960s. Subsequently, a variety of drug counselling and other helping agencies has become established.

A 1995 survey of 10–15-year-olds in the United Kingdom showed that 39.8 per cent of girls and 45 per cent of boys had used illicit drugs (Miller and Plant, 1996).

As illicit drug use is illegal, it is in some ways harder to chart its epidemiology than to delineate patterns of alcohol or tobacco use. Nevertheless, there have been a number of surveys of self-reported drug use and there is other evidence on trends in drug-related problems.

Surveys have mainly focused on groups of adolescents and young people in specific localities or institutions, such as schools and colleges. These have been reviewed in detail elsewhere (Edwards and Busch, 1981; Berridge, 1990; Plant and Plant, 1992; Strang and Gossop, 1994). Such surveys may, of course, be flawed by under- and over-reporting. Even so, they do indicate that a growing minority of young people have at least limited experience of illicit drug use. Drug use

Figure 8.6a

Alcohol-related mortality trends by sex, England and Wales, ages 15–44

Standardised to 1981, rate per 100,000

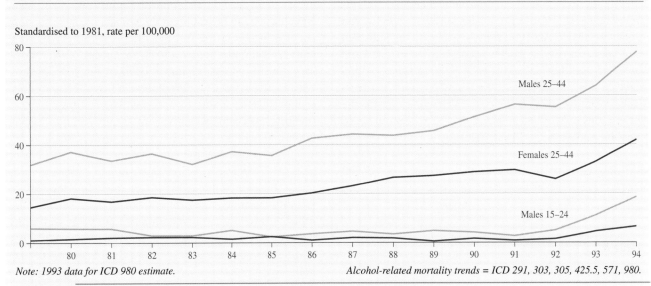

Note: 1993 data for ICD 980 estimate.   *Alcohol-related mortality trends = ICD 291, 303, 305, 425.5, 571, 980.*

Figure 8.6b

Alcohol-related mortality trends, by sex, England and Wales, ages 45 and over

Standardised to1981, rate per 100,000

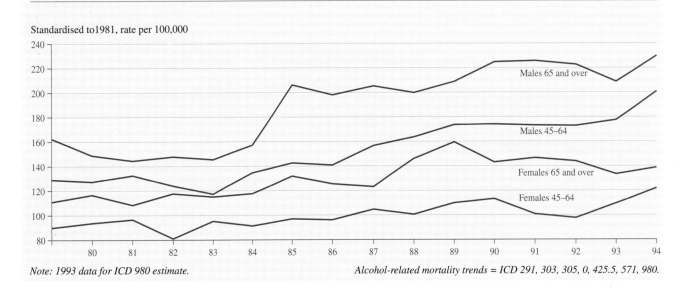

Note: 1993 data for ICD 980 estimate.   *Alcohol-related mortality trends = ICD 291, 303, 305, 0, 425.5, 571, 980.*

surveys have only been conducted in Britain since the 1960s. A number of early studies indicated levels of self-reported drug use, mainly related to cannabis. For example, Binnie and Murdock (1969), found that 9 per cent of a study group of students in Leicester had used some type of drug. McKay *et al.* (1973), reported that 14 per cent of medical students in Glasgow had taken drugs. A British Crime Survey was conducted in 1981. This indicated that 16 per cent of those aged 20–24 in England and Wales had used cannabis. The corresponding proportion in Scotland was 19 per cent (Chambers and Tombs, 1984; Mott, 1989). A national survey of 15–21-year-olds indicated that cannabis was by far the most commonly used drug and it had been tried, in various areas of Britain, by 13–28 per cent of this age-group. Regional variations in other drug use were also reported: amphetamines 3–10 per cent, glues and solvents 1–4 per cent, barbiturates

2–16 per cent, LSD 2–8 per cent, heroin less than 0.5–7 per cent and cocaine 1–3 per cent (NOP Market Research Ltd, 1982).

Williams (1986) conducted a survey of 2,417 secondary school and college students in England and Wales. This indicated that 17 per cent had used cannabis, 6 per cent had used glues or solvents and 2 per cent had used heroin. Pritchard *et al.* (1986) concluded that 19 per cent of a sample of teenagers in Bournemouth and Southampton had used drugs, most commonly cannabis, glue, gas, typewriter fluid and amphetamines. Other studies of various groups of young people have reported levels of drug use in the range 5–40 per cent. Cannabis has universally been found to be the most widely used substance. Other drugs taken have included 'magic mushrooms', crack (smokable cocaine) and a variety of analgesics (Plant *et al.*, 1986; Parker *et al.*, 1988; Coggans *et al.*, 1989; Bagnall, 1991).

Recently the use of Ecstasy (3,4-methylenedioxymethyl-amphetamine or MDMA) has been noted as widespread (Anderson, 1992). The 1992 British Crime Survey indicated that 17 per cent of respondents aged 16–59 in England and Wales had used illicit drugs. This suggested that 4 million people in this age-group had done so (Mott and Mirrlees-Black, 1995). A 1994 survey of 13–16-year-olds in the Western Isles of Scotland indicated that 22 per cent had used cannabis (Anderson and Plant, 1996).

Most drug users do not come to the attentions of 'official agencies' as a result of their drug use, which is mainly very

Table 8.2

Narcotic addicts known to the Home Office, 1970–95

Year	Males	Females	Total	% change over previous years*
1970	1,051	375	1,426	–
1971	1,133	416	1,549	+9
1972	1,195	421	1,616	+4
1973	1,370	446	1,816	+12
1974	1,458	509	1,967	+8
1975	1,438	511	1,949	– 1
1976	1,387	487	1,874	– 4
1977	1,466	550	2,016	+6
1978	1,703	699	2,402	+19
1979	1,892	774	2,666	+11
1980	2,009	837	2,846	+7
1981	2,732	1,112	3,844	+36
1982	3,124	1,247	4,371	+14
1983	3,601	1,478	5,079	+16
1984	4,133	1,736	5,869	+15
1985	4,952	2,100	7,052	+20
1986	5,929	2,515	8,444	+20
1987	7,766	2,950	10,716	+27
1988	9,093	3,551	12,644	+18
1989	10,479	4,306	14,785	+17
1990	12,807	4,948	17,755	+20
1991	15,138	5,682	20,820	+17
1992	18,241	6,462	24,703	+19
1993	21,036	6,940	27,976	+13
1994	25,389	8,561	33,952	+21
1995	28,097	9,067	37,164	+9

* *Rounded to nearest per cent.*
Note: 1970–86 figures indicate addicts notified on 31 December
each year; 1987–95 figures indicate addicts notified during year.
Source: Home Office 1979–96

restricted. Some individuals are convicted of drug offences. Trends in such convictions are influenced by a number of factors and, accordingly, should not be taken as a precise measure of trends in general population drug use. Nevertheless, an indication of the probable increase in drug use is provided by the fact that, in 1945, 230 people were convicted of offences relating to opium, cannabis or manufactured drugs. Opium accounted for 206 of these. Between 1981 and 1994 the numbers of persons found guilty, cautioned or dealt with by compounding for drug offences (mainly related to cannabis) rose from 17,921 to 86,961 During the period 1981–91 the rates of drug seizures per 1,000,000 population rose from 296 to 1,087. In 1991 these rates ranged from 304 in North Yorkshire to 2,956 in the area covered by the Metropolitan Police, including the City of London. It should be emphasised that these rates are influenced by police organisation and policy as well as by the extent of regional drug use. The overwhelming majority of drug offenders are men. In 1994 only 9.4 per cent of such individuals were women. Most are also relatively young. In 1994 only 20 per cent were aged 30 or over (Home Office, 1985, 1992, 1995).

Most illicit drug use appears to be very limited and harmless. Even so, some people use illicit drugs heavily and with adverse consequences. The latter have been accentuated by the advent of HIV/AIDS, since one of the major means of HIV transmission is through the sharing of infected injecting equipment.

8.3.2   Drug-related diseases

It has long been acknowledged that drug use sometimes gives rise to serious health consequences. These include dependence or 'addiction', as well as overdoses and a number of other harmful conditions. These harmful conditions, in the case of injecting drug users, include the transmission of hepatitis and HIV/AIDS. Ghodse (1994), has noted that it is not easy to chart the extent of drug-related ill health with precision:

Hepatitis for example, at one stage in the UK, appeared to be a reliable indicator of heroin dependence, but for a variety of reasons became a much less certain marker.

During the nineteenth century the Registrar General recorded suicides and accidental deaths associated with narcotics. Berridge (1979), reviewing this evidence, has shown that in the period 1863–1900 the annual total of such deaths ranged from 90 to 206. From 1904 this mortality fell from an annual total of 164 to 43 in 1919. Most of these deaths involved laudanum. Eighty laudanum-related deaths were recorded in 1880. The number of deaths related to other drugs were as follows: opium 27, soothing syrups 6, chlorodyne 11 and morphine 7.

The Home Office publishes details of 'known addicts' on an annual basis (Home Office, 1979–94). These are individuals who are notified by medical practitioners as being dependent upon opiates or other illicit drugs. Between 1935 and 1955 the number of such notified addicts declined from 700 to fewer than 400. Since the publication of the second Brain report in 1965, there has been a steady increase in the numbers of notified addicts, rising to 1,426 in 1970. Since that date, the number of notified addicts has climbed to 37,164 in 1995. Trends between 1970 and 1995 are shown in Table 8.2.

In 1995 the proportion of notified addicts who were dependent on heroin fell from 82 per cent in 1990 to 66 per cent, whereas those dependent on methadone increased from 28 per cent to 47 per cent. Fewer than 10 per cent were reported to be dependent on cocaine. It should be noted that many individuals were recorded as dependent upon two or more drugs.

Most notified addicts are relatively young. In 1995 the average age of newly notified addicts was 26.3 years for men and 25.8 years for women. Women accounted for one quarter of newly notified addicts in that year. The average age of notified addicts has changed little in the last decade. Notified drug addicts are prone to high rates of premature mortality. Between 1984 and 1994 the number of individuals dying from poisoning who had at some time been notified addicts rose from 94 to 113. During the same period the number of deaths with an underlying cause described as drug dependence or non-dependent abuse of drugs rose from 99 to 489. (It is further noted that in Glasgow alone in 1994 more than 80 drug user deaths were reported.)

The pattern of drug-related deaths has been changing. The total number of individuals who died in 1988 was 1,212. By 1994 this had risen to 1,620. The first 'official' AIDS-related deaths in this group were noted in 1985 and had risen to 112 in the year 1994. As already noted, the sharing of infected injecting equipment has been an important factor in HIV transmission, and it has been reported that this has been especially evident in cities such as Edinburgh and Dundee (Robertson, 1987; Strang and Stimson, 1990). Injecting drug users are one of the groups most severely affected by AIDS.

As shown in Table 8.3 the numbers of AIDS-related deaths recorded in the United Kingdom rose from 119 in 1985 to 1,191 in 1995. Injecting drug users accounted for only one such death in 1985, but for 119 or 9.9 per cent of the total in 1995. For women they accounted for more than a third of such deaths.

The number of deaths involving people who have previously been notified as drug addicts has been rising in association with the increase in numbers of addict notifications (see Table 8.2). Trends in such deaths between 1985 and 1990 are indicated by Table 8.4. As this shows, the numbers of such deaths, excluding 'therapeutic addicts', increased from 166 to 325 in this period.

Many drug users, even if their use is heavy or problematic, are not notified to the Home Office as being 'addicts'. The scale of drug-related morbidity and mortality extends beyond notified addicts. Between 1980 and 1990 the number of drug-related deaths increased steadily. This is shown in Table 8.5. As shown, the numbers of deaths with an underlying cause of death recorded as drug dependence or non-dependent abuse of drugs rose from 99 to 294. Data produced since 1988 also include deaths from poisoning in which a controlled drug was mentioned. Total drug-related deaths, including these deaths, rose from 1,206 in 1988 to 1,263 in 1990. The involvement of specific types of drug in mortality has been examined by staff in the Research and Statistics Department in the Home Office. Details of this analysis for the years 1980 and 1990 are shown in Table 8.6.

One point to note from Table 8.6 is that it includes no deaths related either to cannabis or to hallucinogens (such as LSD). In addition only one amphetamine-related death was cited (in 1990). By far the two biggest subgroups of fatalities in 1990 involved volatile substances (e.g. glues and solvents) (112 deaths) and drugs of the morphine type, including heroin and other opiates (91 deaths). Trends in deaths associated with volatile solvents are monitored regularly by Taylor *et al*. (1995). There is no separate ICD9 code for such deaths. They are, however, included under ICD codes 304.6 (drug dependence) and codes 981, 982, 983 and 987 (toxic effects). In 1991 the number of deaths caused by volatile substance abuse (VSA) (solvents) had risen to 122 in the United Kingdom but has since fallen to 73 by 1993. VSA is most common in boys in their early to mid-teens. From 1971 to 1993, over 70 per cent of all those who died from VSA were aged less than 20, and nearly 90 per cent were less than 25. Eighty eight per cent were male.

The trends in deaths associated with volatile solvents are shown in Figure 8.6. As indicated, these types of deaths are a relatively recent problem.

Further details of recent trends in drug-related deaths are presented in Figures 8.9 and 8.10. As shown in Figure 8.9, most drug-related deaths involve overdoses. The most notable change in recent years has been caused by the advent of AIDS-related deaths which are increasing and may continue to do

Table 8.3

Deaths of reported AIDS cases by year of death, United Kingdom

	1990	1991	1992	1993	1994	1995
Injecting drug users						
Males	26	54	69	83	83	92
Females	8	25	13	24	29	27
Total	34	79	82	107	112	119
All AIDS deaths						
Males	722	914	1,015	1,136	1,195	1,051
Females	35	76	66	127	127	140
Total	757	990	1,081	1,263	1,322	1,190

Source: Home Office (1992–96, Table 21)

Table 8.4

Number of deaths of drug addicts previously notified to the Home Office, 1985–90

All persons	1985	1986	1987	1988	1989	1990
Under 20	6 (1)	10	1	6	9	4
20 and under 30	71 (1)	94	130	112	122	150
30 and under 40	75 (2)	100 (1)	100	130 (2)	115 (1)	121 (1)
40 and under 50	11 (1)	18 (1)	13	19 (1)	38 (1)	40
50 and over	3 (15)	8 (5)	13 (9)	10 (11)	6 (9)	10 (5)
Unrecorded	– (1)		1	1		
Total all ages	166 (21)	230 (7)	257 (9)	278 (14)	291 (11)	325 (6)
Average age	30.9	31.7	31.8	32.1	32.4	32.3

Note: The figures on the left exclude addicts with theraputic origin for their dependence.
Some of these details may not be drug-related.
Source: Home Office (1992)

Table 8.5

Summary of drug-related deaths by year of registration of death, United Kingdom, 1984–94

	Number of deaths (previously notified addicts **)										
Underlying cause of death	1984	1985	1986	1987	1988	1989	1990	1991	1992	1993	1994
Drug dependence and non-dependent abuse of drugs*	133	190	195	228	222	245	294 (70)	307 (85)	345 (108)	322 (39)	489
Deaths from poisoning where a controlled drug was mentioned †											
Accidental					191	202	233 (88)	255 (91)	327 (137)	358 (37)	442
Suicide					478	433	440 (3)	433 (7)	400 (11)	340 (6)	334
Undetermined					302	279	262 (23)	295 (32)	274 (39)	252 (13)	243
AIDS§	0	4	9	11	19	32	55 (17)	79 (26)	82 (11)	107 (27)	112
Total	NA	NA	NA	NA	1,212	1,191	1,284 (201)	1,369 (241)	1,428 (306)	1,379 (122)	1,620

*   *Includes solvents and other non-controlled drugs such as alcohol.*
†   *Excludes Northern Ireland.*
§   *By year of death.*

** *Not available before 1990 or after 1993.*
Source: Home Office (1996)

so for at least some time. As indicated by Figure 8.10, most drug-related deaths involve relatively young people, with the peak age being in the range 20–30 years of age.

Drug-related deaths in England and Wales have increased significantly since 1979. As shown by Figure 8.11, this rise has been especially marked among men.

8.4 Conclusion

It should be emphasised that morbidity and mortality associated with both alcohol and illicit drugs are influenced by the general misuse patterns of such substances. The effects of any psychoactive drug, licit or illicit, are influenced by interaction between the chemistry of the substance, the characteristics (e.g. age, gender) of the user and the environment in which misuse occurs. Some alcohol/drug-related diseases are strongly influenced by the fact that heavy drinkers may also be smokers and that, among younger people in particular, the misuse of illicit drugs is often also accompanied by heavy drinking and tobacco smoking. Drinking habits and styles of drug use are often associated with a constellation of demographic and lifestyle factors, some of these, such as diet, exerting a powerful influence over health.

Table 8.6

Deaths* with underlying cause described as drug dependence or non-dependent abuse of drugs by type of drug and age, 1980 – 94

Type of drug and year		Age				
		Under 20	20–24	25–29	30–34	35 and over
Morphine type	1980	3	16	15	7	3
	1994	21	72	62	53	40
Cocaine	1980	–	–	–	–	–
	1994	–	–	2	2	2
Cannabis	1980	–	–	–	–	–
	1994	1	–	–	–	–
Hallucinogens	1980	–	–	–	–	–
	1994	–	–	–	–	–
Amphetamine type	1980	–	–	–	–	–
	1994	2	8	3	1	–
Barbiturate type	1980	1	5	1	3	2
	1994	5	14	7	3	6
Volatile substances	1980	4	–	–	–	–
	1994	21	7	8	–	3
Morphine with other	1980	4	2	1	1	–
	1994	1	1	7	3	5
Combinations	1980	–	–	2	–	–
excluding morphine	1994	–	1	–	1	2
Unspecified	1980	–	6	10	7	–
drug dependence	1994	3	8	15	11	11
Antidepressants	1980	–	–	–	–	–
	1994	1	–	–	1	–
Other, mixed, unspecified	1980	1	1	1	1	2
non-dependent abuse	1994	2	16	12	13	22
All drugs	1980	8	28	35	18	10
	1994	57	127	116	88	101

* *Excludes alcohol and tobacco.*
Source: Home Office (1992)

There are ongoing debates about which policies should be adopted to prevent or to curb alcohol- and drug-related problems. Many of the therapeutic responses to alcohol- and drug-related problems have not been evaluated. As this review has indicated, alcohol consumption, and its associated adverse effects (and apparent benefits), are far more commonplace than the use of illicit drugs. Even so the latter appears to be increasing rapidly, together with a rising toll of health problems. There appear to be no simple solutions to the morbidity and mortality reviewed in this chapter. It is probable that, whenever the recreational use of a psychoactive drug is popular, there will be associated dependence, accidents, illnesses and premature deaths.

Acknowledgements

This chapter was written with assistance from John Charlton of the ONS. Special thanks are due to Dr Moira Plant of the Alcohol Research Group (ARG) of the University of Edinburgh. Thanks are also due to Duncan Verall of the ARG, Dr Virginia Berridge of the London School of Hygiene & Tropical Medicine and the staff of the Research and Statistics Department of the Home Office and Mrs Janet Witheridge of the Brewers and Licensed Retailers Association. The ARG receives support from the Portman Group, the Alcohol Education and Research Council and a number of agencies such as charities and government departments.

Figure 8.7

Deaths from VSA by age, United Kingdom, persons

Number of deaths

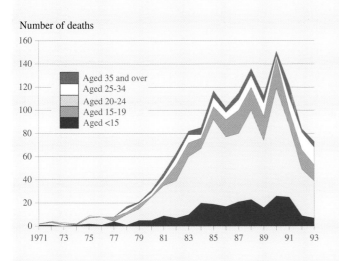

Figure 8.8

Average death rates from volatile solvents per million population by region, ages 10–24, 1984–93

Death rate per million

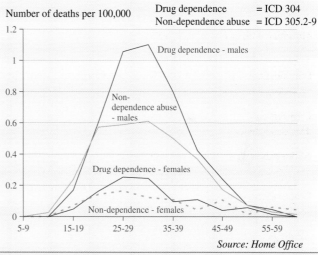

Source: Taylor et al. (1995)

Figure 8.9

Deaths of notified drug addicts, United Kingdom, 1985–92

Number of deaths

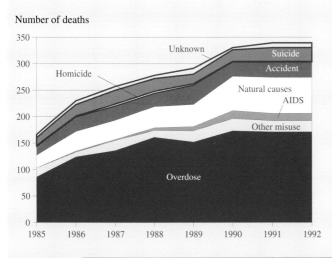

Figure 8.10

Drug dependence and abuse, average rates, England and Wales, 1988–92

Number of deaths per 100,000

Drug dependence = ICD 304
Non-dependence abuse = ICD 305.2-9

Source: Home Office

Figure 8.11

Deaths from causes linked to drugs*, rate per 100,000, England and Wales

Age-standardised rate

Males

Drug dependence = ICD 304 (excluding 304.6)
Non-dependent drug abuse = ICD 305.2-9

Females

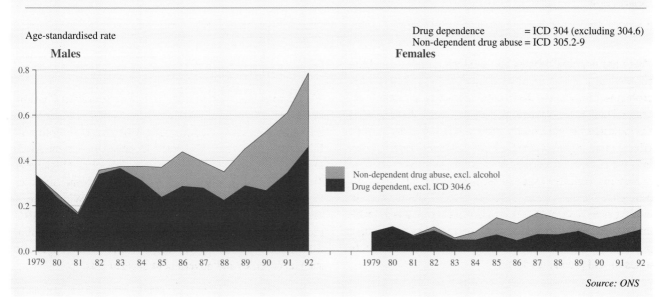

Source: ONS

Chapter **9**

Trends in mortality from smoking-related diseases

By
Richard Doll, Sarah Darby and Elise Whitley

Summary

- Tobacco use by men was well established by 1841. It increased up to the end of the Second World War, when it fell slightly before stabilising. After the 1960s it fell substantially. Between 1890 and 1950 cigarettes largely replaced other tobacco products. Use by women commenced in the mid-1920s and, with few exceptions, was limited to cigarettes. It increased rapidly in the Second World War and continued to increase until the 1970s when it began to fall.

- Tobacco is not the only cause of smoking-related diseases. Changes in the prevalence of other causative agents resulted in the trends in smoking-related diseases differing. Other factors that affect trends in mortality are changes in the efficacy of therapeutic and prophylactic treatment, medical terminology, disease classification and diagnostic efficiency.

- Smoking is much the most important cause of lung cancer. Trends in the sex- and age-specific mortality rates accord with trends in tobacco consumption, when allowance is made for the effect of duration of smoking and the type of cigarette smoked. The relative effects of changes in the prevalence of other factors (notably atmospheric pollution by the combustion of fossil fuels and the use of asbestos) are too small to be clearly detectable.

- The trends for lip cancer are confounded by those for the effect of outdoor work and efficacy of treatment; those for oropharyngeal, oesophageal and laryngeal cancer by trends in the consumption of alcohol; those for oropharyngeal and oesophageal cancer by changes in nutrition; those for laryngeal cancer by changes in the efficacy of treatment; and those for oropharyngeal and laryngeal cancer by other unknown factors.

- The trends for bladder cancer in men accord with those for lung cancer, apart from an early reduction in mortality due to a reduction in occupational hazards; those in women are mostly unexplained. The trends for pancreatic cancer are confounded with changes in diagnostic efficacy.

- The trends in chronic obstructive lung disease are confounded with changes in social conditions in the early decades of the century and a later reduction in pollution from the combustion of coal.

- Much of the increase in mortality attributed to aortic aneurysm is an artefact of classification, but in the elderly some of it reflects past increases in smoking.

- Trends in mortality from ischaemic heart disease require adjustment to reflect changes in medical diagnosis. The adjusted rates have been affected by changes in the prevalence of the many behavioural risk factors and by recent improvements in medical prophylaxis and treatment. The incidence of the disease is reduced quickly after smoking is stopped, and reduced smoking has contributed to the reduction in mortality at all ages in the last 20 years.

9.1 Introduction

Smoking tobacco introduces some 4,000 different chemicals into the body which, in one way or another, help to cause more than 20 diseases and to protect against the development of some others. All the diseases caused by smoking have other causes that, in some instances, are more important than tobacco and some have been found to respond to new forms of therapy introduced during the period studied. The trends in mortality from tobacco-related diseases may, therefore, have been influenced by many factors other than the trend in tobacco consumption, and it is unlikely that there will be any clear relationship between the trends unless smoking has a major influence on the incidence or fatality of the disease. With one exception we have, therefore, limited our examination to the trends in mortality from diseases that are strongly or moderately related to smoking. For this purpose we have defined diseases as strongly related to smoking if the mortality attributed to them has been regularly reported to be at least 10 times higher in heavy cigarette smokers than in life-long non-smokers, and as moderately related to smoking if the mortality in heavy cigarette smokers has usually been three to nine times higher. The exception is ischaemic heart disease which is moderately related to smoking (as defined above) only under 55 years of age, but which is related to smoking to some extent at all ages and is such a major cause of death that even a 50 per cent increase in the mortality rate attributed to it would result in tens of thousands of extra premature deaths.

The diseases examined are listed in Table 9.1, as are the numbers of deaths they were certified as causing, and the proportion of all deaths that they constituted in men and women in Britain (i.e. England, Wales and Scotland) in 1992. The codes of the International Classification of Diseases (ICD) (World Health Organisation, 1948, 1957, 1967, 1977) used to define them are given in Appendix I. The relationships of these diseases to smoking, as observed in the 40-year follow-up of British doctors with known smoking habits, reported by Doll *et al.* (1994), are shown in Table 9.2. For bladder cancer the mortality rates found in this study do not quite satisfy the criteria listed above, because the mortality rate in smokers of 25 or more cigarettes per day is slightly less than three times that in non-smokers. Higher increases have, however, been reported in many other studies (see IARC, 1986, for details).

Table 9.1.

Importance of diseases examined as the certified cause of death (Britain, 1992)

Cause of death	Males		Females	
	Number of deaths	% of all deaths	Number of deaths	% of all deaths
A. Strongly related to smoking – causal*				
Cancer of lung	25,429	8.5	12,541	3.9
Chronic obstructive lung disease	18,588	6.2	11,793	3.7
Subtotal	44,017	14.6	24,334	7.7
B. Strongly related to smoking – causal and confounding†				
Cancer of lip	29	0.01	16	0.01
Cancer of oral cavity and pharynx *(less salivary glands and nasopharynx)*	998	0.3	537	0.2
Cancer of oesophagus	3,668	1.2	2,427	0.8
Cancer of larynx	782	0.3	215	0.1
Subtotal	5,477	1.8	3,195	1.0
C. Moderately related to smoking – causal*				
Cancer of pancreas	3,218	1.1	3,419	1.1
Cancer of bladder	3,803	1.3	1,813	0.6
Aortic aneurysm	6,037	2.0	3,518	1.1
Peptic ulcer	2,135	0.7	2,674	0.8
Subtotal	15,193	5.1	11,424	3.6
D. Other diseases studied				
Ischaemic heart disease and related conditions§	89,939	29.9	78,754	24.8
Total	**154,626**	**51.4**	**117,707**	**37.0**

* Relationship reflects contribution of smoking to the causation of the disease.
† Relationship partly reflects contribution to the causation of the disease and partly confounding between smoking and some other causative factor.
§See text for explanation of diseases included.

Two diseases that have been found to be strongly related to smoking (peripheral vascular disease and pulmonary heart disease) and two found to be moderately related to smoking (pulmonary tuberculosis and cirrhosis of the liver) are omitted. The first two are seldom described as the underlying cause of death on death certificates and the mortality attributed to them bears little relation to their true incidence. The fatality of pulmonary tuberculosis is increased by smoking, but the fatality and incidence of this disease are so much more closely related to socioeconomic conditions and the availability of medical treatment that the relationship to smoking, though of clinical importance, is of little aetiological interest. The mortality from cirrhosis of the liver is mainly (if not wholly) related to smoking incidentally, through the confounding of smoking with the consumption of alcohol (Doll *et al.*, 1994).

None of the diseases that are made less lethal by smoking (including cancer of the endometrium, Parkinsonism, ulcerative colitis and toxaemia of pregnancy) is included in the review, as the mortality due to these diseases in heavy smokers is not less than a third of that in life-long non-smokers.

In Figure 9.1, age-standardised rates in 5-year calendar intervals for each of the 11 smoking-related diseases are displayed, separately for men and women, as multiples of the rate for the period 1951–55. It can be seen that, for many of the diseases, large changes have taken place, both upwards and downwards, in some cases by a factor of almost 10, and that the trends in men and women are often different.

In examining and interpreting these trends we have had to take account of changes in the classification of causes of death with the various revisions of the ICD and of changes in nosological 'fashion'. We have, therefore, also noted trends in a number of other causes of death with which the cause of interest might be confused; these are discussed in association with each of the diseases strongly or moderately related to smoking. In the case of diseases that may be confused with ischaemic heart disease, changes in nosological fashion seem likely to have been so important that we have added their mortality rates (or part of them) to ischaemic heart disease *per se*.

Table 9.2

Mortality rates from smoking-related diseases among British male doctors, 1951–1991 (after Doll *et al.*, 1994)

Annual mortality rate* per 100,000 men

| Cause of death | Number of deaths | Non-smokers (never smoked regularly) | Smokers smoking only cigarettes | | | | | | Other smokers | |
| | | | Ex-smokers | Current | Current daily smoking | | | | | |
					1-14	15-24	≥25		Ex	Current
A. Strongly related to smoking – causal										
Lung cancer	893	14	58	209	105	208	355		59	112
Chronic obstructive lung disease	542	10	57	127	86	112	225		40	51
B. Strongly related to smoking – causal and confounding										
Cancer of lip	0	-	-	-	-	-	-		-	-
Cancer of oral cavity and pharynx (*less salivary glands and nasopharynx*)	65	1	1	14	7	9	32		5	12
Cancer of oesophagus	172	4	19	30	17	33	45		14	23
Cancer of larynx	33	0	2	9	5	8	16		3	3
C. Moderately related to smoking – causal										
Cancer of pancreas	205	16	23	35	30	29	49		11	24
Cancer of bladder	182	13	21	30	29	29	37		13	21
Aortic aneurysm	331	15	33	62	38	74	81		22	43
Peptic ulcer	134	8	12	24	11	33	34		12	15
D. Other diseases examined†										
Ischaemic heart disease	6,438	572	678	892	802	892	1,025		676	653
Myocardial degeneration†	841	61	88	125	122	109	173		96	85
Arteriosclerosis†	232	22	18	40	31	38	72		28	23

* *Standardised for age and calendar period.*
† *See text for reasons included.*

Figure 9.1

Trends in age-standardised mortality rates from smoking-related diseases for males and females in Britain

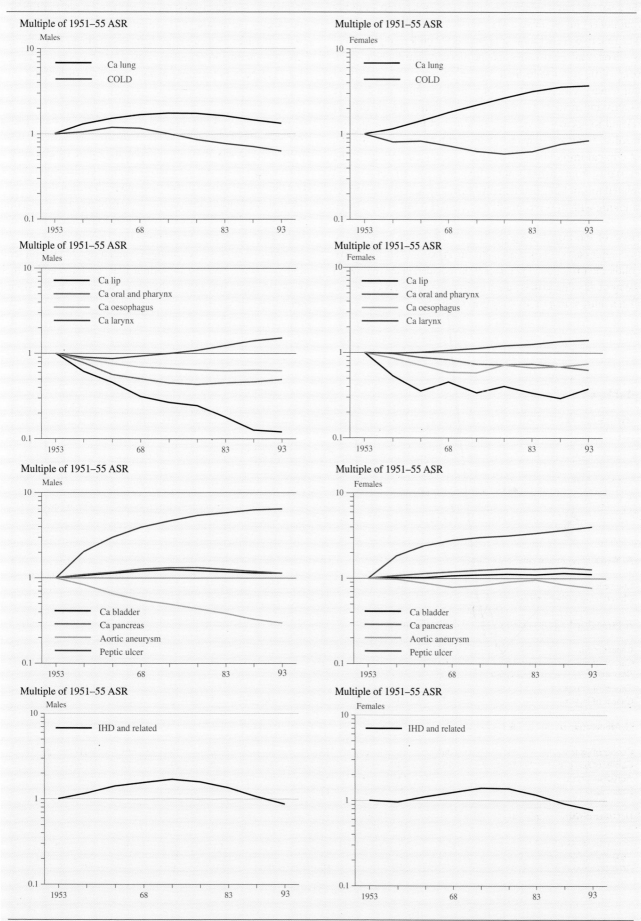

In each calendar period (1951–55, 1956–60, 1986–90, 1991–92) the age standardised rate ASR has been calculated directly standardised to the 1991–92 population of Britain, and divided by the corresponding rate for Britain in 1991–92

In subsequent sections we examine the evidence relating to the trends in mortality from each of the selected diseases under the following nine headings:

- Proportion attributable to tobacco
- Relationship to different products and tar content
- Causes other than smoking
- Changes in fatality
- Changes in ICD codes (where these have affected recorded mortality rates)
- Changes in diagnostic competence and fashion
- Trends in other diseases that may be confused with the disease of interest
- Trends in age-specific mortality
- Discussion

In discussing changes in fatality, survival rates for cancers in the early 1960s have been taken from Waterhouse (1974), whereas those for the early 1980s are taken from data published by the Cancer Research Campaign (1988).

Summary data for each disease are given in figures and tables accompanying the text. More detailed data, including numbers of deaths and mortality rates for individual calendar years and also separately for England and Wales and Scotland, are available from the ONS (previously OPCS).

With this analysis it is not possible to deduce the trends in the total mortality attributable to smoking. They have, however, been examined by Peto *et al.* (1994) who used a technique similar to that adopted by the Health Education Authority (1992) and concluded that the death rate per 100,000 attributable to smoking was as follows:

Men aged 35–69 years	651	in 1955
	732	in 1965
	622	in 1975
	379	in 1990

Men aged 70–79 years	1,310	in 1955
	2,160	in 1965
	2,640	in 1975
	1,890	in 1990

Women aged 35–69 years	55	in 1955
	96	in 1965
	135	in 1975
	153	in 1990

Women aged 70–79 years	93	in 1955
	191	in 1965
	363	in 1975
	635	in 1990

9.2 Trends in smoking

9.2.1 Smoking by men

Tobacco use was well established among men before the twentieth century, and it is estimated that in 1871 average annual consumption of all tobacco products per person (aged 15 years or more) was 2.6 kg (see Figure 9.2). Consumption rose continually, apart from a slight fall at the end of the First World War, until the early 1940s, when it stood at 5.3 kg per annum. Since the Second World War consumption has fallen, erratically at first, but steadily since the late 1960s, so that by 1987 it was estimated to be 2.4 kg per annum, slightly lower than in 1871.

The overall amount of tobacco consumed is not necessarily a good indicator of the resulting burden of disease, because different products cause different disease risks. During the nineteenth century most of the tobacco sold was smoked in pipes, although the figures also include some that was used for cigars, snuff and chewing. Cigarettes were smoked only

Figure 9.2

Trends in tobacco consumption in Britain

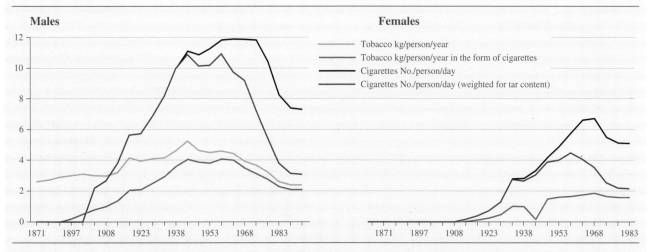

Plotted points are 5-year averages taken from data published by Wald and Nicolaides-Bouman (1991). Figures for all tobacco and cigarettes are based on a combination of sales and survey data and compiled by the Tobacco Advisory Council. Figures for cigarettes include both manufactured and hand-rolled cigarettes.

rarely, and at the beginning of the twentieth century the average per head consumption of tobacco in the form of cigarettes by men aged 15 years or over is estimated to have been 0.5 kg per annum, accounting for only one sixth of total tobacco consumption. During the first half of the twentieth century, however, this increased rapidly so that in the early 1940s it had risen to 4.1 kg, accounting for nearly 80 per cent of all the tobacco that men consumed. Ever since the 1940s cigarettes have accounted for between 83 per cent and 91 per cent of men's tobacco consumption.

Until the early 1960s the number of cigarettes smoked per day was a good reflection of the weight of cigarette tobacco smoked per person. However, during the 1960s, the increasing use of filters meant that there was a reduction in the amount of tobacco per cigarette. As a result there was a reduction in tobacco consumption by weight, despite the fact that the number of cigarettes smoked remained relatively stable (see Figure 9.2). In the late 1970s men were still smoking an average of 10.5 cigarettes per day, only just lower than the value of 10.9 for the late 1940s, but consumption in terms of weight of tobacco was almost 30 per cent lower. During the 1980s the number of cigarettes smoked per day by men fell progressively, to an average of 7.3 in 1987.

In considering the incidence of disease due to smoking, it is not sufficient just to measure cigarette consumption. Methods of manufacture may also have an effect. Since the mid-1960s, the tobacco industry has attempted to reduce toxicity by reducing the amount of tar delivered when a cigarette is smoked in a standard way. However, reducing the tar yield has to some extent reduced the nicotine yield, so that low-tar cigarettes tend to be inhaled more deeply or more often than high-tar cigarettes, at least by addicted smokers; this is done to extract the same amount of, or almost as much, nicotine from them because compensation does not seem to be quite complete (Parish *et al.*, 1995). The impact of a switch to low-tar cigarettes may, therefore, vary for different diseases, depending on the extent to which the depth of inhaling influences the risk of developing the disease, as well as the possible role of less variable components than tar yield and nicotine.

The earliest figures for the yield of tar per cigarette relate to the late 1930s, and indicate an average value of 33 mg per cigarette. Average tar yields tended to decrease slightly during the 1940s and 1950s. They then reduced considerably, to 26 mg per cigarette, in the early 1960s as a result of the switch from plain to filter cigarettes (see Figure 9.3). Since then (mostly as a result of voluntary agreements between industry and government), further changes in cigarettes have continued to decrease tar yields, so that, in 1990, the average tar yield per cigarette was 13 mg. If it is assumed that tar yields up to the late 1930s were roughly constant and, if subsequent cigarette consumption is weighted for tar yield relative to these early values, tar-weighted cigarette consumption by men was approximately constant at about 10.5 tar-weighted cigarettes per day during the 1940s and 1950s and has declined steadily since the early 1960s to 3.1 tar-weighted cigarettes per day in 1987, similar to consumption shortly before the First World War (see Figure 9.2).

Pipe smoking accounts for most of the tobacco consumed other than by cigarettes. At the end of the nineteenth century, men were consuming over 2 kg of pipe tobacco per head per year, but as cigarettes grew in popularity in the first half of the twentieth century, so pipe smoking declined (see Figure 9.2). By 1950, annual per head consumption was down to about 0.8 kg, and pipe smoking accounted for less than one fifth of total tobacco consumption. Its popularity has declined steadily since then, and by 1987 only about 5 per cent of men were pipe smokers.

9.2.2 Smoking by women

Consumption of tobacco by women has been almost exclusively in the form of manufactured cigarettes. As is shown in Figure 9.2, women did not start smoking on a large scale until the mid-1920s. Thereafter, consumption rose steadily, both in terms of weight of tobacco smoked and in terms of number of cigarettes per day, until the late 1970s, when women were consuming on average 1.9 kg of tobacco annually and smoking about 6.8 cigarettes per day. Since then tobacco consumption by women has fallen somewhat, to 1.6 kg per annum or 5.1 cigarettes per day in 1987. When tar weighting is taken into account, consumption by women started to fall about 5 years earlier, and the fall has been more substantial, so that in 1987 it averaged 2.2 tar-weighted cigarettes per woman per day, about half its peak of 4.5 tar-weighted cigarettes per day in the late 1960s.

Although cigarette consumption in women has always been lower than in men, their consumption as a proportion of that in men has been steadily increasing ever since they started to smoke. In the early 1930s consumption by women in terms

Figure 9.3

Sales-weighted tar yields of British cigarettes

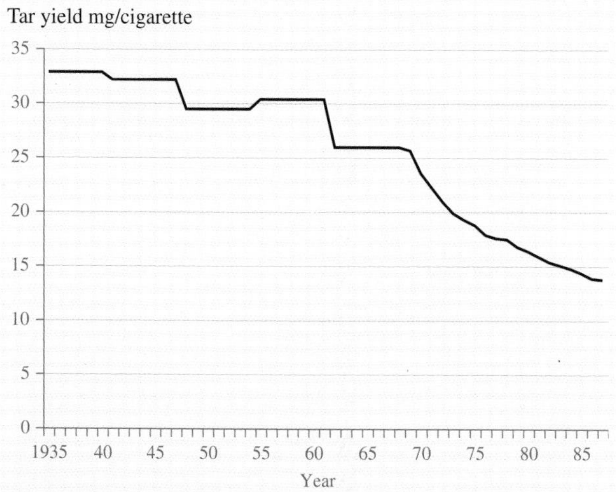

Tar yield mg/cigarette

Figures are taken from Wald & Nicolaides-Bouman (1991) and based on Wal et al. (1981) analyses by the laboratory of the Government Chemist and brand share data published in the journal Tobacco.

of tar-weighted cigarettes per person per day was only 9 per cent of that in men, whereas in the early 1950s it was 30 per cent. In the early 1970s it had risen to 56 per cent and in 1987 stood at around 70 per cent.

9.3 Trends in diseases strongly related to smoking

9.3.1 Lung cancer

The great majority of all lung cancers are caused by smoking in the sense that, in the absence of smoking, the incidence of the disease is consistently low. Comparison with rates in non-smokers indicates that, at the height of the epidemic in the United Kingdom, some 95 per cent of cases in men were attributable to tobacco, whereas in women the proportion is now about 85 per cent and still rising. These high percentages do not mean that only 5–15 per cent can be attributed to other causes, because smoking acts synergistically with at least some other agents, so that these agents may also be considered to cause some of the same cases that can be attributed to tobacco. This is the case with both asbestos and radon and, perhaps, also general atmospheric pollution.

The chief risk of lung cancer comes from smoking cigarettes rather than other tobacco products, as has been clearly demonstrated in case-control and cohort studies, where the relative risk of mortality is about five times greater among those who smoke only cigarettes than among smokers of pipes and cigars, even though risks in the second group are several times greater than those of life-long non-smokers (IARC, 1986). Condensates from low-tar cigarettes are no less mutagenic than condensates from the high-tar cigarettes that were manufactured in the past (Sorsa, 1986), but the amount delivered per cigarette is less and low-tar cigarettes are associated with a somewhat lower risk of lung cancer in humans, as was shown by the results of the two massive cohort studies carried out by the American Cancer Society in the early 1960s and early 1980s (Surgeon General, 1989). In these studies, in the later period, male cigarette smokers under 45 years of age, who had smoked low-tar cigarettes for most of their smoking lives, had a lower risk of lung cancer than their predecessors, whereas among the older men, those in the later period had a higher risk than their predecessors, because they had been smoking cigarettes consistently for longer.

Many other causes of lung cancer are known, including radon, asbestos, atmospheric pollution from carcinogenic polycyclic aromatic hydrocarbons produced in the combustion products of fossil fuels, some species of nickel and hexavalent chromium, bischloromethyl ether, arsenic and mustard gas. The last five have caused only localised excesses in specific industries, but the first three may have caused increased risks in large sections of the population.

Changes in exposure to residential radon over time are unlikely to have been great, and studies indicate that installation of double glazing, reduction in the prevalence of open fires, and changes in building techniques are unlikely to have caused more than about a 20 per cent increase in average population exposures in Britain (Gunby et al., 1993). Major changes, however, have occurred in exposure to asbestos and the combustion products of fossil fuels. From a few thousand tonnes at the beginning of the century, asbestos was used in progressively greater amounts to over 170,000 tonnes in the mid-1970s (Acheson and Gardner, 1979). In spite of the enormous reduction in its use since then and the stricter control of exposure within asbestos industries, the number of cases of lung cancer in which asbestos plays a part is unlikely to have decreased much as yet because the latent period between exposure and the appearance of the disease is typically of the order of 10–20 years. Exposure to air pollution in the form of combustion products of fossil fuels was, in contrast, heavy and declined only slowly in the first half of the century. It began to decline rapidly only with the introduction of the Clean Air Act in 1956 and the substitution for coal of gas, oil and electricity for heating and power in industry and in homes, as a result of which the benzo(a)pyrene concentrations in central London fell from 46 mg/1,000 m^3 in 1949–50 to 1.6 mg/1,000 m^3 in 1974–81 (Waller, 1991). Neither asbestos nor atmospheric pollution causes much increase in risk in non-smokers. However, in conjunction with smoking, atmospheric pollution may have caused some 10 per cent of lung cancers in men in the 1950s (Cederlöf et al., 1978), and asbestos may have contributed to up to 5 per cent in the 1970s (Doll and Peto, 1981).

The 5-year survival rate for lung cancer in the early 1960s was about 4 per cent. Some minor reduction in fatality has occurred with developments in thoracic surgery, but the proportion of surgically curable cases has been too small to have had any large effect on the trend in mortality, and in the early 1980s the 5-year survival rate was still only 7 per cent.

Changes in ICD codes affecting the classification of death due to thoracic cancers have had little influence on the recorded mortality rates, so long as the codes used for the sixth and seventh revisions include both those lung cancers specified as primary and those not specified as either primary or secondary (ICD 162 and ICD 163). Separation of pleural tumours by the eighth revision (operative from 1968) will have had only a minute effect because such cases represented less than 1 per cent of 'lung cancers' at the time.

Techniques for the diagnosis of lung cancer were well established by 1951. They were improved by the introduction of the flexible bronchoscope in the late 1950s, but probably not to the extent of materially affecting the detection rate. Surveys in the 1950s showed that the number of missed cases was approximately equal to the number of cases falsely diagnosed as lung cancer (Bonser and Thomas, 1959).

By 1951, the disease was recognised to be common and changes in diagnostic fashions are unlikely to have had any major effect. A few lung cancer cases however, may, have been misdiagnosed as 'mediastinal tumours' in the next decade and subsequently as pleural mesotheliomas, if there was any evidence of exposure to asbestos. The mortality rates attributed to both these diseases are, however, too low to have materially affected the trend in deaths caused by lung cancer.

The trends in mortality from lung cancer, separately for five 10-year age-groups from ages 30 to 79 years and for age-group 80–84, are shown for each sex in Figure 9.4 and in 5-year age-groups from ages 30 to 84 years in Table 9.3.

In men, the mortality reached a maximum in the early 1950s at ages 30–39 years and in the late 1950s at ages 40–59 years. At older ages it continued to increase for progressively longer periods, reaching a maximum about 5 years later with each 5-year increase in age, so that, in age-groups 60–64 and above the highest mortality rates in men were in the cohort born in and around 1901 and the 80–84 age-group reached a maximum only in the early 1980s. From the maximum the mortality rate has declined by about 70 per cent under 40 years of age, by about 60 per cent at ages 40–49 years, by about a half at ages 50–59 years and by progressively smaller proportions at older ages.

In women the trends provide an almost perfect example of a cohort effect, with the maximum at ages 35–39 years in 1961–65 and occurring 5 years later with each 5-year increase in age. Consequently, the maximum mortality has been in the cohort born in and around 1926. From the maximum, the mortality has declined by about a half at ages under 40 years and between a fifth and a quarter at ages 40–59 years, with no decline having as yet occurred over age 65 years.

The trends in lung cancer mortality can, for the most part, be explained adequately by the trends in the consumption of cigarettes and the variations in the type of cigarette smoked. In the case of men, these were discussed in Section 9.2.1 and illustrated in Figure 9.2.

There is strong evidence from the effect of stopping smoking that cigarette smoke acts as a promoting agent as well as an initiating agent, so that a quick response to a reduction in tar yields is to be expected and provides a partial explanation, in addition to the age-specific reduction in the prevalence of smoking, for the reduction in lung cancer rates for men at ages under 60 beginning after 1961–65. Whether the early reduction in men under 45 years, a large proportion of whom would have served in the Forces during the war, can be accounted for by the drop in cigarette consumption when the war ended, or whether it was contributed to by the reduction in atmospheric pollution, which had accelerated in the late 1950s, is unclear. The fall in atmospheric pollution, however, can have had only a relatively minor effect, because the mortality in older men continued to increase.

Presumably the beneficial effect of the reduction in low-tar yield also affected older men although possibly to a lesser extent than younger men. However, any resulting decrease in lung cancer risk in the early 1960s was obscured by the fact that the rates in older age-groups had not yet started to stabilise and were still increasing in each successive cohort as a result of increases in the number of cigarettes smoked. The cohort with maximum lung cancer rates was born around 1901, and the members would have been in their late teens at around the time of the First World War, when cigarette consumption was increasing very rapidly (see Figure 9.2). It therefore seems likely that this cohort was the first in whom the habit of cigarette smoking became firmly established in early adult life, and it is only in later cohorts that the beneficial effect of tar reduction can be seen.

For women the influence of the Second World War seems to have been similar to that of the First World War for men, because maximal lung cancer rates are observed in women born around 1926 who would have been in their late teens

Figure 9.4

Mortality rates per million in Britain from lung cancer by age, sex and calendar year

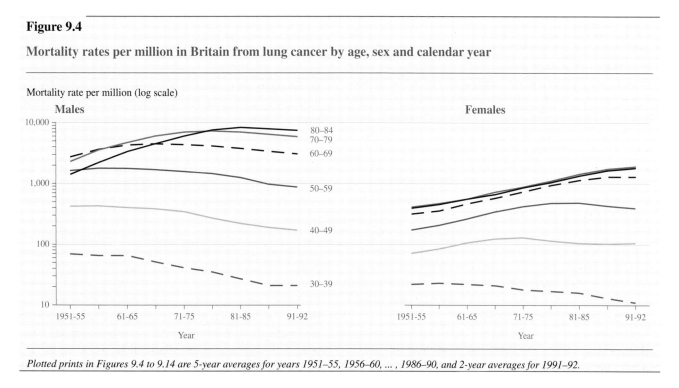

Mortality rate per million (log scale)

Plotted prints in Figures 9.4 to 9.14 are 5-year averages for years 1951–55, 1956–60, ... , 1986–90, and 2-year averages for 1991–92.

during the Second World War, when cigarette consumption was rising rapidly among women (see Figure 9.2). Thus, when lower-tar cigarettes began to be available in the early 1960s, their immediate beneficial effect was seen only in women born around 1931 and aged 30–34, because they were the only age-group in which the habit had already been firmly established since early adult life in a previous cohort. The beneficial effects of tar reduction continued to be apparent in women born around 1931 in succeeding quinquennia, even though it was not until the early 1970s that the tar-weighted average number of cigarettes smoked per woman started to decline (see Figure 9.2).

9.3.2 Chronic obstructive lung disease

The term 'chronic obstructive lung (or pulmonary) disease' was introduced only in the late 1950s. Until then the condition now commonly described in this way was variably described as chronic bronchitis or emphysema, and these terms are still used interchangeably by many doctors. The definition of chronic obstructive lung disease (COLD) is extended here to include all deaths attributed to chronic bronchitis and emphysema. Until 1968, the term 'chronic obstructive lung or (or pulmonary) disease' as a cause of death was categorised, on the rare occasions that it was used, with 'emphysema without mention of bronchitis' and a variety of uncommon or vaguely described respiratory diseases under 'Other diseases of lung and pleural cavity' (ICD6 and ICD7, code

527). In the eighth ICD revision it was still classed under 'Other disease of respiratory system' (ICD 519) whereas emphysema with or without mention of bronchitis was classified separately (ICD 492). Only with the ninth ICD revision was it given a category of its own (ICD 496). Throughout the whole period, chronic bronchitis was given a specific number, irrespective of whether emphysema was mentioned with it. These changes do not, however, result in any sharp discontinuities in the trends in mortality throughout the time period being considered, provided that all three specific conditions (COLD, emphysema and chronic bronchitis) are grouped together, as well as the residual group of other diseases of the respiratory system (see Appendix I for details of the codes used in this chapter).

COLD differs from lung cancer in its relationship to sex and age. The deaths attributed to this group of diseases have been much more concentrated in the oldest age-groups, especially among men in the 1950s. Although mortality rates in men in recent years have been about twice those in women for both lung cancer and COLD, the ratio of male to female age-standardised rates in the early 1950s was less than 3 for COLD whereas it was over 6 for lung cancer. It has been estimated that, in recent years, 80 per cent of deaths from COLD in men, and 70 per cent in women, are attributable to smoking (Health Education Authority, 1992). These estimates are very uncertain because there are very few data relating to the risk from smoking at old ages or in women. It is clear, however, that a very high proportion of deaths in men, other than in the

Table 9.3

Mortality rates per million in Britain from lung cancer by age, sex and calendar year

						Age					
Year	30–34	35–39	40–44	45–49	50–54	55–59	60–64	65–69	70–74	75–79	80–84
Males											
1951–55	37	102	251	591	1,244	2,024	2,564	2,909	2,568	2,026	1,413
1956–60	35	95	256	599	1,262	2,326	3,368	3,944	3,861	3,289	2,221
1961–65	34	95	229	575	1,241	2,319	3,716	4,882	4,974	4,494	3,367
1966–70	26	77	225	540	1,170	2,226	3,719	5,304	6,213	5,933	4,525
1971–75	23	59	180	510	1,081	2,090	3,554	5,195	6,825	7,243	6,058
1976–80	17	54	139	401	1,009	1,908	3,346	4,977	6,692	7,987	7,638
1981–85	13	42	120	322	780	1,731	3,021	4,574	6,336	7,753	8,395
1986–90	8	34	104	276	600	1,350	2,691	4,129	5,850	7,135	7,975
1991–92	9	33	91	250	612	1,135	2,241	3,936	5,312	6,542	7,518
Females											
1951–55	15	28	52	89	139	207	286	352	391	440	398
1956–60	15	31	63	105	171	243	331	387	454	496	459
1961–65	11	32	71	140	219	308	424	518	548	580	564
1966–70	11	31	82	164	286	401	512	653	729	740	671
1971–75	8	28	70	187	339	504	678	807	880	901	868
1976–80	7	27	65	164	374	583	869	1,033	1,112	1,134	1,060
1981–85	7	25	61	147	315	650	992	1,313	1,450	1,462	1,360
1986–90	6	21	63	141	276	583	1,131	1,496	1,757	1,769	1,663
1991–92	4	17	62	147	289	499	1,019	1,608	1,891	1,976	1,827

oldest age-groups, must be attributable to smoking because the ratio of the mortality rates in cigarette smokers to that in lifelong non-smokers in cohort studies has been similar to that for lung cancer (see Table 9.2; see also Surgeon General, 1989). Also, there is strong evidence that the observed association is causal (Fletcher and Peto, 1977). As with lung cancer, the risk from smoking is much greater from cigarettes than from pipe or cigars, although cigars also carry an appreciable risk (Doll and Peto, 1976). The evidence does not suggest that low-tar cigarettes cause lower mortality than high-tar ones, but they do reduce phlegm production and cough (Stellman, 1986). A randomised trial showed no reduction in the severity of cough (Withey *et al.*, 1992).

There are certainly other major causes which, in the main, act synergistically to produce the disease. Air pollution by coal smoke, as was widespread and intense before the implementation of the Clean Air Act of 1956, caused an increased prevalence of cough and dyspnoea, and may have contributed to the development of the disease, but its impact on mortality has been difficult to establish. Local air pollution may have contributed to the steep social class gradient, with mortality rates five times higher in Social Class V than in Social Class I. A more important factor in determining this gradient however, may have been social conditions in infancy and childhood, leading to repeated chest infections and greater susceptibility to the disease in adult life, as illustrated by the close correlation between the infant mortality rate in towns and the mortality rate from bronchitis 50 years later (Barker and Osmond, 1986). The practical elimination of serious infectious disease in childhood and improved treatment of respiratory infections, when they occur, may consequently also have contributed to a reduced prevalence of the disease in later life. A few cases of primary emphysema, a minor component of COLD, are the direct result of a genetic defect leading to a low level of anti-trypsin A, which allows cellular enzymes, secreted in response to infection, to destroy the alveolar membrane and cause progressive emphysema

(Eriksson, 1964, 1965). There is no effective therapy for emphysema once it has been produced.

Confusion has occurred in the past, and still does so to some extent, between the use of 'chronic bronchitis' and 'asthma' as terms to describe the cause of death in someone who has been subject to asthmatic attacks. The confusion erred in one direction before 1958, when any reference to asthma caused the death to be classed as asthmatic, irrespective of concomitant bronchitis, and may have swung in the opposite direction with the seventh revision of the ICD when 'asthma not indicated as allergic with mention of bronchitis' was switched to 'bronchitis'. The switch had a major effect on the number of asthma deaths, but only a small effect on the number attributed to bronchitis, which in old age was already 10 times greater. A greater effect in the oldest age-groups (ages 70 and above) was produced in and after 1984, with the OPCS ruling that deaths attributed to bronchopneumonia should not be classed as such if any other disease was mentioned anywhere on the death certificate. (This ruling was reversed in 1993.)

Among men aged under 55, mortality attributed to bronchitis has been declining steadily since the early 1950s, and the reductions, of five- and tenfold, have been considerably greater than those for lung cancer (see Figure 9.5 and Table 9.4). Among older men the rates were initially increasing slightly and have tended to peak at progressively later time periods for successive cohorts. To this extent they are similar to those for lung cancer; however, the peaks tend to occur earlier following smaller increases, and the subsequent decreases have been greater, so that at all ages except 80–84 years the rates in 1991–92 were lower than they had been in 1951–95.

In women aged over 65, rates fell steadily from the early 1950s to the late 1970s, decreasing by roughly a half. Since then they have increased, but in those aged above 75 they are still below the values in the early 1950s. In younger women rates

---

Figure 9.5

Mortality rates per million in Britain from chronic obstructive lung disease by age, sex and calendar year

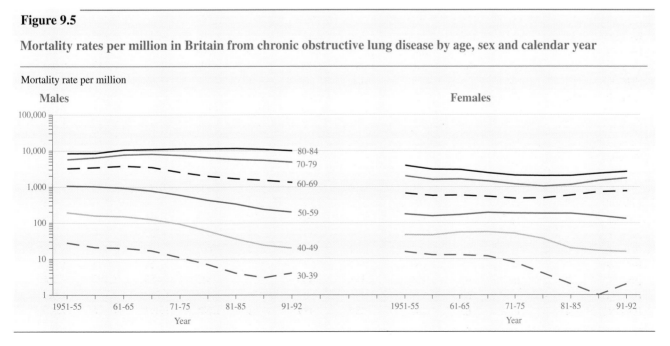

have been decreasing in recent years, with the reductions starting earlier and being progressively more pronounced in younger age-groups. The reductions are greater than those seen in lung cancer, and started earlier in some age-groups.

These complex changes reflect the fact that deaths attributed to the combined category of chronic obstructive lung disease, chronic bronchitis and emphysema are the result of three distinct respiratory diseases, which cannot be separated in certified causes of death because the terms are so often used interchangeably. Primary emphysema is very rare and caused by a genetic abnormality. The other two diseases may be contributed to by smoking, atmospheric pollution and poor social conditions in childhood; however, chronic obstructive lung disease results primarily from smoking whereas chronic bronchitis, which is particularly liable to cause death in old people, may result primarily from pollution and social conditions. The improved social conditions in towns since the first three decades of this century and the reduction in pollution with the combustion products of coal since the mid-1950s certainly account for some of the reduction in mortality in young ages, and all the reduction at old ages in women before the 1970s. The increased consumption of cigarettes by men in cohorts born up to the beginning of the twentieth century accounts for the increased mortality that occurred in men at older ages up to the 1980s. Increased consumption by women at later periods accounts for the recent increase in mortality in women aged over 65. It seems probable that reduction in smoking has contributed to the reduction in mortality of men and younger women in more recent periods and there is no reason to postulate any extra benefit from the introduction of low-tar cigarettes.

9.3.3 Cancer of the lip

Cancer of the lip has long been associated with smoking, but there are few quantitative data for the contribution of smoking. In combination with other factors, smoking is likely to have contributed to the great majority of all cases (see below) but it is not possible to make any precise estimate. No data are available relating to any differential effect of different types of cigarettes or tobacco. Pipe smoking was noted to be associated with lip cancer 200 years ago (Sömmering, 1795), shortly after Pott noted the association of scrotal cancer with employment as a chimney sweep. Case-control studies show that pipes cause a greater risk than cigarettes (Surgeon General, 1979). No data are available for low-tar tobacco. The disease is one of the few types of cancer that is always found to be more common in rural areas than in urban, and in outdoor workers than in those who work under cover. It has been particularly common in sailors, fishermen and agricultural workers (IARC, 1990). Tobacco and ultraviolet light in conjunction cause a high risk, but not separately.

Lip cancer responds well to both surgery and radiotherapy. Progressive improvements in radiotherapy over the last 50 years have reduced the fatality in recent years to less than 10 per cent. The distinction between cancer of the lip proper and

Table 9.4

Mortality rates per million in Britain from chronic obstructive lung disease by age, sex and calendar year

						Age						
Year	30–34	35–39	40–44	45–49	50–54	55–59	60–64	65–69	70–74	75–79	80–84
Males											
1951–55	15	41	102	284	709	1,425	2,502	3,735	4,836	6,293	8,185
1956–60	12	31	90	225	618	1,434	2,660	4,022	5,557	6,927	8,272
1961–65	12	27	77	222	548	1,310	2,798	4,538	6,425	8,595	10,249
1966–70	9	25	65	184	485	1,071	2,378	4,370	6,683	8,987	10,603
1971–75	5	17	47	140	352	823	1,700	3,224	5,793	8,698	10,993
1976–80	4	10	28	91	257	591	1,335	2,497	4,630	7,857	11,078
1981–85	3	6	17	55	164	505	1,090	2,184	4,015	7,140	11,253
1986–90	2	5	13	35	114	358	970	1,983	3,882	6,653	10,604
1991–92	2	6	10	30	109	290	781	1,808	3,291	6,062	9,713
Females											
1951–55	11	21	30	64	116	235	450	830	1,402	2,485	3,819
1956–60	8	17	34	57	104	208	409	698	1,194	1,927	2,973
1961–65	8	19	38	73	125	212	413	722	1,230	1,963	2,931
1966–70	7	16	37	75	147	238	369	671	1,109	1,691	2,367
1971–75	5	11	26	76	135	236	373	549	891	1,420	2,031
1976–80	2	6	17	57	135	229	391	556	797	1,228	1,976
1981–85	2	3	11	30	107	257	443	681	934	1,301	1,994
1986–90	1	2	8	25	81	233	534	864	1,234	1,676	2,300
1991–92	1	3	9	24	66	196	493	986	1,410	1,985	2,582

cancer of the skin, on the one side and cancer of the mouth on the other side, is not always clinically clear, and this may have affected the classification. However the proportions of cancers of facial skin and mouth arising in areas close enough to the lip for confusion are too small for their trends to have had any influence on the trend in mortality from lip cancer.

This mortality has been very low and more or less constant in men under 50 years of age and has fallen rapidly at all ages over 60 years, being approximately halved every 10 years since 1951–55 (see Figure 9.6 and Table 9.5). In women there has been some suggestion of a small increase at ages 50–59 from a very low rate since 1950, and a reduction by a half or more at older ages.

Figure 9.6

Mortality rates per million in Britain from lip cancer by age, sex and calendar year

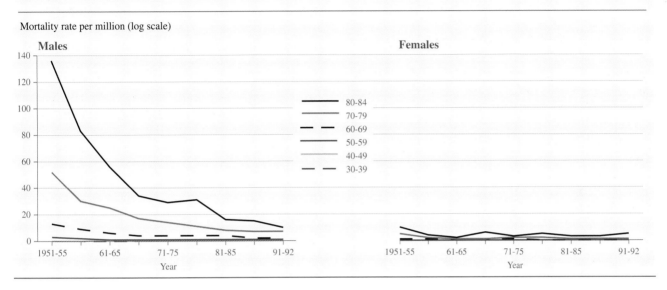

Table 9.5

Mortality rates per million in Britain from lip cancer by age, sex and calendar year

Year	30–34	35–39	40–44	45–49	50–54	55–59	60–64	65–69	70–74	75–79	80–84
Males											
1951–55	0.0	0.2	0.1	0.5	1.3	4.7	8.2	17.6	37.3	67.0	135.9
1956–60	0.1	0.0	0.5	0.4	1.2	2.2	6.3	11.3	20.3	40.3	83.1
1961–65	0.0	0.1	0.2	0.9	0.5	1.6	4.9	7.3	13.4	37.1	55.9
1966–70	0.0	0.0	0.1	0.3	1.0	2.0	3.8	4.9	9.9	23.9	34.0
1971–75	0.0	0.1	0.0	0.7	0.8	1.6	2.7	4.3	7.9	20.9	28.7
1976–80	0.0	0.1	0.4	0.3	0.8	1.3	2.8	4.8	5.7	16.5	31.3
1981–85	0.0	0.0	0.4	0.0	0.4	1.1	2.5	4.5	7.7	9.3	15.9
1986–90	0.0	0.0	0.1	0.0	0.7	0.4	0.6	2.5	4.6	9.2	15.1
1991–92	0.0	0.0	0.3	0.3	1.0	0.4	1.1	2.0	6.1	7.1	9.5
Females											
1951–55	0.0	0.0	0.0	0.1	0.2	0.1	0.7	1.2	4.0	5.3	9.5
1956–60	0.0	0.0	0.0	0.1	0.0	0.4	0.4	1.1	1.2	3.3	4.5
1961–65	0.0	0.1	0.0	0.0	0.1	0.5	0.8	0.5	0.8	2.1	2.2
1966–70	0.0	0.0	0.0	0.0	0.1	0.1	0.5	0.8	0.7	1.5	6.5
1971–75	0.0	0.0	0.0	0.0	0.0	0.1	0.4	0.8	1.3	1.8	2.5
1976–80	0.0	0.0	0.0	0.3	0.1	0.2	0.0	0.3	1.7	1.6	4.6
1981–85	0.0	0.0	0.0	0.0	0.1	0.3	0.2	0.4	1.0	1.7	3.4
1986–90	0.0	0.0	0.0	0.0	0.3	0.4	0.3	0.1	1.5	0.5	3.1
1991–92	0.0	0.0	0.3	0.0	0.3	0.0	0.0	0.3	1.9	0.5	4.8

The trends bear little relation to the trends in cigarette consumption but correspond qualitatively with the trend in pipe smoking. The reduction in mortality has also been contributed to by improved treatment, and this may account for most of the trend in older women. For older men, another major factor is the great reduction in the number of men regularly employed out of doors, such as sailors, fishermen and agricultural workers.

9.3.4 Cancers of oral cavity and pharynx

Cancer of the salivary glands has not been related to smoking, and cancer of the nasopharynx is only weakly related to smoking, so the mortality rates from these two types of cancer have been subtracted from the total for this group. In principle, the remaining cancers of the oral cavity should not be regarded as an entity, because their causes differ depending on the precise site within the mouth in which they occur. They all, however, have major causes in common and it is impracticable to distinguish between most of the sites in national mortality data collected over a long period. They are considered here in conjunction with cancer of the pharynx (other than the nasopharynx), with which they share major causes, because the number of deaths attributed to each category is small. Where important differences between the causes in the two sites occur, attention is drawn to them.

Smoking is an important cause of both oral and pharyngeal cancer. However, because it acts synergistically with other factors in a complex way, the proportion of cases attributable to smoking varies with the prevalence of the other agents. An approximate figure for the late 1980s is 70 per cent (Health Education Authority, 1992). Pipe and cigar smoking cause as great a risk as cigarette smoking (Surgeon General, 1979). Whether low-tar cigarettes cause less risk than the older high-

tar cigarettes is unknown, but they might be expected to do so, because the risk is unlikely to depend on the depth of inhalation. Oral snuff, which has been associated with oral cancer in the USA, has been prohibited in the United Kingdom and chewing tobacco has not been used to any significant extent since the early part of this century. Two causes have been described, other than tobacco use: the consumption of alcoholic beverages and poor nutrition. Alcohol and smoking act synergistically to multiply each other's effect (Doll *et al.*, 1993). Poor nutrition, with a diet lacking in fruit and green vegetables, seems to increase the effects of both tobacco and alcohol (Doll *et al.*, 1993).

Cancers of the oral cavity and pharynx are principally treated by radiotherapy with fair success, the fatality rate being between 40 per cent and 50 per cent. Some small reduction in fatality has occurred as a result of improved techniques. The cancers are easy to diagnose. The only likely source of confusion is with cancers arising in neighbouring sites (nasopharynx, extrinsic larynx and upper end of the oesophagus). Cancers of the nasopharynx and upper end of the oesophagus are uncommon and trends in the mortality from these diseases should not have had any material effect on the trend in mortality from cancer of the pharynx. Trends in the mortality from laryngeal cancer may have had some minor influence on it.

The trends in mortality differ markedly from those for cancer of the lung and to some extent from those for cancer of the oesophagus (see Figure 9.7 and Table 9.6). In men under 55 years of age the trends resemble those for cancer of the oesophagus, showing a substantial increase, particularly in the last 20 years, when those for lung cancer decreased; they differ, however, from those for oesophageal cancer in that the rates in men over 60 remained low after 1965 or continued

Figure 9.7

Mortality rates per million in Britain from cancer of oral cavity and pharynx (excluding salivary glands and naso pharynx) by age, sex and calendar year

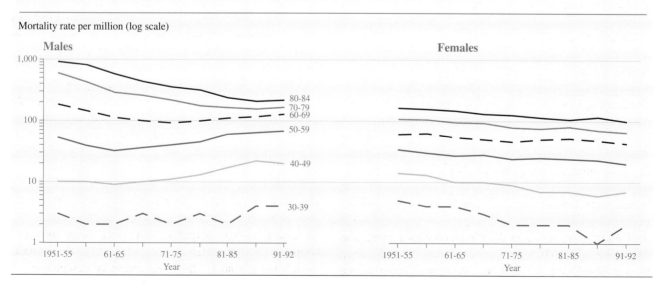

Table 9.6

Mortality rates per million in Britain from cancer of oral cavity and pharynx (excluding salivary gland and nasopharynx) by age, sex and calendar year

Year	30–34	35–39	40–44	45–49	50–54	55–59	60–64	65–69	70–74	75–79	80–84
Males											
1951–55	1.9	4.2	6.8	12.3	29.5	76.0	126.6	231.3	430.5	734.3	897.1
1956–60	1.8	3.1	5.5	13.6	25.1	52.0	98.8	183.4	317.5	516.5	797.1
1961–65	0.7	3.7	7.2	11.0	23.9	40.2	82.4	138.0	218.2	344.0	564.1
1966–70	1.5	4.2	6.2	13.4	27.5	45.4	70.8	123.1	205.5	297.6	423.8
1971–75	0.7	3.3	6.8	15.4	29.7	50.7	68.1	111.7	164.3	258.7	346.7
1976–80	2.3	4.5	8.2	17.9	30.1	59.5	86.2	106.8	144.8	197.8	309.2
1981–85	1.4	3.4	10.5	23.2	46.1	74.0	100.2	115.1	152.1	167.0	231.8
1986–90	2.0	5.4	12.7	31.6	48.2	79.2	102.0	125.6	140.5	162.9	202.6
1991–92	2.6	5.9	13.6	27.2	56.5	78.7	104.5	146.1	159.9	164.3	212.2
Females											
1951–55	3.3	6.1	9.1	18.8	28.0	39.3	50.7	67.2	91.7	117.5	159.2
1956–60	2.3	4.9	9.2	17.4	23.6	35.6	54.9	66.5	84.6	121.4	152.8
1961–65	3.2	4.9	6.4	13.9	20.8	33.1	47.3	59.6	82.3	103.2	144.4
1966–70	1.4	4.1	6.7	13.2	23.7	32.0	38.1	60.3	74.2	107.4	128.0
1971–75	1.6	1.9	6.0	11.6	20.7	27.1	38.4	51.3	64.0	90.5	122.8
1976–80	1.1	2.3	5.4	8.4	20.5	30.4	42.5	55.1	62.7	86.2	111.8
1981–85	1.4	2.3	4.2	9.7	17.8	30.3	43.8	58.4	71.0	88.0	104.2
1986–90	0.8	1.6	4.6	8.0	15.9	29.6	39.8	54.6	67.2	71.2	113.7
1991–92	1.0	3.8	4.6	9.5	14.6	25.4	38.5	46.1	56.2	72.0	97.4

to decrease, so that from 75 years of age and above they became only about a quarter of what they had been in 1951–55. In women the rates have fallen at all ages and, at most ages, progressively throughout the period 1951–52: by more than 70 per cent under 35 years of age, by about half at ages 35–54 years and by a third at older ages.

In young women there is a notable difference in the trends for cancer of the oral cavity and cancer of the pharynx. The mortality from the former fell less and increased slowly after 1965 to the original level or above at ages 35–54 years, whereas the mortality from the latter fell more and continued to fall into the 1990s.

Neither tobacco nor alcohol, nor the two in combination, seems capable of accounting for all the trends in these cancers. The doubling in alcohol consumption between 1950 and 1980 (Brewers and Licensed Retailers' Association, 1994) could have accounted for the recent increase in mortality in young men, but some further major factor is required to account for the continued decrease in mortality in elderly people. Improvements in nutrition may have played a large part in bringing about the decrease in old age, particularly perhaps in women in whom cancer of the hypopharynx was related to poor nutrition resulting in the Plummer-Vinson syndrome (Wynder *et al.*, 1957); other factors however, may, also have been involved. One may have been the virtual disappearance

of tertiary syphilis which caused leukoplakia of the tongue and was thought to be a precursor of cancer (Wynder *et al.*, 1957).

9.3.5 Oesophageal cancer

Smoking is an important cause of oesophageal cancer, but as with oral and pharyngeal cancers. its contribution is affected by the prevalence of other factors with which it interacts. An approximate figure is about 70 per cent (Health Education Authority, 1992). Pipe and cigar smoking cause as great a risk as cigarette smoking (IARC, 1986). Although low-tar tobacco might be expected to reduce the risk, there is no direct evidence either way. Alcohol and poor nutrition are also causes of the disease, with alcohol and smoking acting synergistically. Alcohol may, however, be quantitatively the more important (Breslow & Day, 1980). Poor nutrition, with a diet lacking in fruit, green vegetables and meat, seems to increase the effect of both tobacco and alcohol (Doll *et al.*, 1993).

The disease is nearly always fatal and there has been no material improvement in its treatment. The 5-year survival rate in the early 1980s was still less than 10 per cent. The disease is easy to diagnose. The only likely source of confusion is with cancers of the cardiac end of the stomach, which may extend into the lower end of the oesophagus.

There is some evidence to suggest that cancers of the gastric cardia have been increasing recently, in spite of a reduction in the incidence of cancer of the stomach as a whole. The confusion between adenocarcinomas of the lower end of the oesophagus and adenocarcinomas of the cardia of the stomach could possibly have accounted for a small increase in the mortality attributed to the former. Any such contribution however, could, only have been small.

The changes in mortality, though substantial, have been much smaller than those for lung cancer, and differ from them in many ways (see Figure 9.8 and Table 9.7). In men, the mortality decreased in most age-groups between 1951–55 and

1961–65 and continued to decrease for a further 10 years in old age. Since the early 1960s (or early 1970s for men over 75) there has been a progressive increase in mortality, leading to a doubling of the rate at ages 40–69 years, with no suggestion of a subsequent decrease except under 40 years of age in the most recent period (1991–92). In women the rate was fairly stable until the late 1960s, since when it has decreased under 45 years of age, remained fairly stable at 45–54 years and increased at older ages.

Whether these changes can be accounted for entirely by the differential rates of change in the consumption of tobacco and alcohol is uncertain. The reduction in mortality in men

Figure 9.8

Mortality rates per million in Britain from oesophageal cancer by age, sex and calendar year

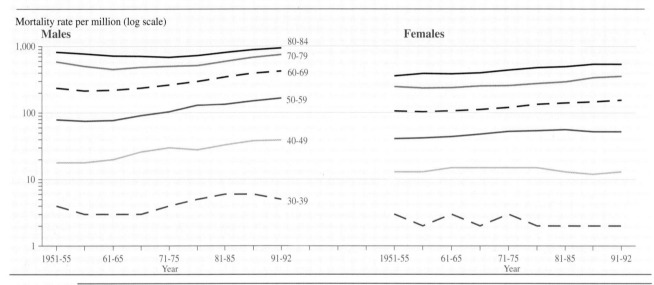

Table 9.7

Mortality rate per million in Britain from oesophageal cancer by age, sex and calendar year

Year	30–34	35–39	40–44	45–49	50–54	55–59	60–64	65–69	70–74	75–79	80–84
Males											
1951–55	2.0	5.9	11.4	23.7	55.6	102.0	182.0	292.1	464.8	714.0	818.6
1956–60	1.6	5.2	11.1	25.8	49.7	100.8	165.0	267.5	416.2	590.6	775.2
1961–65	1.8	5.1	11.0	29.1	57.7	96.7	179.5	264.0	377.4	531.5	721.9
1966–70	1.5	4.9	16.5	34.8	66.9	115.8	184.8	289.2	395.2	576.8	713.2
1971–75	2.5	6.0	17.8	41.3	73.3	135.3	215.4	310.6	437.4	565.6	683.5
1976–80	2.5	7.2	17.7	39.1	100.5	158.6	246.8	346.6	433.3	600.9	725.6
1981–85	3.6	7.9	19.1	46.2	92.4	180.6	281.1	412.3	500.2	681.3	812.8
1986–90	3.1	9.8	21.4	53.8	106.4	197.1	325.9	469.6	627.6	742.2	894.1
1991–92	1.9	7.5	23.7	54.3	124.4	209.1	325.2	529.0	682.9	817.2	950.1
Females											
1951–55	1.6	5.2	9.5	17.3	33.6	49.3	88.5	126.3	208.4	288.9	360.8
1956–60	1.7	3.2	8.4	17.6	32.9	50.7	81.0	126.9	186.7	287.5	389.0
1961–65	2.2	4.1	9.8	20.4	35.5	52.9	86.9	128.6	193.1	284.6	385.6
1966–70	1.5	2.9	9.1	21.1	37.4	58.8	93.1	132.9	202.7	309.3	400.0
1971–75	1.1	4.3	10.4	19.8	37.4	68.4	99.6	142.5	219.3	295.9	441.6
1976–80	1.4	3.4	8.4	21.1	46.0	62.0	111.0	161.7	224.2	331.1	477.2
1981–85	0.8	3.0	7.6	18.0	37.4	73.7	112.9	172.0	243.5	342.0	494.2
1986–90	0.8	3.5	6.3	18.3	37.4	67.5	120.1	173.5	269.2	406.1	542.0
1991–92	1.0	3.2	5.3	19.9	37.3	67.2	122.8	188.7	288.4	420.2	541.2

in the early years can be related to a reduction in the consumption of alcohol from the end of the last century to the 1950s (Brewers and Licensed Retailers Association, 1994), whereas the subsequent doubling in consumption since 1950 may have cancelled out the reduction caused by the reduced prevalence of smoking. Changes in alcohol consumption are likely to have had less impact on the trends in women, and a third factor, which could be improved nutrition, may have contributed to the stability of the rate in older women up to 1965 when the lung cancer rates were rising. Since then, the decreasing rates in young women and increasing rates in older women correspond qualitatively with those for lung cancer.

9.3.6   Laryngeal cancer

Smoking and alcohol are both important causes of laryngeal cancer. It is difficult to make a precise estimate of the contribution of smoking because it acts synergistically with alcohol in a complex way and the proportion varies depending on the extent to which alcoholic beverages are consumed. An approximate estimate for the 1980s is about 70 per cent (Health Education Authority, 1992). Cancer of the glottis, the principal type of laryngeal cancer, is particularly related to cigarette smoking, whereas cancer of the extrinsic larynx, above the glottis and adjoining the pharynx, is equally closely related to tobacco smoking in all forms (Wynder et al., 1956). In principle, low-tar cigarettes should carry less risk of glottic cancer in two ways: by reducing the amount of carcinogens in the smoke and by decreasing the amount of smoke deposited on it. The latter is presumed to occur because the smoke from low-tar cigarettes is relatively low in nicotine and is, in consequence, inhaled more deeply (to provide the same dose of nicotine) and proportionally more of it is absorbed in the alveoli. The quantitative relationship between the relative effects of alcohol and tobacco varies with the site of the cancer within the larynx, with alcohol making a relatively small contribution to cancer of the glottis (Doll et al., 1993).

Laryngeal cancer is effectively treated by both surgery and radiotherapy and improvements in their use have reduced the fatality from about 55 per cent in the 1950s, to about 40 per cent in the 1980s. The disease is easy to diagnose and cannot be confused with any other when it occurs in the glottis. There may, however, be occasions when it is not easy to distinguish between cancers arising in the extrinsic larynx or the pharynx. Trends in the mortality of pharyngeal cancer (which in 1951–55 was somewhat less common than laryngeal cancer in men and slightly more common in women) may have had some minor influence on the trend in the mortality from laryngeal cancer. The mortality from laryngeal cancer has declined progressively since 1951–55 in both sexes and at almost all ages, with only minor variations (see Figure 9.9 and Table 9.8). The decline has been most marked in women under 55 years, in men under 40 years and (less notably) in men over 70 years. The principal variation has been a tendency for the mortality to rise slightly in women over 65 years of age since the late 1960s and early 1970s after falling to about 60 per cent of the rate in 1951–55.

The trends in men contrast sharply with those of the two other cancers that are related to both alcohol and smoking (oral cavity and pharynx, and oesophagus) and also with the trends for cancer of the lung, which is associated only with smoking, in that they show no overall increase at any age. To some extent this can be accounted for by improved treatment and to a relatively small contribution from alcohol to the development of cancer of the glottis, the principal type of the disease. Some additional, but unknown, factor seems to be required to account for the progressive fall in mortality in older men, to about 60 per cent of the 1951–55 level, when lung cancer became two to five times more common in this age-group over the same period. The trends in women are not very different from those for cancers of the oral cavity and pharynx, except that the reduction in young women is more extreme and the mortality in older women showed some slight increase in the last two decades. The reduction for younger women could result from greater improvement in

Figure 9.9

Mortality rates per million in Britain from laryngeal cancer by age, sex and calendar year

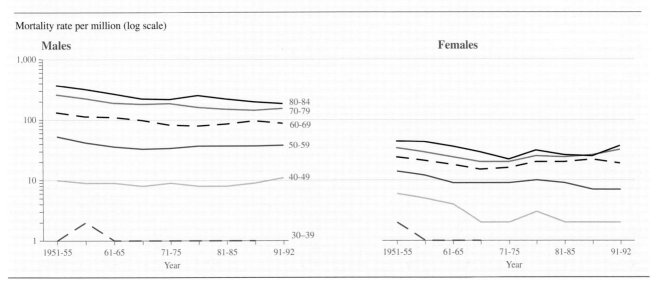

Mortality rate per million (log scale)

Table 9.8

Mortality rate per million in Britain from laryngeal cancer by age, sex and calendar year

Year	Age 30–34	35–39	40–44	45–49	50–54	55–59	60–64	65–69	70–74	75–79	80–84
Males											
1951–55	0.7	1.8	5.7	13.9	33.6	71.4	104.4	158.7	227.7	292.4	370.5
1956–60	1.2	2.9	5.3	13.0	27.0	57.9	95.2	131.3	196.4	254.1	319.6
1961–65	0.2	1.6	4.8	12.6	23.3	48.5	84.8	135.2	171.9	206.8	267.8
1966–70	0.6	1.6	3.8	11.8	23.9	41.4	67.0	129.0	160.8	200.4	222.3
1971–75	0.6	1.3	5.7	11.8	24.3	42.7	67.4	96.6	170.1	202.2	217.2
1976–80	0.5	2.2	4.5	11.1	24.7	49.9	62.5	96.4	136.5	183.8	252.0
1981–85	0.2	1.9	6.1	10.2	25.5	49.1	73.5	95.6	136.7	161.1	220.3
1986–90	0.2	0.8	4.2	13.5	26.1	48.0	79.6	112.1	134.9	151.4	196.9
1991–92	0.2	0.5	4.3	17.4	28.4	46.8	69.4	104.4	135.0	171.4	183.6
Females											
1951–55	0.6	2.9	3.6	8.5	11.1	16.0	19.9	28.3	32.8	35.6	43.5
1956–60	0.6	1.6	3.5	5.5	9.8	14.0	17.3	24.0	25.3	32.4	43.2
1961–65	0.2	1.3	2.4	5.4	8.3	9.9	16.7	19.2	19.1	29.0	36.2
1966–70	0.4	1.0	1.3	2.9	6.2	11.4	14.2	15.2	20.6	19.8	28.7
1971–75	0.2	0.5	1.6	3.4	7.6	9.9	14.0	17.2	20.6	20.3	21.8
1976–80	0.2	0.6	1.4	3.6	7.6	12.4	19.5	19.9	22.5	28.4	31.5
1981–85	0.1	0.0	1.4	2.5	4.3	14.0	19.4	20.0	24.6	23.8	25.6
1986–90	0.2	0.0	1.3	2.4	4.3	10.2	19.4	25.0	24.5	27.7	25.2
1991–92	0.0	0.3	1.5	3.1	5.0	9.8	11.7	25.6	30.2	32.8	37.3

treatment and perhaps a better separation of cancers of the extrinsic larynx and pharynx (some pharyngeal cancers being classed as extrinsic larynx in the 1950s), whereas the trends for older women could reflect a relatively greater dependence on cigarette smoking than on other factors such as nutrition.

9.4 Trends in diseases moderately related to smoking

9.4.1 Pancreatic cancer

It has been estimated that about a quarter of pancreatic cancer deaths in men and a third of deaths in women have been attributable to smoking in recent years (Health Education Authority, 1992). The evidence that pipe or cigar smoking increases the risk of pancreatic cancer is weak and inconsistent (IARC, 1986). There is no evidence from case-control or cohort studies to suggest that changes in tar yield affect the risk. Pancreatic cancer is unusually common in diabetics and in people heavily exposed to ionising radiation. These factors, however, account for only a small number of cases, and smoking is the only established major cause.

The disease is almost invariably fatal and there has been no material improvement in its treatment. The 5-year survival rate in the early 1980s remained less than 5 per cent. The disease is difficult to diagnose and many cases are likely to

have been missed in the past. Improvement in medical services may have caused some increase in the detection rate.

There has been a progressive increase in the mortality attributed to cancers of unspecified sites, some of which are likely to have been pancreatic cancers, and this may have counteracted the increase attributable to improved possibilities of detection.

Mortality rates from cancer of the pancreas have been much more stable over the period considered than many of the other smoking-related diseases and only in the younger age-groups, where the numbers of deaths are small, have changes of over 50 per cent occurred (see Figure 9.10 and Table 9.9). Nevertheless, there have been some changes. In men aged under 50 mortality rates increased until the late 1960s or 1970s and subsequently decreased, so that in recent years they have been somewhat lower than they were in the early 1950s. In older men the rates also increased initially and the increases tended to continue somewhat longer than in younger men. Although there have been decreases in recent years in all age-groups, male rates in those aged over 50 remain higher than they were in the early 1950s. In women aged under 55 the rates at first tended to increase, but have shown decreases in most age-groups in recent years, returning to about the same level as they were in the early 1950s. Among women aged 55–79 the rates initially increased in all age-groups, peaked at various times between the late 1960s and the late 1980s, and have recently shown a decrease in all age-groups, but

Figure 9.10

Mortality rates per million in Britain from pancreatic cancer by age, sex and calendar year

Mortality rate per million (log scale)

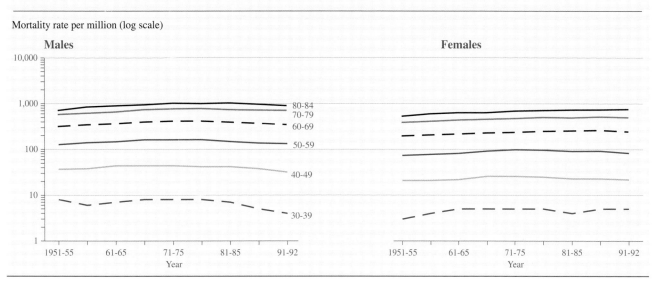

Table 9.9

Mortality rates per million in Britain from pancreatic cancer by age, sex and calendar year

								Age			
Year	30–34	35–39	40–44	45–49	50–54	55–59	60–64	65–69	70–74	75–79	80–84
Males											
1951–55	4	12	26	48	91	163	265	375	509	660	715
1956–60	3	10	25	52	98	181	286	412	556	688	851
1961–65	5	9	28	60	104	191	289	445	603	722	903
1966–70	5	11	28	60	117	207	318	479	659	829	949
1971–75	6	10	28	59	117	207	324	508	682	865	1,024
1976–80	4	13	25	58	119	207	343	493	686	888	1,006
1981–85	4	11	27	57	103	192	314	478	653	831	1,038
1986–90	3	7	24	51	96	178	303	441	642	805	971
1991–92	1	7	20	45	96	170	280	415	620	807	904
Females											
1951–55	2	4	13	29	56	92	149	244	332	440	532
1956–60	2	6	16	27	54	102	159	253	352	464	600
1961–65	3	7	12	32	62	103	174	257	382	490	636
1966–70	2	7	19	33	71	113	184	273	391	515	636
1971–75	3	7	17	35	74	124	178	292	409	533	690
1976–80	3	6	16	34	70	124	198	298	414	583	711
1981–85	3	5	14	32	67	115	205	301	419	553	728
1986–90	3	7	14	32	64	121	214	307	452	568	734
1991–92	2	7	12	31	60	106	196	288	424	562	752

still remain above their levels in the early 1950s. Among women aged 80–84 the rates have risen steadily throughout the time period considered.

Trends in mortality resemble those for lung cancer only weakly, and cannot easily be interpreted. The changes were much smaller and the increases persisted longer than for lung cancer in men up to the age of 75. This would be compatible either with improvements in medical services leading to a higher detection rate, or with the smoking risk being more closely linked to total cigarette consumption than tar-weighted consumption. In contrast, the maxima for women tended to occur at the same time or slightly before those for lung cancer, possibly as a result of sex differences in the trends in the detection rate.

9.4.2 Bladder cancer

It has been estimated that 45 per cent of these deaths in men and 30 per cent in women have been attributable to cigarette smoking in recent years (Health Education Authority, 1992). There is only weak and inconsistent evidence that smoking cigars or pipes increases the risk of bladder cancer (IARC, 1986). There is no evidence from case-control or cohort studies to suggest that changes in tar yield affect the risk from smoking cigarettes (IARC, 1986). Several chemicals belonging to the class of aromatic amines used in the manufacture of dyes have been shown to cause bladder cancer (IARC, 1974, 1982, 1987). By far the most important has been 2-naphthylamine because of its potency and widespread use and its presence as an impurity in chemicals used in the rubber industry. Another that has been important in Britain is benzidine. The manufacture of 2-naphthylamine ceased in the United Kingdom in 1949, but small amounts continued to be imported for 20 years; benzidine was withdrawn from use in 1969. Occupational exposure to these chemicals was estimated to have caused some 5 per cent of bladder cancers in men and 2 per cent in women in the early 1970s (Davies, Somerville and Wallace 1976) but the peak latent period after exposure was relatively short (less than 20 years; Case *et al.*, 1954) and they must have caused higher proportions in earlier periods from both occupational and general environmental exposure. Other established causes include some anti-cancer drugs, notably cyclophosphamide, and ionising radiation, but neither has caused sufficient cases to have had a detectable effect on the mortality rate.

The management of bladder cancer may have improved slightly, but there has been no qualitative change in the method of treatment. The disease is easy to diagnose and there is no reason to suspect any change in the detection rates. In the early years some cases will have been classified as benign or of uncertain behaviour, which would have been classified as malignant if they had occurred more recently. This shift in

nosological fashion may have affected incidence rates, but will have had little effect on mortality rates. No other fatal disease is likely to have been confused with bladder cancer as a cause of death.

In men aged 60 and over the mortality rates have peaked in precisely the same quinquennia as those for lung cancer, but neither the preceding rise nor the subsequent fall has been as great (see Figure 9.11 and Table 9.10). In men aged 55–59 rates have been decreasing since the early 1970s, and have fallen by about a third. In younger men the rates have been decreasing ever since 1951–55, with a few exceptions that can be attributed to random variation of small numbers; by the late 1980s they were about half what they had been in 1951–55. In women aged under 50 the rates tend to have decreased, but they have been low throughout and consequently unstable. In women aged 50–54 and 55–59 mortality remained relatively stable until 1976–80 and 1981–85 respectively, and since then has decreased by about 30 per cent. In older women mortality has risen and fallen as in men, but to a smaller extent, more irregularly and with peak rates some 10 years later.

The early reduction in mortality in men aged 45–54, when there had only been a small reduction in the tar-weighted cigarette consumption, and before any apparent decrease in lung cancer mortality, may have been contributed to by the reduced use of 2-naphthylamine from the mid-1940s. This factor may also have affected older age-groups, but the progressive shift of the maximum rate in each age-group to older ages with the passage of time accords with the cohort effect that would be expected from the increase in cigarette smoking in the first part of the century. In men the similarity of the pattern with that for lung cancer suggests that the introduction of low-tar cigarettes may also have led to a reduced risk, after tar-weighted cigarette consumption in males started to decline, but before 1971–75 when a reduction in total male cigarette consumption first took place. The

Figure 9.11

Mortality rates per million in Britain from bladder cancer by age, sex and calendar year

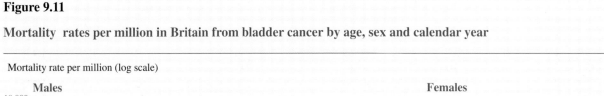

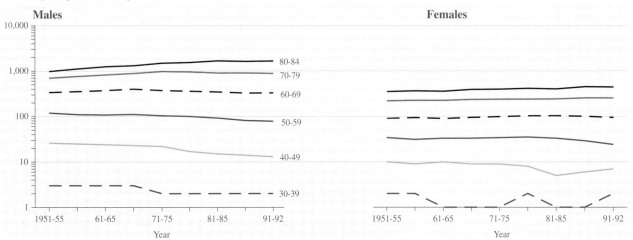

patterns of bladder cancer mortality in women are not clearly related to trends in cigarette consumption, although the decreases seen in recent years in all but the oldest age-groups may partly reflect the recent changes in smoking.

9.4.3 Aortic aneurysm

The Health Education Authority (1992) estimated that in recent years about 30 per cent of these deaths had been attributable to smoking (44 per cent in men and 15 per cent in women). In the Health Education Authority's estimate, the small number of peripheral vascular disease deaths were combined with the much greater number attributed to aortic aneurysm. There is no evidence to suggest that pipe or cigar smoking would have had any material effect on the risk of the disease. No data are available specifically for low-tar cigarettes and their effect cannot be predicted because it is not known which constituents of smoke are responsible. Other factors that contribute to the production of vascular atheroma must contribute to the development of the disease. As with peripheral vascular disease, however, many of these factors other than smoking that contribute to ischaemic heart disease, such as lack of physical exercise, are likely to be less important, if they are of any importance at all.

Rupture of an aortic aneurysm is usually fatal and the only effective treatment is prophylactic. Surgical repair before rupture has been increasingly common, but has made little impact on the fatality of the disease because it is seldom diagnosed early enough.

Changes in the classification of deaths attributed to aortic aneurysm have had major effects in the recorded mortality rates. Before 1958, deaths were classified according to the sixth revision of the ICD and were attributed to what is now simply called 'aortic aneurysm' only if they were specified as non-syphilitic or dissecting aneurysms; the rest were classified with syphilitic vascular disease. With the seventh revision, which came into effect in 1958, aortic aneurysms specified as abdominal were also classed as non-syphilitic, but unspecified aortic aneurysms continued to be regarded as syphilitic. Only with the eighth revision, which came into effect in 1968, were thoracic and all unspecified aortic aneurysms classed in the generic category of aortic aneurysms (ICD 441), with only those specified as syphilitic being classed with syphilitic vascular disease (ICD 093).

The disease is not difficult to diagnose as a cause of death, so long as it is considered as a possibility and cases of sudden death are subjected to postmortem examination. The disease

Table 9.10

Mortality rates per million in Britain from bladder cancer by age, sex and calendar year

Year	30–34	35–39	40–44	45–49	50–54	55–59	60–64	65–69	70–74	75–79	80–84
Males											
1951–55	2	5	13	38	86	152	263	397	570	789	954
1956–60	1	5	16	34	69	152	263	429	612	880	1,089
1961–65	1	6	14	33	71	145	281	449	683	921	1,219
1966–70	1	4	12	34	71	151	279	506	731	1,004	1,285
1971–75	1	4	11	33	68	141	268	463	788	1,124	1,455
1976–80	1	4	10	25	65	135	248	457	726	1,143	1,507
1981–85	2	3	8	22	58	126	243	436	702	1,065	1,633
1986–90	1	2	7	21	49	113	230	410	708	1,065	1,590
1991–92	1	3	9	18	53	103	224	421	682	1,044	1,618
Females											
1951–55	2	2	5	14	26	42	66	112	172	260	345
1956–60	1	3	6	12	22	40	67	118	175	268	359
1961–65	0	2	7	13	23	42	69	109	173	272	352
1966–70	0	2	5	13	22	44	70	118	184	282	387
1971–75	1	2	6	13	26	43	75	121	186	287	392
1976–80	1	3	5	10	26	45	80	124	185	289	409
1981–85	1	2	3	7	21	46	77	129	195	284	398
1986–90	1	2	3	8	17	42	75	126	197	309	447
1991–92	1	3	4	11	19	30	67	121	201	303	438

was not recognised to be common in the 1950s and some cases of sudden death due to a ruptured aneurysm may have been overlooked in that period.

Aortic aneurysms can be arteriosclerotic or syphilitic in origin. The former usually affect the abdominal aorta, whereas the latter are limited to the ascending aorta (in the thorax). There is no difficulty in distinguishing the two conditions clinically, but confusion has arisen because of the use of the term 'aortic aneurysm' without aetiological qualification. Before the Second World War, arteriosclerotic aneurysms were rare and syphilitic aneurysms were common, so that unqualified aortic aneurysms were regarded as syphilitic. Now the term is used as synonymous with the arteriosclerotic disease. In consequence, many more deaths were attributed to syphilitic aneurysms of the aorta in 1950 than to arteriosclerotic aneurysms. Deaths attributed to the syphilitic aneurysms subsequently decreased and by the late 1950s the situation was reversed. The decrease continued throughout the 1960s and 1970s and had almost disappeared by the early 1980s, corresponding to the introduction of penicillin for the treatment of syphilis 30 years before. In 1958 and 1968 the decline was accelerated by the introduction of the seventh and eighth revisions of the ICD (see above).

The mortality attributed to aortic aneurysm increased rapidly at all ages and in both sexes between 1951–55 and 1966–70, doubling in most sex- and age-specific groups (except under 40 in men and under 50 in women where the numbers of deaths were small) and increasing sixfold in old men (see Figure 9.12 and Table 9.11). Examination of the trends by single calendar year showed large increases in 1952, 1958 and, to a lesser extent, 1968. From 1966 to 1970 the mortality in men under 60 years of age changed very little, but it continued to increase at older ages, and was still increasing in 1991–92 at ages 65 years and over. In women, the pattern has been similar.

Much of the increase in mortality between 1950 and 1970 is an artefact of classification. The sharp increases in 1958 and 1968 corresponded to the introduction of the seventh and eighth revisions of the ICD and were accompanied by complementary declines in the deaths attributed to cardiovascular syphilis. The increase in 1952 cannot be explained by a reduction in cardiovascular syphilis and may have resulted from some change in the application of the rules for determining the underlying cause of death when an aortic aneurysm was referred to. Nevertheless there was some progressive increase in other years which could have been real. The increased prevalence of smoking is likely to have contributed to the enormous increase in older men and women. If, however, there has been any benefit from reduced smoking at younger ages it has been counteracted by other factors. There is certainly no evidence of any benefit from the switch to low-tar cigarettes.

9.4.4 Peptic ulcer

The Health Education Authority (1992) has estimated that, in recent years, about a fifth of all peptic ulcer deaths were attributable to smoking. Pipe and cigar smoking are less closely related to peptic ulcer than cigarette smoking (Doll and Peto, 1976; Surgeon General, 1979). There is no evidence relating to the effect of tar yield on the risk of the disease. Knowledge of the causes of peptic ulcer is far from complete, but there are certainly several major causes other than cigarette smoking. Infection with *Helicobacter pylori* is the major cause of duodenal ulcers and of some gastric ulcers. Aspirin and other non-steroidal anti-inflammatory drugs are other causes of a small proportion of gastric ulcers. What was responsible for the great increase in the incidence of duodenal ulcer in the first half of this century is, however, unknown, as is the reason for the progressive decrease in both types of

Figure 9.12

Mortality rates per million in Britain from aortic aneurysm by age, sex and calendar year

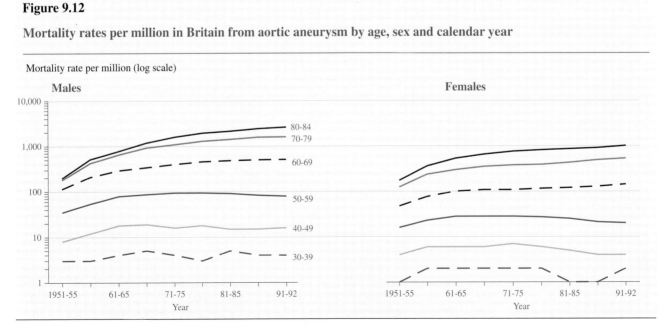

peptic ulcer in the second half of the century unless, perhaps, it is a reduction in the prevalence of *helicobacter* infection brought about by improved social conditions and reduced overcrowding.

The fatality of peptic ulcer has been greatly reduced by improvements in treatment and is now low. Improved surgical care and the treatment of infection reduced the fatality of gastric operations in the 1950s, and improved medical treatment and clearer indications for surgical intervention reduced the fatality from bleeding ulcers. The introduction of histamine H_2-receptor antagonists in the early 1970s transformed medical treatment and it has been improved further in the last decade by antibiotics that eliminate *helicobacter* infection. The disease is easy to diagnose and there is no reason to suspect any change in its recognition as a cause of death. No other diseases are likely to be confused with peptic ulcers.

The mortality from peptic ulcer has declined steadily in both sexes and at all ages under 75 years since 1951–55 and in 1991–92 it was only about 10 per cent of what it had been in men under 60 years of age and about 20 per cent of what it had been in women under 50 years (see Figure 9.13 and Table 9.12). In old age (75 years and above) the decline in men started 5–10 years later and has not yet started in women over 80 years of age.

The decline in mortality results from both improved treatment and a reduction in the prevalence of the disease (see Chapter 22). The reduced prevalence of smoking in men and young women will have contributed to the reduction in the prevalence, whereas the increased prevalence of long-term smoking in elderly women will have helped to prevent a fall in mortality.

9.5 Trends in ischaemic heart disease and related conditions

Ischaemic heart disease is related to smoking at all ages. The relationship, however, gets progressively weaker with increasing age and it is only under 55 years of age that it is moderately related to smoking according to our definition. It is, however, such a major cause of death and accounts for such a high proportion of all deaths attributed to smoking, that it has also been included in this study. According to the Health Education Authority (1992), the proportion of IHD deaths attributable to smoking at all ages combined is about 18 per cent. The relationship with smoking is specific for cigarette smoking (Doll and Peto, 1976; Surgeon General, 1979) because the risk of the disease appears to be dependent on deep inhalation and the absorption of noxious chemicals from the alveoli. According to Stellman (1986), the risk is unaffected by tar yield, but Parish *et al.* (1995) have found a small reduction with cigarettes yielding low levels of nicotine.

Many other factors determine the risk of ischaemic heart disease, which become relatively more important, in comparison with cigarette smoking, as age advances. The most important are elements of the diet. The precise importance of the different elements (saturated fat, different types of unsaturated fat, antioxidant micronutrients, salt and total calories) is, however, still controversial. Other avoidable factors are hypertension (itself determined by diet), lack of exercise, alcohol (which is protective provided consumption is moderate) and possibly psychological stress. The treatment of hypertension, which improved greatly in the late 1950s; the spread of screening for hypertension, once it was realised that long-term treatment of hypertension was likely to be beneficial; and the introduction of coronary bypass surgery, which was taken up slowly in the United Kingdom in the late 1960s and spread rapidly a decade later, will all have

Figure 9.13

Mortality rates per million in Britain from peptic ulcer by age, sex and calendar year

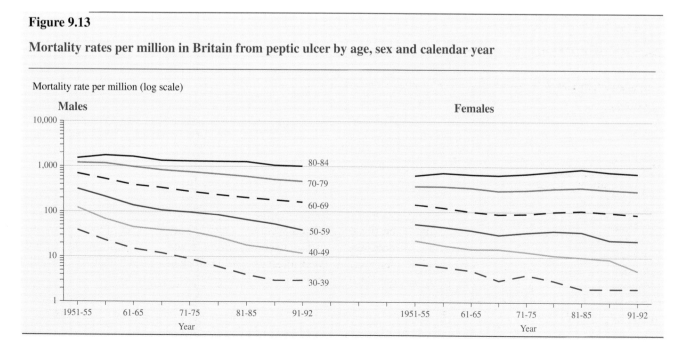

Mortality rate per million (log scale)

Table 9.11

Mortality rates per million in Britain from aortic aneurysm by age, sex and calendar year

Year	30–34	35–39	40–44	45–49	50–54	55–59	60–64	65–69	70–74	75–79	80–84
Males											
1951–55	2	4	5	10	23	46	89	138	169	190	196
1956–60	3	4	8	15	36	71	146	273	391	453	511
1961–65	3	6	10	26	48	110	203	379	572	719	770
1966–70	4	5	14	25	59	115	245	433	756	1,081	1,179
1971–75	3	6	10	22	56	132	264	531	866	1,298	1,582
1976–80	3	4	12	25	55	133	314	594	1,043	1,517	1,931
1981–85	4	6	9	21	51	132	303	656	1,139	1,662	2,118
1986–90	2	5	9	20	43	124	320	677	1,254	1,866	2,406
1991–92	3	5	10	22	42	116	309	701	1,280	1,890	2,593
Females											
1951–55	1	2	2	6	10	22	36	57	100	147	174
1956–60	1	2	4	8	16	29	56	95	178	293	359
1961–65	1	2	4	8	20	36	71	128	230	363	530
1966–70	1	2	4	8	18	37	78	138	252	449	650
1971–75	1	3	4	9	18	37	75	142	270	480	751
1976–80	1	3	4	8	16	38	76	155	283	490	808
1981–85	1	2	3	7	13	36	80	160	316	541	855
1986–90	1	1	3	6	14	28	77	180	379	599	901
1991–92	1	2	3	6	14	25	79	207	396	664	1,002

Table 9.12

Mortality rates per million in Britain from peptic ulcer by age, sex and calendar year

Year	30–34	35–39	40–44	45–49	50–54	55–59	60–64	65–69	70–74	75–79	80–84
Males											
1951–55	26	51	88	159	263	374	560	837	1,045	1,345	1,511
1956–60	18	27	50	86	153	271	415	634	982	1,347	1,749
1961–65	10	19	33	58	93	184	302	479	804	1,142	1,634
1966–70	8	15	26	51	72	142	238	436	677	980	1,340
1971–75	6	11	27	44	71	124	203	353	612	892	1,307
1976–80	5	7	17	37	60	109	178	291	502	848	1,283
1981–85	3	6	13	22	43	88	156	253	437	760	1,265
1986–90	2	4	10	19	37	69	132	230	379	643	1,057
1991–92	2	4	7	16	27	50	120	203	338	599	1,009
Females											
1951–55	5	10	18	28	44	63	111	177	293	440	632
1956–60	4	7	13	23	35	56	86	159	268	458	724
1961–65	4	6	9	20	29	48	76	124	262	416	670
1966–70	2	5	11	19	24	39	66	111	206	380	646
1971–75	3	5	9	17	28	41	65	115	219	388	698
1976–80	2	3	9	14	32	44	77	125	229	432	785
1981–85	2	3	7	13	28	44	78	134	244	449	882
1986–90	1	2	7	11	16	31	75	120	230	397	764
1991–92	1	3	3	7	14	32	58	116	209	373	705

contributed substantially to a reduction in the incidence of the disease in the older age-groups.

Changes in the treatment of acute ischaemic heart disease (that is, myocardial infarction) made little impact on the fatality of the disease until the discovery of the beneficial effects of anti-thrombotic and fibrinolytic agents in the 1970s, although the new treatments were not used extensively until the late 1980s. Before then the fatality was probably reduced to a small extent by the provision of specialised coronary care units from the late 1950s. Most deaths, however, occurred acutely, before admission to a specialist unit was possible.

Major changes have occurred in the classification of deaths attributed to heart disease, which complicate analysis of the trends attributed to ischaemic heart disease. In particular, the broadening of the category 'arteriosclerotic heart disease including coronary disease' (ICD 420) from the sixth and seventh revisions to 'ischaemic heart disease' in the eighth revision (ICD 410–414) in 1958 brought in some deaths previously classified as 'other myocardial degeneration'.

The term 'coronary heart disease' was a relatively new concept in the 1920s. In the following decades it became used progressively more often until it began to be displaced by the term 'ischaemic heart disease'. From the 1930s on, relatively non-specific terms such as myocardial degeneration, cardiovascular degeneration and arteriosclerosis began to be abandoned, and were progressively displaced by the more specific coronary artery disease and ischaemic heart disease.

Mortality attributed to 'other myocardial degeneration' (code 422 in the ICD7) or 'other myocardial insufficiency', which replaced it in the ICD8 (code 428), has declined steadily since 1951; in 1991–92 the rates in men and women over 50 years were less than 10 per cent of those recorded 40 years earlier. Arteriosclerosis, as the description of the cause of death,

suffered a similar, although less sharp, decline until 1991–92 when the rates attributed to it in men and women over 50 years of age were less than 20 per cent of those recorded 40 years earlier. Much of the decline in these two 'causes of death' is likely to have arisen from a change in medical diagnostic habits and skills, resulting in the increased use of 'ischaemic heart disease' to describe what would previously have been described less specifically. Examination of a sample of death certificates using the term 'arteriosclerosis' as a cause of death showed that about equal numbers also referred to associated cardiac and cerebrovascular conditions (R Doll, personal observation). We have, therefore, calculated mortality rates for 'ischaemic heart disease and related diagnoses' rather than for ischaemic heart disease alone; this is obtained by adding the recorded rates for ischaemic heart disease and myocardial degeneration and half the rates for arteriosclerosis. These are shown in Figure 9.14 and Table 9.13. Rates for the three component diseases (ischaemic heart disease, myocardial degeneration and arteriosclerosis) are also shown individually in Table 9.14.

Further confusion may have arisen from a change in the attribution of deaths from myocardial infarction associated with hypertension from 'hypertension' to 'myocardial infarction'. There is no way of estimating how big such an effect has been, but it may be that some of the reduction in mortality from hypertension has been at the cost of artificially increasing the mortality attributed to myocardial infarction and hence 'ischaemic heart disease'.

Mortality from ischaemic heart disease and related diagnoses (as defined above) in men under 65 years of age showed a small increase to progressively later dates with increasing age (to 1961–65 for men aged 30–34 years and 1976–80 for men aged 55–64 years) and then progressive decreases to rates a little below those in 1951–55 (see Figure 9.14 and Table 9.13). At older ages the initial increase was very small (14 per cent at ages 65–69 years) or non-existent. Mortality then

Figure 9.14

Mortality rates per million in Britain from ischaemic heart disease and related conditions by age, sex and calendar year

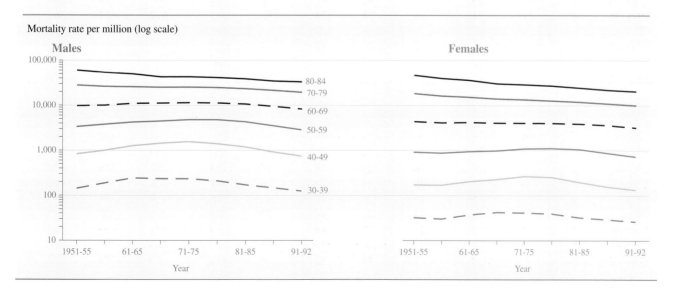

decreased, starting in the late 1970s for men aged 65–74 years or in the late 1950s for older men, reducing the rates in 1991–92 to below the initial level and almost halving the initial level in the oldest age-group. The trends in women were very similar, save that the increases under 65 years of age were slightly less and the decreases (with the sole exception of ages 30–34 years) slightly more.

The continuing increase in mortality in men under 65 years until the early 1960s or late 1970s cannot have been caused by tobacco, the consumption of which had stabilised some time earlier; it seems likely to have resulted instead from a continuing change in those factors that had caused the great increase in earlier years, the nature of which is still largely controversial, but which included decreasing physical effort. The subsequent decreases in mortality will have been contributed to by the reduced prevalence of smoking, but the greater part of the reduction must have been caused by the therapeutic and prophylactic measures described above, to the increased consumption of alcohol since 1950 and recently to the reduction in the consumption of saturated fats. The trends in women and the reasons for these trends are broadly similar to those in men, save that they will have been affected less by changes in physical effort and alcohol and will have been affected by the increase in smoking in women under 60 years of age, as, for this disease, the reduction in tar yield is modest (Parish *et al.*, 1995).

Table 9.13

Mortality rates per million in Britain from ischaemic heart disease and related conditions by age, sex and calendar year

						Age					
Year	30–34	35–39	40–44	45–49	50–54	55–59	60–64	65–69	70–74	75–79	80–84
Males											
1951–55	80	206	506	1,152	2,430	4,285	7,469	12,573	21,094	36,279	61,671
1956–60	96	281	638	1,349	2,700	4,874	7,862	12,773	20,681	33,151	55,231
1961–65	111	374	832	1,682	3,095	5,384	8,935	13,691	21,051	31,915	51,026
1966–70	110	359	953	1,908	3,361	5,588	8,941	14,067	20,994	30,666	43,884
1971–75	111	355	987	2,124	3,733	5,860	9,123	14,355	21,342	30,650	43,974
1976–80	95	326	872	1,918	3,664	5,921	9,229	13,888	20,794	30,088	42,255
1981–85	86	256	714	1,653	3,159	5,462	8,650	13,229	19,790	28,121	39,544
1986–90	71	223	555	1,278	2,511	4,530	7,636	11,852	18,077	25,901	35,441
1991–92	56	194	473	1,008	2,046	3,693	6,422	10,590	16,115	23,796	34,051
Females											
1951–55	20	45	97	247	559	1,263	2,859	6,157	12,616	25,046	47,916
1956–60	20	41	105	235	521	1,223	2,758	5,725	11,487	21,902	40,744
1961–65	21	54	130	278	578	1,306	2,876	5,787	11,206	20,156	37,132
1966–70	24	60	155	302	648	1,315	2,833	5,549	10,432	18,310	31,047
1971–75	22	60	169	362	721	1,455	2,894	5,466	10,048	17,594	29,689
1976–80	22	56	160	345	735	1,471	2,930	5,343	9,613	16,398	27,902
1981–85	19	45	118	275	665	1,435	2,793	5,178	9,149	15,272	25,045
1986–90	16	42	90	220	517	1,215	2,635	4,797	8,586	13,878	22,487
1991–92	15	37	85	181	428	1,018	2,228	4,348	7,618	12,945	20,999

Table 9.14

Mortality rates per million in Britain from ischaemic heart disease, myocardial degeneration and arteriosclerosis by age, sex and calendar year

The category "ischaemic heart disease and related conditions", shown in Table 9.13, has been obtained by adding the recorded rates for ischaemic heart disease and myocardial degeneration and half the rates for arteriosclerosis.

						Age					
Year	30–34	35–39	40–44	45–49	50–54	55–59	60–64	65–69	70–74	75–79	80–84

a) Ischaemic heart disease

Males

Year	30–34	35–39	40–44	45–49	50–54	55–59	60–64	65–69	70–74	75–79	80–84
1951–55	71	191	475	1,093	2,268	3,904	6,543	10,391	15,827	24,102	35,194
1956–60	92	272	623	1,314	2,620	4,664	7,366	11,508	17,388	25,166	36,559
1961–65	105	363	817	1,655	3,043	5,267	8,634	12,936	19,012	26,709	38,004
1966–70	106	351	942	1,890	3,325	5,515	8,759	13,578	19,633	27,143	35,435
1971–75	108	350	979	2,114	3,709	5,808	9,014	14,048	20,487	28,312	38,043
1976–80	91	322	864	1,907	3,643	5,874	9,134	13,656	20,160	28,364	37,714
1981–85	83	251	705	1,640	3,134	5,413	8,558	13,023	19,312	26,902	36,449
1986–90	67	219	547	1,267	2,489	4,488	7,560	11,718	17,774	25,256	33,893
1991–92	53	189	467	998	2,029	3,665	6,367	10,483	15,920	23,375	33,035

Females

Year	30–34	35–39	40–44	45–49	50–54	55–59	60–64	65–69	70–74	75–79	80–84
1951–55	12	30	72	186	433	1,003	2,213	4,612	8,515	14,874	24,699
1956–60	15	33	91	206	466	1,086	2,423	4,856	9,043	15,511	24,977
1961–65	17	47	121	260	541	1,228	2,678	5,251	9,626	15,834	25,861
1966–70	21	57	149	289	622	1,269	2,716	5,214	9,396	15,441	23,573
1971–75	20	58	163	353	705	1,425	2,812	5,261	9,398	15,666	24,502
1976–80	21	53	155	336	722	1,444	2,867	5,194	9,135	14,993	23,836
1981–85	17	42	113	267	650	1,411	2,741	5,055	8,813	14,275	22,116
1986–90	14	39	86	213	508	1,197	2,596	4,714	8,362	13,334	20,973
1991–92	12	34	82	177	423	1,002	2,202	4,289	7,478	12,575	20,017

b) Myocardial degeneration

Males

Year	30–34	35–39	40–44	45–49	50–54	55–59	60–64	65–69	70–74	75–79	80–84
1951–55	8	15	29	54	148	344	821	1,892	4,535	10,397	22,741
1956–60	4	8	14	32	71	186	420	1,055	2,719	6,528	15,350
1961–65	7	10	14	23	45	94	236	573	1,525	3,915	9,936
1966–70	4	8	10	16	30	57	130	337	941	2,424	5,938
1971–75	3	4	7	8	18	37	72	196	543	1,474	3,786
1976–80	4	4	7	10	17	35	65	149	401	1,104	2,978
1981–85	3	4	9	12	22	39	71	151	330	825	2,089
1986–90	3	4	7	9	20	35	59	97	202	419	962
1991–92	4	5	5	8	14	24	45	85	132	280	658

Females

Year	30–34	35–39	40–44	45–49	50–54	55–59	60–64	65–69	70–74	75–79	80–84
1951–55	8	15	24	58	120	242	590	1,396	3,655	9,047	20,599
1956–60	5	7	13	28	51	125	299	752	2,073	5,431	13,420
1961–65	4	6	8	17	33	67	164	435	1,247	3,407	8,942
1966–70	3	3	6	12	23	38	95	258	758	2,080	5,485
1971–75	2	3	5	8	14	24	62	147	440	1,289	3,445
1976–80	1	3	4	8	10	22	47	108	334	965	2,764
1981–85	1	3	4	8	13	20	41	95	250	722	2,094
1986–90	2	3	3	6	7	15	33	64	164	382	1,035
1991–92	2	2	3	3	4	15	23	46	107	263	666

Table 9.14 - *continued*

Year						Age					
	30-34	35-39	40-44	45-49	50-54	55-59	60-64	65-69	70-74	75-79	80-84

c) Arteriosclerosis

Males

Year	30-34	35-39	40-44	45-49	50-54	55-59	60-64	65-69	70-74	75-79	80-84
1951-55	1	1	4	9	29	74	208	578	1,464	3,557	7,469
1956-60	0	1	3	6	18	47	151	419	1,148	2,914	6,640
1961-65	0	1	3	6	14	46	129	362	1,028	2,581	6,168
1966-70	0	0	2	4	12	32	104	303	839	2,196	5,019
1971-75	0	0	1	3	11	29	74	221	623	1,726	4,290
1976-80	0	0	2	3	9	23	59	166	468	1,238	3,125
1981-85	0	0	1	2	6	20	42	108	294	786	2,010
1986-90	0	0	1	3	5	13	33	73	200	450	1,169
1991-92	0	0	1	2	5	9	21	43	123	279	715

Females

Year	30-34	35-39	40-44	45-49	50-54	55-59	60-64	65-69	70-74	75-79	80-84
1951-55	1	1	2	4	12	35	111	298	890	2,247	5,234
1956-60	0	1	1	2	8	24	73	233	740	1,917	4,692
1961-65	0	0	1	2	7	20	67	202	666	1,830	4,657
1966-70	0	0	0	1	7	16	46	154	555	1,576	3,977
1971-75	0	0	1	2	5	13	39	118	418	1,277	3,482
1976-80	0	0	1	2	5	10	30	83	287	880	2,601
1981-85	0	0	0	1	2	7	20	56	173	549	1,669
1986-90	0	0	1	1	2	6	12	39	120	324	959
1991-92	0	0	0	1	1	2	7	25	66	214	630

9.6 Conclusion

Trends in mortality from smoking-related diseases show, for the most part, only little correlation with the consumption of either all tobacco products or cigarettes. This is because of various combinations of major changes in the prevalence of other, sometimes more important, aetiological agents, in the efficacy of treatment and in the classification and nomenclature of disease. For most diseases these changes mask the effect of trends in smoking, particularly at old ages, when the relative effects of smoking are generally less important. With the exception, however, of cancers of the oral cavity, pharynx and larynx in men and cancer of the oesophagus in both sexes (which are closely related to the consumption of alcohol) all show a reduction in mortality in both men and women under 60 years of age over the last 20 years, corresponding to a reduction in the prevalence of smoking. For lung cancer, which is principally caused by smoking, the trends correlate well, once allowance is made for cohort effects and for the beneficial effect of the reduction in the delivery of tar.

Appendix 1

Codes of the International Classification of Diseases (ICD) used to define the diseases examined

ICD Revision

Disease	6th	7th	8th	9th
A Strongly related to smoking - causal				
Lung cancer	162-3	162-3	162	162
Chronic obstructive lung disease	502, 527	502, 527	491-2, 519	491-2, 496, 519
B Strongly related to smoking - causal and confounding				
Cancer of lip	140	140	140	140
Cancer of oral cavity (less salivary gland)[a]	141, 143-144	141, 143-144	141, 143-145	141, 143-145
Cancer of pharynx (less nasopharynx)[a]	145, 147-148	145, 147-148	146, 148-149	146, 143-145
Cancer of oesophagus	150	150	150	150
Cancer of larynx	161	161	161	161
C Moderately related to smoking - causal				
Cancer of pancreas	157	157	157	157
Cancer of bladder	181	181	188, 189.9	188, 189.3-9
Aortic aneurysm	451	451	441	441
Peptic ulcer[b]	540-1, 784.5	540-1, 784.5	531-3. 784.5	531-3, 578.0
D Other diseases studied				
Ischaemic heart disease[c]	420, 422.1	420, 422.1	410-414	420-414
Myocardial degeneration[c]	422.0, 422.2	422.0, 422.2	428	429
Arteriosclerosis[c]	450	450	440	440

a,c   *Diseases are grouped together for analysis, see text for explanation.*
b   *Codes 784.5 and 578.0 omitted from Scottish data.*

Chapter 10

Housing-related disorders

By
Sonja Hunt

Summary

- In the mid-nineteenth century, urban and rural poor alike were generally in cramped and insanitary housing.

- Around the beginning of the twentieth century, provision of adequate housing became recognised as the responsibility of local and national government.

- Early public housing stock was of good quality but this declined in the 1950s and 1960s. Owner-occupation increased from the 1950s.

- Building and repair of public housing decreased following the right-to-buy policy of the 1980s, leading to a severe shortage of good quality accommodation for those on low incomes.

- Special surveys are needed to examine relations between health and housing conditions, but some disorders are clearly housing-related.

- Dampness, inadequate heating and overcrowding are among the factors affecting general ill health and respiratory disorders, heart disease, accidental injury and emotional problems.

- The adverse effects on children of poor housing can continue into adulthood.

- Homelessness, including the use of temporary accommodation, is related to illness, with each being a contributory cause of the other.

We live in muck and filthe, we aint got no priviz no dust bins, no drains, no water splies and no drain or suer in the hole place . . . we all of us suffur and the numbers are ill, and if the colera comes Lord Help us.

Letter in the *London Times*, 7 March 1849,
signed by 54 of the city's poor

10.1 Introduction

There are a number of factors associated with housing which might be expected to have an adverse effect on physical and mental health, both directly and indirectly. The need for adequate shelter is regarded as a basic human requisite and by 'housing' is meant, here, those more or less fixed attributes of a dwelling such as structure, fabric, state of repair, insulation, ventilation, heating arrangements, size and number of rooms, and sanitary cooking facilities. Consideration will also be given to the effects of having no permanent shelter at all, as in varying states of homelessness. Individual behaviours within a dwelling which may affect indoor air quality or risk of accidents, such as smoking, will not be dealt with here except in so far as they may be considered to be contributory or confounding variables.

A dwelling may harbour pathogens which can produce allergies and infections in the occupants. Lack of sufficient space, light, ventilation and sanitation may encourage the growth and spread of harmful organisms. Individuals may have inadequate shelter from the elements because of poor building construction, lack of repair or because they have no permanent accommodation at all. Dwellings may be unsafe, insecure and unsuitable, thus creating emotional strain in the occupants and increasing the risk of accidents.

In the past 150 years the focal points of housing in relation to health have shifted from the spread of infections and overcrowding in relation to mortality, to the climatic conditions within a house and their implications for morbidity and to the mental health implications of inappropriate and unpleasant housing conditions. However, a common theme has been the controversy over whether it is the dwelling that is primarily to blame or the occupants themselves. The individual mechanistic approach of Western medicine has tended to minimise the contribution of social factors to ill health. The very close associations of bad housing, poverty and social disadvantage have proved difficult to disentangle and it has only been in the past few years that it has proved possible to show that housing conditions can make an independent contribution to the state of health.

There are few topics in the medical field which are not subject to political pressures of some kind. The housing and health debate cannot be divorced from the political climate of the time, a fact as true today as in 1841. Many of the same arguments, methodological and ideological, recur throughout the years.

10.2 Housing and health 1841–1960

The population of Britain virtually doubled between 1801 and 1851, to about 18 million, largely as a result of an increased birth rate and a lowered mortality rate. This rapid growth meant that there were far fewer dwellings than the number needed. It has been calculated that by 1851 there were almost 2 million people who were surplus to the housing stock (Mitchell and Deane, 1962). A Report from the London Statistical Society in 1847 described a street in St Giles where, in 1841, 27 houses with an average of five rooms had 655 occupants. By 1847, the same houses contained 1,095 people. Some of this increase was attributed, ironically, to 'improvements' such as pulling down dwellings to widen the streets. In Liverpool, it was estimated that there were 40,000 individuals living in cellars which were frequently polluted with the overflow from privies above. The average life expectancy of these individuals was calculated at 15 years (Chadwick, 1842).

Chadwick described the grossly overcrowded, insanitary, decaying, damp and cold dwellings of town dwellers, with the poorest accommodation, not surprisingly, being occupied by the poorest people, mostly day labourers. Such dwellings lacked light and space, fresh water or any means of refuse disposal and were likely to be adjacent to open sewers and piles of rotting animal and vegetable waste. There was nowhere to keep food. Apart from a few philanthropic or prudent employers, there was no interest in building homes for the poor, because many builders were themselves constantly in debt and had no incentive to construct dwellings upon which they would never see a return. Consequently, people flocking into the towns in search of work and fortune had to find what meagre shelter they could, usually by moving into an already crowded space. Subdivision of existing accommodation led to further overcrowding.

London, Manchester and other large towns contained common lodging houses, often known as 'rookeries' – inhabited by migrant workers and others of no fixed abode. These 'rookeries' were tenement blocks which had once housed the families of rich merchants, since moved away from the noisome and crowded urban areas. They became rooming houses where 12 people to the room was not unusual. The same bed was often shared by strangers of both sexes and had a stream of occupants. An outbreak of typhus in 1851, in Leeds, was thought to emanate from such a lodging house. At that time there were 222 such houses, with almost 3,000 inhabitants and an average of 2.5 people to a bed, 4.5 to a room (Harrison, 1971). Interestingly, this was the first category of housing to come under legislation, possibly because of the association of such houses with crime, drunkenness and licentious behaviour.

Although rural areas were less crowded, there were still whole families, often more than one, living in a single room. A Report on Women and Children in Agriculture, published in

1843, describes a dwelling in Somerset with 29 people under one roof and a sleeping space of just 100 square feet for the adults. Such rural cottages had no privies and no storage space, no water and often no heat or light. Outbreaks of cholera, malaria, scarlet fever, typhus and typhoid were common; tuberculosis and other respiratory diseases were rife. An enquiry into rural housing in 1864 surveyed 821 parishes and found that less than 5 per cent of dwellings had more than two rooms and 40 per cent had only one (Smith, 1876).

Chadwick produced some of the earliest evidence for the continuing social class gradient associated with mortality rates. Table 10.1 shows a comparison of death rates for different social groups in different locations in 1839 (Flinn, 1965).

In the 1840s typhus was endemic and tuberculosis was the major cause of death, accounting for about a quarter of all deaths annually. Although many writers of the time were inclined to blame Irish immigration, the fecklessness of the poor or an 'act of God' for this, there was some agreement that overcrowding, insanitary and squalid housing conditions, and malnutrition were the most likely culprits.

Engels, writing in 1844, described the stinking streets, where 'pale, narrow-chested, hollow-eyed ghosts' walked through offal and excrement, and the swarming tenements where 'sick and well' slept in the same room and, often, in the same bed. In 1847 Gavin wrote of the lack of ventilation, fetid air, lack of drainage, ubiquitous sewage, filthy and crowded dwellings, and hazardous occupations which were the fate of the poor and had no hesitation in attributing to this the high mortality rate in towns.

Much of the evidence for the effects of housing on health came from the investigations and observations of Medical Officers of Health. For example, an address to the Sanitary Institute in 1894 contained the information that infant and overall mortality from tuberculosis was 50 per cent higher in back-to-back houses than in those with through ventilation (Public Health, 1895). Work by members of the Statistical Society of London succeeded in linking housing conditions with the incidence of typhus.

The Select Committee on the Health of Towns, reporting in 1840, specifically linked the sickness and misery of the population to the construction and type of dwellings of poor people, and the Public Health Act of 1848 was the first attempt at some form of sanitary action. For the first time Public Health became recognised in law and the welfare of citizens was established as a responsibility of governments. This Act enabled local authorities to gain access to inspect and regulate insanitary dwellings (Burnett, 1978). Unfortunately, it was largely ineffective because it targeted mortality in relation to housing and the authorities had powers only in towns where mortality exceeded 23 per 1,000. It also had the effect of embedding the notion that housing should be bad enough to kill someone before there was a need for remedial action (Gauldie, 1974).

The 1848 Act was followed by a string of Acts aimed at improving housing conditions. Although it may have been the economic and social costs of bad housing which prompted these reforms, rather than ill health and misery, it was a local Building Act of 1846 that authorised Liverpool Corporation to appoint the nation's first Medical Officer of Health (Frazer, 1947).

Early understanding of the link between housing and health tended to be based upon miasma theory where disease was associated with noxious smells. This did have the consequence of improvements in ventilation and refuse disposal, but did nothing about the overcrowding itself.

10.2.1 Health and overcrowding

The census information of the period was mainly concerned with the number of persons in a room and a dwelling. Examination of the returns for the nineteenth century and the first half of the twentieth show that the average number of persons in a house declined from 5.6 to 5.4 between 1801 and 1861, but the number of families to a house remained virtually the same at 1.2, possibly reflecting a decline in the size of families.

Table 10.1

Average age at death (years) in three urban areas and one rural area for three groups in 1839

	Professional persons & gentry	Tradesmen	Labourers
Manchester	38	20	17
Liverpool	35	22	15
Bethnal Green	45	26	16
Rutland	52	41	38

Source: Flinn (1965)

Table 10.2

Average number of occupants in a one-roomed dwelling by town; 1911

	Persons per room
Birmingham	1.64
London	1.92
Liverpool	2.09
Edinburgh	2.71
Glasgow	3.18

Source: ONS

Between 1861 and 1881 the population of London grew by almost 50 per cent and in the 90 years between 1801 and 1891 the density of population in Britain expanded from 153 to 497 persons per square mile. This included those living in 'barns, sheds, caravans, tents and the open air' of whom more than 16,000 were counted. In 1891, the average number of persons per room was 2.2 in a one-roomed dwelling, 1.7 in a two-roomed dwelling, 1.4 in a three-roomed dwelling and 1.2 in a four-roomed dwelling; 11 per cent of the population lived in overcrowded conditions but this varied from 41 per cent in Gateshead and over 30 per cent in Newcastle and Sunderland to 2 per cent in Portsmouth and Leicester. The greatest overcrowding was in Northumberland and County Durham and in some London boroughs, such as Shoreditch and Bethnal Green, a state of affairs that has lasted until the present day, albeit on a much smaller scale. There was much variation between urban areas, as shown in Tables 10.2 and 10.3.

Figure 10.1 shows the decline in the number of people living at a density of more than two to a room between 1891 and 1951.

By 1931 only 3.9 per cent of dwellings were officially overcrowded but there were still over 60,000 families living more than four to a room.

The Sanitary Law Amendment Act of 1874 and the Public Health Act of 1890 controlled the construction and conditions of new dwellings but simultaneously discouraged builders and increased overcrowding by removing houses. Moreover, most towns had large numbers of people without regular wages whose criteria for a dwelling were that it should be as cheap as possible and that time to pay the rent would be granted. This meant that landlords were still able to fill filthy and hazardous dwellings to bursting point. Those 'unlucky' enough not to be able to find even this standard of accommodation had to occupy buildings which were legally unfit or would live anywhere they could for free, in sheds, storehouses or derelict buildings (Gauldie, 1974).

Occasionally, a few philanthropists would finance the building of superior houses as in the 'cottage movement' where model cottages with two bedrooms and adequate light and ventilation were built for farm workers. However, there were some who thought these cottages far too good for the labouring classes and fears were expressed that they would keep potatoes in the extra bedroom (Garnier, 1895). This sentiment was echoed 50 years later in relation to slum clearance, when residents moved to council estates were widely believed to keep coal in the bath.

Even such subsidised dwellings were too expensive for the poor but they did have the effect of demonstrating that it was possible to construct sanitary accommodation on a relatively large scale without incurring a huge cost. They thus paved the way for local authority housing provision (Wohl, 1983), and the Housing of the Working Classes Act in 1900 enshrined the idea of the provision of housing by local and national government. However, it was not until after the First World War and the demand for 'homes fit for heroes' that state housing provision really began (Byrne et al., 1986). In fact, the basis of our present minimum standard for housing has its origins in the 1919 Manual on unfit homes and unhealthy areas, put out by the newly formed Ministry of Health. The 1920s produced some of the best local authority housing for low-income workers and the following quote illustrates that the association between housing and health was taken into account by at least some architects, even if their information was not strictly accurate:

Table 10.3

Percentage of children under 10 years of age living in accommodation with more than two persons per room; 1911

	Percentage
Newcastle-upon-Tyne	48.3
London	32.8
West Ham	24.3
Leeds	20.0
Bradford	18.5
Birmingham	16.7
Liverpool	16.4
Kingston-upon-Hull	14.0
Sheffield	13.9
Manchester	12.3
Bristol	9.8
Nottingham	8.2

Source: ONS

Figure 10.1

Percentage of the population living more than two people per room, 1891–1951

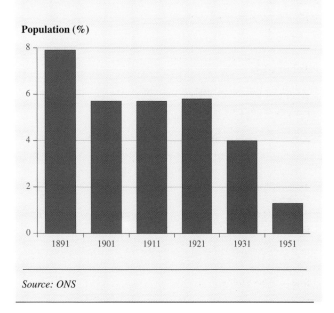

Source: ONS

Mr. Parker (the architect) has always before his mind the following facts: a tuberculosis germ will live for two years out of the direct rays of the sun. A typhoid germ has the same life out of the sun and two minutes in the sun. He regards a through living room – i.e. one with a window at each end – as essential.

Weaver (1926)

Infectious diseases declined 92 per cent between 1850 and 1901 and McKeown (1979) estimated that 86 per cent of the reduction in overall death rates between 1800 and 1971 was attributable to this decline. It is easy to show a correlation between the decline in death rates from infectious diseases and the decline in overcrowding over the same time period. However, it is impossible, with the data available, to attribute the one to the other directly. There were parallel improvements in sanitation and hygiene and the facilities for the storage and preparation of food. However, it seems highly probable that better housing conditions were a significant factor in the decline in mortality and morbidity rates.

10.2.2 Tuberculosis

One problem that proved particularly intransigent was tuberculosis and this gave rise to a number of epidemiological and other studies. The controversies over the main contributory factors to tuberculosis and its control and prevention illustrate very well both the shortcomings of routine data and the methodological issues that still pertain today.

Tuberculosis declined considerably in most European countries in the 100 years between 1850 and 1950. The relationship between tuberculosis and socio-economic factors, including housing, had been supported by a number of epidemiological studies as well as by medical opinion (Bryder, 1988; Smith, 1988). The general improvement in living standards was assumed to be a factor in this decline. However, in Glasgow the pattern was markedly different from the rest of Britain. By the end of the First World War, Glasgow had a lower rate of respiratory TB than other comparable cities, but by 1938 the death rate from pulmonary TB was higher than any city in England and by 1949, notification rates were the highest since 1910 (McFarlane, 1989).

Death rates in the poorer parts of the city were up to six times as high as those in the more affluent areas. Investigations into the reasons for this tended to focus upon overcrowding and malnutrition. As McFarlane (1989) noted, it was possible for researchers using the same data to come to entirely opposite conclusions stating, with confidence, that pulmonary TB was not related to housing (McKinlay, 1947) and that it was (Stein, 1952).

Lack of sunlight and poor ventilation combined with overcrowding in Glasgow's tenement flats and vennels narrow alleyways between buildings were held to lower resistance to the TB bacillus and McMillan (1957) concluded that overcrowding certainly increased the risk of the disease spreading. An examination of the links between overcrowding

and TB cases notified for wards where the incidence was low showed a high correlation between incidence of TB and the average number of rooms in a house, as well as the average number of persons per room and the percentage living more than two persons to a room. However, these correlations were not present where the incidence of the disease was high, suggesting that other factors were in operation. For example, although there was a lower incidence where there was less than one person to a room, Brett and Benjamin (1957) concluded that there was no simple direct relationship between TB and overcrowding, and that it was economic and social conditions that encouraged TB.

On the other hand, Stein (1952), using a definition of overcrowding as the average number of persons per room per ward and of 'ordinary crowding' as the average number of persons per house per ward, found high correlations between notification rates and mortality rates in conditions of ordinary crowding and overcrowding. These were said to be higher than associations with unemployment and poverty, although Stein concluded that these latter contributed to the overall rates. Crowding accounted for 60–70 per cent of the variance in TB mortality as compared with poverty and unemployment which accounted for 5–15 per cent. Nevertheless, Stein stated that the incidence of TB and mortality rates must be regarded in the context of the 'social complex' where different factors played interacting contributory roles.

Many of the discrepancies in the reported associations between overcrowding and tuberculosis and the resulting controversy arose from the fact that the indices of housing conditions in official statistics were insufficiently refined. Important variables were not taken into account, because they were not available, because they required special surveys or because they were not, at the time, regarded as contributory factors. For example, respiratory TB was most prevalent in the age group 16–30 years. Thus, to compare overcrowding in the entire population with TB rates was inappropriate. The indices of overcrowding often had irregularities and official statistics were regarded as so complex as to be unhelpful in solving the mystery of links between housing and health. Moreover, different investigators used not only different indices of overcrowding but also different ways of representing TB, for example, by mortality rates, by incidence estimates and by case finding. Many of these issues remain important in contemporary investigations of links between housing and health and can only be resolved by special studies that gather sufficient relevant data.

The 1930s constituted a period of major epidemiological research and housing was identified as a key factor for investigation in the health of the population, even if its exact role could not be specified. After the Second World War the local authority was the normal means of providing new houses for many families. Much of the housing stock of this time was of a high standard in construction and design and a high proportion were semidetached with gardens. It was not until 1954 that owner occupation came to be seen as a desirable goal (Byrne *et al.,* 1986) a change which in the 1980s started to have undesirable repercussions.

10.3 Housing and health: 1961 to the present day

It's very noisy being right by the motorway but we couldn't open the windows anyway, because of all the break-ins. The walls are running with damp and there's mould on our walls, our clothes and shoes. It's freezing cold most of the time and in winter we all huddle into the one room. The kids are always sick and I'm at my wits end.

> Interview with a resident of a Merseyside housing estate (March, 1989)

The year 1955 saw the beginning of mass housing schemes, high-rise flats built to house the victims of 'slum clearance', which appears to have been more often in the interests of commercial exploitation of land than the health of the citizenry (Dunleavy, 1981). Families rehoused in the 1950s and 1960s sometimes found themselves in worse accommodation than their peers of the previous generation, because in spite of improvements in design and heating, the developments were characterised by shoddy workmanship and inferior materials, as well as social isolation, thus paving the way for future health problems, both physical and mental.

By the mid-1960s some of the less desirable effects of demolition and rehousing were becoming evident and there was a move towards the improvement of existing dwellings. However, by this time the scale of the problems had become too large to be corrected without huge investment. For example, a survey of house conditions of England and Wales in 1967 revealed 1.8 million dwellings to be unfit for habitation. Nevertheless, overall there had been enormous improvements in basic housing standards with respect to light and space, sewage disposal, indoor plumbing and the availability of hot water, as well as regular refuse collection.

The 1991 Census shows only a small proportion of dwellings having more than 1.5 persons per room and the vast majority of Britons are now provided with indoor washing and toilet facilities (OPCS, 1993). However, according to the English House Conditions Survey (DOE, 1991), 7.4 per cent of dwellings are still unfit for human habitation. Of these, 38 per cent are inadequate in terms of repair and/or facilities for food preparation, 25 per cent have no bath or shower, 22 per cent are damp, 19 per cent have an inadequate WC, 18 per cent have insufficient heat and 12 per cent have inadequate ventilation. These figures are probably an underestimate because of the criteria used to establish inadequacy. The greatest absolute number of these dwellings is in the owner-occupied sector. However, it is the privately rented sector which is in the worst condition with 20 per cent of all such accommodation failing the standard on one or more counts. The bulk of unfit property was built before 1850 but 2.2 per cent, representing 143,000 dwellings, was built after 1964.

There is still a substantial quantity of substandard accommodation, particularly in north-east England and Scotland. The building of high-rise flats in the 1960s with little supervised space for children to play still has its legacy.

The increase in the number of people in temporary accommodation, which is often insanitary and overcrowded, and the number of people whose home is the pavement, keep the topic of housing and health a current one. In addition, increasing crime rates have highlighted the importance of feelings of security in relation to mental health, especially for elderly people.

After the decline of TB the health aspects of housing received little attention. The abolition of the post of Medical Officer of Health in 1974 meant that there was no single official charged with monitoring links between housing conditions and illness in the community.

The 1980s Housing Act encouraged the sale of council houses under the 'right to buy' banner and restricted local authorities in the amount of money they could spend on renovations and new building. This, together with other legislation, paved the way to the present shortage of accommodation for the lower income groups and young people and consequent increases in homelessness.

10.3.1 Social inequalities, housing and health

If interest in housing *per se* declined in the 1960s, there was an upsurge of interest in the continuing problem of social inequalities in health. Significant changes in housing, education and other standards failed to level the gradient of mortality and morbidity associated with social class. Various explanations have been put forward for this from genetics to 'lifestyle' (Brotherston, 1976). As low income and poor health have been shown to be linked regardless of place or period, it would seem that the explanation must lie in consideration of what it is that the poor have in common across time and location. One major characteristic among others is, of course, the inability to afford good quality housing. It is known that the gradient of health status is also affected by area of residence. Thus, sickness rates indicate that the health experience of people living in a deprived area is worse than that of people in a non-deprived area, regardless of social class (Neligman *et al*, 1974; Skrimshire, 1978). A study linking childhood mortality with housing density and housing amenities found that housing characteristics had a highly significant association with mortality rates, independent of social class and unemployment (Brennan and Lancashire, 1978) and the authors concluded that much of the difference in mortality between groups in different social circumstances and in different locations could be attributed to housing.

However, in order to clarify the issue of the precise contribution housing makes to health, a number of methodological problems need to be addressed.

10.3.2 Methodological issues

As adverse housing conditions are rarely found in isolation from other factors known to be associated with ill health, the nature of links between the two has, until very recently, been uncertain. In fact, there has been surprisingly little scientific research on housing and health. Only in the last 10 years, in Britain, Scandinavia and Canada, have there been significant advances in our understanding of the precise nature of the links between ill health and housing conditions.

There have been methodological problems in disentangling the role of housing from poverty, unemployment, working conditions, behavioural factors believed to be more prevalent in low-income groups such as smoking, as well as the selection of people in poor health into poor housing and disadvantaged areas. Council tenants, for example, tend to have higher rates of illness than owner-occupiers, to die at younger ages and to report greater distress in their daily lives (Hunt *et al.*, 1985; Whitehead, 1987). Fox and Goldblatt (1982) demonstrated that in 1971–75 there was a gradient in standardised mortality rates relating to tenure, and reported an SMR of 91 for owner-occupiers compared with 114 for local authority tenants. By 1981–89, analyses from the same Longitudinal Study suggested that differences across tenure groups had increased in relative and absolute terms, particularly for those aged under 65 (Filakti and Fox, 1995). A similar gradient was found for morbidity (McCormick *et al.* 1995) – people living in council or other rented accommodation were more likely to consult their GP for serious illnesses, a finding that was confirmed by multivariate analyses adjusted for social class, unemployment and numerous other socio-economic conditions. A higher proportion of people aged 16–64 renting accommodation consulted than those in owner-occupied premises for diseases in every ICD chapter of illness apart from neoplasms. The differences were most pronounced for mental diseases, but were also large for circulatory, digestive and musculoskeletal diseases. Tenure could be regarded as an indicator either of low income or of unhealthy housing. However, such a link is culture bound, because, in other countries, such as Germany and the United States of America, where owner occupation is less common and less prized, rented accommodation is generally of good quality and inhabited by those on high and middle incomes as well as those on low.

There are issues concerned with the ways in which health problems are defined. There has been a preference for a case-finding approach where a pre-existing diagnosis (for example, tuberculosis or asthma, can be linked to housing. However, some diagnoses are controversial, as is the case with asthma) and diagnoses and diagnostic categories are subject to fads and fashions (Heasman and Lipworth, 1966; Allander and Rosenquist, 1975). Moreover, diagnosis requires a doctor and it is known that a great deal of illness is self-treated and symptoms must pass some threshold of severity or 'normality' before they are seen as needing medical attention (see Chapter 2). It follows from this that those individuals who experience symptoms on a regular basis may be less likely to seek attention. For example, a recent study of several thousand adults and children in Canada found a much closer relationship between clinically confirmed respiratory symptoms and dampness/mould than between dampness and doctor-diagnosed asthma (Dales *et al.*, 1991a).

Reliance on diagnostic instrumentation, such as measures of respiratory function or other indicators of physiological function, is misplaced unless their application can be rigidly controlled with respect to timing, place and observer error. Instruments are notoriously subject to error both in their readings and in the way that they are read (Grasbeck and Saris, 1969; Bradwell *et al.*, 1974; Hall *et al.*, 1976). In addition, many people are reluctant to comply with intrusive measures and lowered response rates lead to inevitable bias. Thus, a case-finding approach, although useful in some instances, may well underestimate the extent of ill health in a community.

Although it is difficult and expensive to gather information in special surveys, routinely recorded information such as that provided by the ONS General Household Survey can do no more than point to areas of investigation. The only way to obtain precise data is to conduct investigations upon specific individuals in specific houses and use the appropriate controls.

The bulk of contemporary work on housing and health has tended to focus on overcrowding in relation to infections and the effects on mental health of lack of space and privacy. Dampness, mould growth and dust mites have received increasing attention, as have cold indoor temperatures, noise and accidents in the home. The health of the homeless also gives cause for concern. Almost all this work has been conducted using special surveys rather than routine data, because of the need to control for confounding variables not collected in census and national surveys.

10.3.3 Overcrowding now

Population density is conventionally defined as the number of persons per unit space. The ratio of persons to space in dwellings has been calculated from census statistics since 1931, using the Registrar General's formula of two persons per habitable room, i.e. bedrooms and living rooms. Maximum allowable levels of density in dwellings, as laid down in the 1957 Housing Act and repeated in the 1985 Housing Act, follow this convention, counting children aged 1–10 years as half a person and making no allowance for infants. This formula does not take into account conditions that may affect the habitability of rooms. For example, in some substandard dwellings, rooms may become uninhabitable in the winter months because they are too expensive to heat to an adequate level. Where bedrooms suffer from dampness and mould, children may have to share the parents' bedroom or the family may live entirely in one room, even though there are other notionally 'habitable' rooms in the dwelling. On the other hand, the Housing Act does not consider that some rooms defined as 'non-habitable', such as kitchens, can be and often are used for socialisation and other leisure activities.

Figure 10.2 shows that the number of persons living at densities greater than 1.5 persons to a room declined steadily from 1951 to 1991 as a result of a greater number of dwellings and smaller families. In 1991, the number of households with more than 1.5 persons per room was only 0.4 per cent of the total in England and Wales, representing 109,302 households. Overcrowding is greatest in rented furnished accommodation and almost four times as great in Scotland as in England and Wales. Northumberland and Durham remain the most crowded areas in England, whereas the rural counties of Buckinghamshire, Cambridgeshire and Cheshire are the least crowded. The policy of putting homeless people into temporary accommodation in bed-and-breakfast hotels has been responsible for an upsurge in local overcrowding. Some controversy exists concerning the relation between available space and risk of infection. Many common infections are spread through contamination of the air. These include measles, mumps, chickenpox, diphtheria and most respiratory conditions, including pulmonary tuberculosis (Riley, 1974; Mayon-White, 1992). The common cold, which can be transmitted directly by droplet contact and through the air (Burge, 1989), may be more easily spread when a room is shared with others (Jaakola *et al.*, 1990).

Skin infections, such as scabies, which are passed on by physical contact, are likely to be more common in crowded conditions. Early studies of overcrowding and infection reported strong positive associations between them. However, these associations were mediated by poverty and poor living conditions. Currently, very little is known about the independent effects of overcrowding on physical health.

Transmission of infection within a dwelling is affected by more than just the ratio of people to rooms. Patterns of contact between household members and between them and other people play a part, including the sharing of beds, intimate contacts between adults and play contact between children. Sanitary conditions and general hygiene and cleanliness, including shared amenities such as kitchens and toilets, will affect risk. Infectious diseases, especially the childhood diarrhoeas, are now common in bed-and-breakfast accommodation where facilities for storage, cooking and toiletting are all shared and where responsibilities for cleaning are ambiguous (Connelly *et al.*, 1991). Using data from the General Household Survey, Haynes (1991) found that the highest age-standardised level of for acute illness was for women living in multiple occupation dwellings in the inner city.

Although the question of causation must remain open, a number of recent studies have suggested strong associations between overcrowding in childhood and adult risk of disease. A follow-up of a national sample of over 5,000 men and women from birth to age 36 years showed that overcrowding (more than two persons per room) at the age of 2 years was one of four factors independently associated with adult respiratory disorder (Britten *et al.*, 1987). Short stature and adult heart disease have also been linked to overcrowding in the childhood home (Barker and Osmond, 1986; Kuh and Wadsworth, 1989). Using data from death certificates in England and Wales over a 10-year period and census data

from place of birth, Barker *et al.* (1990) found deaths from stomach cancer to be significantly linked to domestic crowding in childhood and suggested that this may have been a consequence of small houses lacking food storage facilities – this could possibly be linked with *Helicobacter pylori* (see Chapter 15). Williams (1991), using ONS data, found that mortality rates from cancer, circulatory disease, respiratory illness, accidents and violence to women increased as persons per room exceeded one. However, the explication of associations such as these must wait upon more precise investigation.

10.3.4 Damp and cold housing

Twin problems which have attracted interest in recent years are the effects of cold and damp housing on health. These problems are a consequence of poor quality construction, cheap materials and inappropriate renovations, with lack of insulation and adequate ventilation, combined with expensive and inappropriate heating systems. There has also been a rise in the cost of fuel relative to income, which has created fuel poverty estimated to affect some 8 million households (Boardman, 1991). In Glasgow, in 1991, the families with the lowest incomes spent 24 per cent of their household budget on heating compared with the 3.2 per cent spent by the wealthiest households (Satsangi and MacLennan, 1991). In Scotland about 33.4 per cent of public sector housing stock is subject to dampness, with figures being much higher in parts of Glasgow (City of Glasgow, 1989; Scottish Development Department, 1978, 1984). About 22 per cent of English housing is damp, most of such houses being in the north (DOE, 1991).

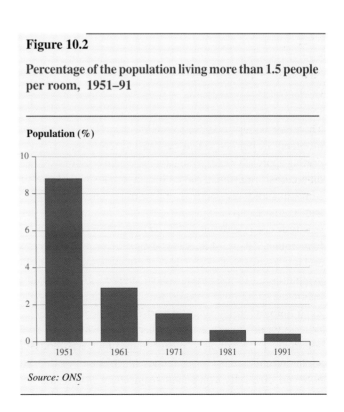

Figure 10.2

Percentage of the population living more than 1.5 people per room, 1951–91

Population (%)

Source: ONS

10.3.5 Dampness, mould growth and health status

Damp conditions in a dwelling encourage the presence of several agents which might be damaging to health. Viruses that give rise to infection are more common in damp houses (Buckland and Tyrell, 1962; Hatch *et al.,* 1976). Bacteria, too, thrive in moist conditions, although very little work has been done in relation to their presence in domestic dwellings (Kingdom, 1960).

Damp conditions, particularly condensation, are conducive to the growth and proliferation of fungal spores, which thrive on the organic material on walls and in cavities, such as plaster, wallpaper and wallpaper paste. Once present, mould spreads easily to carpets, furniture and clothing. Fungal spores can give rise to three types of reactions: allergies, infections and toxic effects. Moulds have long been known to be a source of respiratory allergens and there are case studies describing reactions so severe as to require hospitalisation (Solomon, 1974; Kozak *et al.,* 1980; Torok *et al.,* 1981; Pedersen and Gravesen, 1983; Fergusson *et al.,* 1984).

Several larger-scale investigations have indicated that mould may be responsible for respiratory conditions which are a consequence of allergic reactions, such as asthma, rhinitis and alveolitis (Maunsell, 1954; Hosen, 1978; Fergusson, *et al.,* 1984; Strachan and Elton, 1986; Burr *et al.,* 1988). Fungi of the genera *Alternaria, Cladosporium, Penicillium* and *Aspergillus* appear to be the most significant in causing allergic reactions. *Aspergillus fumigatus* and other *Aspergillus* species can produce bronchial aspergillosis, which is characterised by asthma and pulmonary eosinophilia and can give rise to acute illness with severe symptoms, typically fever and wheezing, sometimes superimposed upon the chronic form of the disease (Wardlaw and Geddes, 1992). All these genera have been found in domestic dwellings (Hunter *et al.,* 1988; Hunt and Lewis, 1989).

Responses to the inhalation of fungal spores can range from mild through acute and severe, with 'flu-like' symptoms, to irreversible changes in lung function after chronic exposure (Tobin *et al.,* 1987). Certain fungi produce metabolites which can be toxic. These mycotoxins are contained in the spores of toxigenic fungi and have been established as causes of illness in humans and animals (Smith and Moss, 1985). Reports of human reactions have been mainly associated with ingestion rather than inhalation. However, food may become contaminated by fungi in domestic dwellings and spores may well be swallowed with mucus especially where, in the presence of respiratory problems, there is a tendency for breathing to be done through the mouth. Mycotoxins are readily absorbed through the membranes in the respiratory tract and enter the bloodstream causing damage to other parts of the body. Their presence in the lungs may interfere with immunity and contribute to diffuse alveolitis (Northup and Kilburn, 1978). As mycotoxins can affect the immune system they may also contribute to the severity of allergies and infections.

The development of reactions to fungi requires repeated exposure, which can be expected to occur where dwellings are perpetually or recurrently damp. As the severity of the effects may be related to the vulnerability of the person, young children, elderly people and those who are already ill are particularly at risk.

A double-blind study carried out in Edinburgh, involving independent assessments of housing conditions and the health status of the occupants, found significant links between aches and pains, diarrhoea, headaches and respiratory complaints and the presence of visible mould in the house. This study also showed that the damp conditions could not be attributed to the behaviour of the inhabitants, but rather were related to the type and location of the building and, in some cases, to the types of renovations which had been carried out (Hunt *et al.*, 1986; Martin *et al.*, 1987).

A much larger, double-blind study by the same team (Hunt *et al.*, 1988; Hunt and Lewis, 1989; Platt *et al.*, 1989) carried out in three cities, showed significant and severe effects associated with the presence of mould on walls and in the air, including symptoms of allergy and infection such as fever, sore throat, headache and respiratory complaints, aching joints, nausea and breathlessness. There was a dose-response relationship between mould and symptoms, that is, the greater the extent of mould on the walls and the higher the air spore count, the more symptoms were reported for both adults and children. These results were independent of income, smoking, unemployment, cooking and washing facilities, and the presence of pets. The authors were also able to rule out investigator, respondent and selection bias in the explanation of the findings.

The findings from the previous two studies were strongly supported by a Canadian investigation of over 13,000 children and 15,000 adults, which found that the prevalence of respiratory symptoms in homes with mould and damp was greater than in those homes that were dry, with an odds ratio for adults of 1.56 for asthma, 1.62 for lower respiratory complaints and 1.50 for upper respiratory problems, adjusted for smoking, age, sex, heating system and location of the dwelling (Dales *et al.*, 1991a.,b).

A study by Hyndman (1990) of dwellings in Tower Hamlets, which used subjective and objective measures of both health status and housing conditions, also found strong associations between dampness/mould and respiratory symptoms, diarrhoea, vomiting, depression and general health.

In probably the largest longitudinal study of its kind, residents on a housing estate in Glasgow were interviewed before and after the installation of a new heating system in some of the dwellings. There was a general decline in health status in the area during the period of the study, but the results showed convincingly that children living in the warmer homes were protected from those symptoms which previous studies had shown to be associated with dampness/mould, i.e. wheeze, sore throat, headaches and persistent cough (Hopton and Hunt, 1996).

These investigations succeeded in controlling for relevant confounding variables such as income, other household characteristics and behavioural factors, and indicate the feasibility of combining social epidemiological investigations with independent environmental monitoring.

It could be argued that the evidence with respect to domestic mould and symptoms of ill health now meets most of the nine criteria set out by Bradford Hill (1965) for the interpretation of data as indicative of causation, that is, the associations are very strong, particularly with respect to respiratory symptoms; the findings are consistent, even in different countries; the associations are specific and the mouldy conditions pre-date the development of symptoms; there is a biological gradient as represented by a dose-response curve; and the findings are biologically plausible and coherent. Although it is not possible to carry out true experiments, information obtained before and after remedial actions which removed mould is indicative of causation and removal of an affected person from a mouldy house clears up the symptoms.

10.3.6 House dust mites

Dampness also encourages the house dust mite population which increases dramatically in damp conditions (Voorhorst *et al.*, 1969; Maunsell *et al.*, 1970). Mites flourish in 40 per cent or more humidity (Korsgaard, 1979), and their debris, particularly faecal pellets, act as allergens (Reed, 1981). The major problems caused by house dust mites are respiratory, especially wheeze and they are thus of particular concern in asthma (Dorward *et al.*, 1988). There is seasonal fluctuation with the greatest infestation occurring towards the end of the summer months. Faecal pellets of the mites *Dermatophagoides pternonyssinus* and *D. farinae* have been associated with asthma (Platt-Mills and Chapman, 1987) whereas allergens contained on the body of mites are thought to be of relevance in eczema (Carswell and Thompson, 1987).

A graded dose-response relationship has been found between mite-specific IgE levels and asthma (Shibasaki *et al.,* 1988) and most young asthmatic individuals show skin sensitivity to allergens from house dust mites. Experiments involving the direct inhalation of dust mites have detected significant bronchial reactivity in asthmatic people (M'Raihi *et al.,* 1990; Ostergaard *et al.,* 1990). Removal from exposure to dust mite allergens leads to a decline in symptoms (Kerrebijn, 1970; Platt-Mills and Chapman, 1987). Thus, there is evidence that house dust mites are one of the causative elements in asthma but it has not proved possible to define levels at which people are at risk of disease. Exposure during the first year of life may be an important factor in later occurrence of asthma (Sporik *et al.,* 1990) but this has yet to be confirmed.

10.3.7 Cold

Investigations by Hunt *et al.* (1988) and Hopton and Hunt (1990) in Scotland revealed that over 70 per cent of respondents from deprived areas reported that their dwelling was 'too cold'. A survey of 1,000 dwellings in Scotland found mean whole house temperatures of 14°C compared with an average of 16°C in England and Wales, 18°C in France and 21°C in Sweden (Hunt and Gidman, 1982). Murie (1983) suggested that any health problems associated with cold housing were more likely to be a consequence of insufficient income to heat the house adequately, not a direct result of the characteristics of the house. However, although the ability to maintain adequate indoor temperatures depends upon the climate, the expectations and the disposable income of the occupants, it is also closely related to the available heating system, its cost, how quickly heat is lost to the outside and the position and structure of the building.

10.4 Health implications of cold housing

An excess number of winter deaths has been noted for some time. Mortality tends to increase after a cold spell, particularly from myocardial infarction, strokes and respiratory conditions (Bull and Morton, 1978). There were 50,000 extra deaths between October 1985 and March 1986 compared with the previous six summer months (OPCS, 1988).

It is not easy to establish minimum temperatures below which risks to health arise, because of ethical barriers to experimentation. The World Health Organisation (1987) recommended a minimum air temperature for sick, handicapped, very old and very young people of 20°C, but reached no conclusion about the average indoor temperature necessary to maintain health in the general population.

Elderly persons are particularly at risk because they are more likely to have a sedentary life, not to be in employment, to spend more time at home and to have low incomes. They are also at a physiological disadvantage by reason of age-related illnesses, a diminishing body mass, greater immobility and the taking of medication. It has been suggested that elderly people are also more likely to live in energy-inefficient homes with low average temperatures (Boardman, 1991).

People who live in homes that are hard to heat, where heating is expensive and especially where household income is low, are inclined to heat one room to a comfortable temperature (if possible) and to economise by partially heating, or not heating at all, other rooms. In this case the temperature in bedrooms and bathrooms can fall so low as to constitute a serious health hazard. In 1972 a national survey found that 90 per cent of 1,000 elderly people had morning living room temperatures below the recommended level and 47 per cent did not heat their bedrooms at all (Wicks, 1978).

10.4.1 Hypothermia

Hypothermia is most common in elderly people and infants. It increases with low external temperatures, and has been linked to indoor temperatures below 16°C, although it makes a relatively small contribution to excess winter mortality (Sainsbury, 1983; Collins, 1986). It is possible that the death rate is higher than that officially recorded because of failure to diagnose the condition in some cases.

With the exception of investigations of hypothermia in elderly people there have been no systematic studies of the impact of cold housing *per se* on health status. The evidence for such a relationship is currently indirect.

10.4.2 Cold and respiratory function

Exposure to severe cold gives rise to increased pulmonary flow resistance and a decreased forced expiratory volume in sensitive people (Martin, 1967). Cold air can act as a direct trigger of bronchospasm (Strachan and Sanders, 1989) and Rasmussen *et al.* (1991) found cold to be linked with impaired lung function in men as measured by forced expiratory volume; the findings being independent of smoking. A rapid change in temperature produces greater respiratory effects than a gradual one. Thus, moving between warm and cold rooms, e.g. as at bedtime, is particularly stressful.

A report of the World Health Organization indicated that chilling of the body was associated with increased risk of upper respiratory tract infections and that the breathing of cold air increases the risk of respiratory problems in babies (WHO, 1982). Collins (1986) estimated that diminished resistance to respiratory infections occurred at indoor temperatures below 16°C.

A study by Blackman *et al.* (1989) in Belfast linked recurrent illness to reports that the respondent had been unable to keep warm the previous winter. Hyndman (1990) in her study of Bengalis in East London showed that both measured and reported low temperatures in the home were closely associated with symptoms of 'hidden asthma' and that people in cold homes were twice as likely to have poor chest health. It has also been suggested that cold affects the prevalence of viruses, because influenza epidemics often occur after a particularly cold spell (MacFarlane, 1977). The effects of temperature variations on health are discussed in some detail in Chapters 12 and 13.

10.4.3 Cold and risk of heart disease

In Sweden, mortality from ischaemic heart disease is related to the degree of cold exposure experienced in an area (Gyllerup, 1987). Several countries show a north-south gradient, with deaths from ischaemic heart disease increasing in the more northerly direction as the climate becomes colder (West *et al.*, 1973; Pyorala *et al.*, 1977; *British Medical Journal*, 1980; Akerblom, 1987; Balarajan *et al.*, 1987;

Tunstall-Pedoe, 1989). Daily deaths in England and Wales increase from 4.9 to 6.9 per million for myocardial infarction and from 3.2 to 4.8 per million for strokes when the minimum daily temperature falls from 17°C to -5°C (Bull and Morton, 1978). A recent investigation established that in one Scottish region 25 per cent of excess winter deaths from cardiovascular diseases occurred in the community rather than in hospital (Douglas and Rawles, 1989).

Two important risk factors for heart disease – hypertension and elevated fibrinogen levels – are associated with low temperatures. It has been suggested that the cardiovascular changes which perpetuate hypertension may result from peaks or acute surges in blood pressure rather than from sustained high levels (*Lancet,* 1983). Thus, repeated exposure to cold could be a factor in the development of essential hypertension, especially in predisposed individuals.

The risk of ischaemic heart disease is related to plasma fibrinogen levels and the general viscosity of the blood. Several epidemiological studies have produced prospective data on fibrinogen concentrations and cardiovascular events at a later time (Wilhelmsen *et al.,* 1984; Stone and Thorp, 1985; Meade *et al.,* 1986; Kannel *et al,* 1987). Fibrinogen concentration is positively correlated with other risk factors such as age, hypertension, smoking, diabetes, body mass index and low levels of physical exercise. Nevertheless, fibrinogen appears to be an independent risk factor for cardiovascular disease. Recent studies have established that fibrinogen levels are raised before transient ischaemic attacks (Qizilbash *et al.,* 1991; Coull *et al.,* 1991). Cold increases the number of circulating platelets, the packed cell volume and the blood viscosity (Keatinge *et al.,* 1984). A recent study of elderly people found seasonal changes in fibrinogen and plasma viscosity, with fibrinogen being significantly and negatively related to measures of environmental temperature. The authors concluded that the variation in plasma fibrinogen was large enough to increase the risk of both myocardial infarction and stroke during the winter months (Stout and Crawford, 1991).

Controversy exists as to whether the link between respiratory and heart conditions and cold is in relation to the external or internal temperature: going out into the cold with inadequate protection or inhabiting a dwelling that is consistently below a minimum temperature. These explanations are not, of course, mutually exclusive and there is evidence to support both views. Woodhouse *et al.* (1993) have shown that a decrease in internal temperature of only 1°C was associated with a rise in both systolic and diastolic blood pressure in persons over 65 years of age.

The figures for 1976–79 show an average rise in deaths in February of 24 per cent in Britain, 6 per cent in France and Sweden, and 8 per cent in the United States of America. All have cold winters. Sweden and parts of the USA have much lower winter temperatures but also have better insulated and heated homes (Wicks, 1978). On the other hand, excess deaths are not confined to those living in cold homes (Keatinge *et al.,* 1984).

Data from Finland have suggested that the decline in heart disease in that country is closely associated with improvements made to the housing stock, such as adequate affordable heating, increased insulation and appropriate ventilation (Salonen *et al.,* 1983; Tuomilheto *et al.,* 1986).

10.5 Poor housing and mental health

Adverse influences on mental health may stem from a number of housing conditions, such as dampness and mould, cold, noise, crowding and lack of play space, poor repair and feelings of insecurity.

At least two studies have shown that people who live in 'difficult to let' housing experience poorer emotional well-being than people in 'better' areas (Keithley *et al.,* 1984; Blackman *et al.,* 1989). In the latter study, men in poor housing areas were three times as likely to have symptoms of emotional distress and women twice as likely compared with people in better housing areas. In the MSGP4 study the largest morbidity differences by tenure were for mental health (McCormick *et al.,* 1995).

In relation to specific conditions, noise, particularly unpredictable, intermittent and uncontrollable noise, such as that emanating from noisy neighbours or traffic, can have deleterious psychological effects (Gloag, 1980). Sleep disturbance as a consequence of noise can impair performance on cognitive tests and lead to irritability, poor concentration and slower reaction times (Bastenier *et al.,* 1975). A survey of dwellings built in the 1970s showed that nearly half failed the performance standards laid down in the Building Regulations (Sewell and Scholes, 1978). In London these regulations do not apply at all. Therefore, it is likely that a significant proportion of the population is suffering the effects of noise, although a sound epidemiological study remains to be carried out.

Brown and Harris (1978) found damp housing to be associated with depression in women, and Hyndman (1990) also reported a strong association between both objective and subjective measures of dampness and reported depression. Data from over 800 women in local authority housing in Glasgow, Edinburgh and London showed significant relationships between damp housing and scores on the General Health Questionnaire (GHQ) (Goldberg, 1972) which indicated severe emotional distress (Platt *et al.,* 1989). This finding was independent of social class, employment status and household income. Using these and other data, Hunt (1990) showed that, as the number of housing problems (independently assessed) increased, so did scores on the GHQ as well as other symptoms of mental distress such as 'bad nerves', 'feeling low' and feeling irritable. These findings were replicated in the study by Hopton and Hunt (1990) which also controlled for age, sex, long-term illness and housing benefits.

Crowding is known to have deleterious effects on mental health. Enforced social contact can lead to irritability and tension and creates emotional disturbance in children, such that interaction with other children is limited and social development may be affected (Hartup, 1978). Being in the continual presence of others has been shown to impose mental strain on both children and adults and can impair the potential for satisfactory social relations (Wolfe and Golan, 1976). There is some evidence that children from more densely populated homes display more aggression and have poorer educational attainment and mental adjustment (Murray, 1974; Rutter, 1974).

The amount of internal space interacts with access to external space. This will also be affected by climate, with people in warmer parts of the country having more options for spending time outside than those in colder and wetter areas. An important factor in crowding is the availability of 'escape routes' so that individuals do not feel psychologically trapped. The ability to gain easy access to the outside has been shown to be a crucial variable in whether or not people feel crowded (Wilner *et al.,* 1969).

If children can 'play out', the mother can gain respite and privacy and the children can indulge in a greater range of behaviours than they could indoors. However, the availability of a garden, yard or play area does not guarantee that it can or will be used, as this will depend, to some extent, on weather conditions and on actual and perceived dangers, such as being located near a busy road or in an area of high crime. Several studies have found that there is a reluctance to allow children living in high-rise flats to go outside without supervision (Marcus, 1974).

Fanning (1967) found that young wives living in flats were more likely to consult a doctor with emotional symptoms than comparable women who lived in houses. A study by Stewart (1970) confirmed this and it was concluded that mothers with young children living in tower blocks were more likely to suffer from social isolation and psychiatric disturbance compared with those living in houses. However, two well controlled studies indicated that the underlying reason for this was dissatisfaction with living conditions, i.e. the findings were reflective of emotional distress rather than mental illness (Ineichen and Hooper, 1974; Richman, 1974). This explanation is given weight by the fact that living in high-rise dwellings is more common in some countries and appears to have no deleterious effects. The most important conclusion would seem to be that circumstances which suit some people may be distressing for others and that young families, elderly people and those who are handicapped may suffer from isolation and feelings of being 'trapped' if they are housed in multi-storey accommodation.

An investigation in New Zealand combined several housing 'stressors' such as noise, cold, presence of pests and state of disrepair, and found that living in a substandard dwelling represented an independent and additive source of stress (as measured by the GHQ) for low-income urban dwellers (Smith *et al.,* 1993).

The OPCS Survey of Psychiatric morbidity in Great Britain, conducted for the Department of Health in 1993 found that symptoms of psychological distress were more prevalent in people in rented accommodation (Meltzer *et al.*, 1995):

Compared with women who owned their own homes, women who rented from an LA or HA were more than twice as likely to have depression, depressive ideas, and panic. The same comparison among men showed that those who rented from an LA or HA were more than twice as likely to have experienced worry, depressive ideas, poor concentration and forgetfulness, somatic symptoms, compulsions, phobias and panic. Depressive ideas were about three times more prevalent among LA and HA renters than among those who owned their homes outright. Renters in the private sector were also more likely to have any symptom of emotional distress than owner-occupiers.

These findings were confirmed in a multivariate analysis that simultaneously allowed for the effects of sex, age, ethnicity, marital status, terminal age of education, educational level, employment status, social class, family unit type, type of accommodation, region and locality. When the prevalence of clinically confirmed psychiatric disorders was analysed by housing tenure it was found that the prevalence of panic disorders, generalised anxiety disorders, mixed anxiety/depression, functional psychoses and drug dependence were significantly greater among those renting their accommodation, even when all the other factors described above were controlled for.

10.6 Accidents

Accidents in the home are a significant cause of death and injury. About 5,000 fatal accidents and 3 million accidents requiring medical attention occur in Britain each year. Over 40 per cent of deaths are attributable to falls (DTI, 1989). These occur predominantly in elderly people because they are particularly vulnerable to injury if they do fall (OPCS, 1988). A high proportion of falls in the home have been attributed to inadequate lighting and it has been estimated that 60 per cent of British homes have insufficient light for ordinary purposes (Mant and Muir Gray, 1986). Other features of a dwelling can contribute to serious and fatal falls, for example, long, straight flights of stairs, lack of stair handrails and doors that open on to stairs.

Poor housing also contributes to the likelihood of death and injury from fire by faulty electric wiring and dangerous cooking and heating facilities, by limiting the ease of escape and by giving rise to toxic fumes (Chandler et al, 1984). The relative risk of fatality from fire in houses in multiple occupation compared with those housing a single family is about 50:1 (Acheson, 1991).

About a quarter of a million children are admitted to hospital each year following an accident at home mainly as a consequence of burns and scalds (Page, 1986).

10.6.1 Cooking and heating appliances

Gases given off by cooking and heating appliances, especially nitrogen dioxide and carbon monoxide, can pose risks to health. The bulk of studies on the topic have been epidemiological. For example, a national survey on the use of gas cookers, which can pollute indoor air with nitrogen dioxide, found some relationship between gas appliances and respiratory problems in children (Melia *et al.*, 1979). However, such studies have often failed to take into account a sufficient number of confounding and interacting variables. Special surveys have found elevated indoor levels of nitrogen dioxide in homes with inadequately vented gas appliances, associated with pulmonary oedema, bronchoconstriction and increased infection rates (Spengler and Sexton, 1983; Samet *et al.*, 1987).

Raised carbon monoxide levels can result from gas cookers, particularly when they are used for heating a room. This is not an uncommon practice in low-income families, especially elderly people, where the dwelling is hard to heat, and there can be effects on oxygen uptake in the blood. In extreme cases unvented gas fires have resulted in death from carbon monoxide poisoning (Spengler and Sexton, 1983). However, reviews of the relatively large number of epidemiological investigations in Britain and elsewhere have failed to find consistent results where circumstances are not unusual and have concluded that, if there is an effect from cooking and heating appliances, it is likely to be too small to be a health hazard at concentrations encountered in most homes (ECAO, 1982; Samet, *et al.*, 1988).

10.7 Homelessness

Local authorities in England and Wales accepted 133,328 households as homeless in 1991. This represents almost half a million individuals and is almost certainly an underestimate both because of the limitations of the qualifying criteria (one being that a person is 'unintentionally' homeless) and because of the considerable discretion with which the criteria are applied. The percentage of acceptances in relation to enquiries ranges from 24 per cent in south Somerset to 67 per cent in Lincoln, and the Audit Commission (1989) found that 'discretion' accounted for 20–25 per cent of the variation between local authorities. Clearly, many more people feel themselves to be effectively homeless than are accepted as being so by the statutory authorities. An investigation in Scotland found that figures from the Scottish Office on homeless families had seriously under estimated the true numbers (Johnston, 1991).

The relationship between homelessness and health is complicated by a number of factors, not least the fact that ill health can be a cause of homelessness; for example, discharge from psychiatric hospital without adequate provision of alternative shelter (Marshall, 1989), inability to keep up mortgage repayments because of loss of employment (Ford, 1988), or because of the disadvantage experienced by disabled and ill people in finding suitable accommodation (Smith, 1990).

However, there is evidence that homelessness itself may give rise to ill health as a consequence of three main factors: the environment inhabited, health-related behaviour and access to health care, of which only the first will be considered here.

10.7.1 Environmental factors

Homeless people may be literally 'roofless', that is, living in the streets, occasionally finding a night's accommodation in common lodging houses, or they may be in temporary accommodation such as a 'bed and breakfast' hotel. In both these situations individuals are likely to be exposed to hazards associated with housing in their most extreme form: inadequate shelter, cold, dampness, overcrowding, sharing inadequate facilities with unrelated others, noise, insecurity and risk of accidents.

In March 1991, 37,971 London households were in temporary accommodation. A national survey of such accommodation showed that a substantial proportion of bed and breakfast hotels provided unsuitable accommodation, with an average of 16 people sharing a bath or shower and 20 sharing one WC. Twenty six per cent of the hotels were found by Environmental Health Officers to be lacking or inadequate in the provision of drinking water, food storage and cooking facilities (Thomas and Niner, 1989). A survey in London found 61 per cent of bed and breakfast accommodation to be overcrowded, with two or more people to a room. Almost half posed a risk of fire with inadequate escape routes (BABIE, 1989).

There is considerable evidence for the relatively poor health of the homeless, in particular, susceptibility to infectious diseases such as pulmonary tuberculosis (Shanks and Carroll, 1982, 1984). They are at increased risk of musculoskeletal conditions and dermatological complaints (Shanks, 1988; Toon *et al.*, 1987). Homeless women are vulnerable to problems during pregnancy (Conway, 1988) and their children are prone to behavioural disturbance, high levels of illness and infection, and are at increased risk of accidents (Boyer, 1986; Lovell, 1986; *British Medical Journal*, 1987; Richman *et al.*, 1991). At least two investigations have found higher than average rates of use of hospital services by the 'temporarily' homeless (Victor *et al.*, 1989).

Given that many homeless people have undergone stressful experiences before their homelessness, that homelessness in itself may give rise to harmful behaviours, such as excessive smoking and alcohol consumption, and that accessibility to health care for the homeless is recognised to be inadequate, it is difficult to disentangle cause and effect. However, it seems reasonable to conclude that, whatever health problems may have existed before the experience of homelessness, the additional health hazards posed by it are likely to exacerbate existing conditions and give rise to new ones. In particular, the long-term effects on children's health give cause for serious concern.

10.8 Conclusions

There is no doubt that over the past 150 years improvements in health have paralleled improvements in housing conditions. To what extent the latter has contributed to the former is impossible to answer. There are few diseases which are not multi-causal. The TB bacillus is the proximate cause of tuberculosis but measures such as proper sanitation, reasonably hygienic conditions, light and space affect the ability of the bacillus to spread and survive. Not everyone exposed to the TB bacillus will contract tuberculosis; like most other medical conditions it will tend to be found more frequently among those who have become vulnerable. One factor in this vulnerability will be environmental circumstances, lack of warmth, overcrowding, emotional and physical discomfort. Thus a dwelling may both contain pathogens and have other characteristics which enhance susceptibility to those pathogens.

The persisting links between low income and ill health have led some observers to doubt the role of housing in creating ill health. However, this would seem to beg the question of what it is about low income that makes individuals ill. Part of the answer must surely lie in the inability of disadvantaged individuals to gain access to good quality housing. Moreover, housing conditions may well interact with other factors which are also more common in low-income families, such as unemployment, hazardous occupations and smoking vulnerability.

Although the nature of substandard housing has changed in the last 15 decades, as has the nature of the health problems, some things have not changed. The most obvious is that the financially worst off, by and large, get the worst housing, sometimes none at all. Thus, those who need the most protection tend to get the least. Low-income households must spend a greater proportion of their time, money and energy in trying to make their homes habitable than those who are more affluent. In 1996, as in 1841, interest in building good quality homes for the poor is minimal or non-existent. The provision of housing by local authorities did much to get the poor off the streets and out of cellars, barns, hovels, overcrowded tenements and insanitary back-to-backs and into decent homes. Both the health statistics and the housing statistics reflect the beneficial effects of this policy. The 1991 Census shows the effects of the 'Right to Buy' policy. There are now on average 8.8 per cent fewer council dwellings in England and Wales than there were in 1981, but this hides extremes of 43 per cent fewer in the City of London, 25 per cent in Merseyside and 23 per cent in Tower Hamlets (Forrest and Gordon, 1993). Thus the availability of housing for low-income families is declining, a fact also endorsed by the rising figures for homelessness.

A further common theme is the tendency to blame those unlucky people who have inadequate homes or no homes for their own fate; an unpleasant characteristic which also shows itself with respect to ill health. This stratagem puts the responsibility for misfortune on the shoulders of the unfortunates themselves and absolves the rest from taking remedial action.

Routine figures have always been inadequate to disentangle the various factors that surround the issue of housing and health because important confounding variables are not recorded. Moreover, the type of information gathered and the tendency for epidemiology to focus upon the quantity of life has led to an unwarranted emphasis, in this country, on longevity and cause of death. An over emphasis on specific diseases and diagnoses has overshadowed the quality of people's lives and the sheer misery which can be a consequence of living day after day after day in adverse conditions. Although it is important to increase our understanding of ways in which specific housing conditions affect health, we should also place more emphasis on ways in which housing factors are intertwined in the whole fabric of social and environmental influences on health.

The growth of knowledge is rarely sudden and dramatic, rather it is the slow accumulation of information from different sources that persuades in such a way as to make something 'self-evident'. Historical and contemporary evidence clearly presents a case for housing as both a direct and an indirect cause of health problems. The issue now is how to integrate housing conditions into the mainstream of primary, secondary and tertiary prevention and to get it a place on the agenda of health policy.

Chapter 11

Family and household structure: the association of social support and living arrangements with health

By
Mike Murphy and John Charlton

Summary

- The importance of social support factors for health were examined by Farr in 1858. Marital status, role strain, social networks and geographical variations are strong themes of current research about living arrangements and health.

- Changes in household living arrangements, and perhaps attitudes, between 1841 and 1991 have accompanied changing patterns of marriage, divorce and workforce participation. Changing attitudes towards privacy and social mixing may also have been factors in the spread of infection and the development of some chronic diseases.

- We have examined the impact of family and household structures on health mainly using routine data sources, where coverage is almost complete. Special data collection studies are needed to investigate these social processes in more detail.

- The recording of marital status at death began early this century in Britain. Standardised mortality ratios for single, married, widowed and divorced people for ages 15–74 show the protection of the married, and that married men may be more protected than women.

- Hospital admissions data by age and marital status are available from the 1960s in Britain. Census population data, hospital discharge data and GHS data taken together provide an ambiguous picture of variation in hospitalisation and hospital usage. Caution must be observed in interpreting the results of such estimates because of methodological difficulties in computing the variables used in the definition of rates.

- Detailed information about morbidity in relation to marital status and living arrangements is available from the second, third and fourth studies of morbidity in general practice. The fourth national study introduced multivariate analysis to look at the impact of living arrangements on consultation rates.

- Measurements of self-reported health in ONS surveys have produced different associations with marital status and household characteristics. This may be due to variations in survey question wording. Evidence from the General Household Survey and Longitudinal Study data suggest that marital status and the presence of a partner independently affect a number of measures of health.

The family is the social unit; and it is founded in its perfect state by marriage. The influence of this form of existence is therefore one of the fundamental problems of social science. A remarkable series of observations, extending over the whole of France, enables us to determine for the first time the effect of conjugal condition on the life of a large population ... If unmarried people suffer from disease in undue proportion, the have-been-married suffer still more ... This is the general result: Marriage is a healthy estate. The single individual is more likely to be wrecked on his voyage than the lives joined together in matrimony. In what respect do the married among the masses of the people differ from the unmarried classes?

William Farr, 1858. The Influence of Marriage on the Mortality of the French People

11.1 Introduction

This chapter examines the reciprocal association between the social structure of families, households and, to a very limited extent, neighbourhoods, with health. The physical structure of housing and the economic position of households are also important; socio-economic trends are dealt with in Chapter 6, and changes in housing in Chapter 10. The socio-economic determinants of health will be the subject of a further ONS decennial volume. More general socio-economic influences on health, including material wealth and disposable income, are particularly difficult to disentangle from the influence of social support mechanisms within families, households and neighbourhoods (see Figure 6.14), and conclusions about the effects of social support as such may be difficult to draw.

Farr, in the mid-nineteenth century, was among the first to examine the importance of social factors for health (Farr, 1858). His discussion of the reasons for his findings is extensive, as is that of a contemporary, Rigoni-Stern, who investigated the relation of cancer incidence to marital status in Italy (Rigoni-Stern, 1842; Griffiths, 1991). Rigoni-Stern did not mention any possible influences of childbearing on the cancers he discussed, though we now believe them to be important. It is not only scientific understanding that has changed over the period we are considering, however, but attitudes, beliefs and meanings. 'Nubile' to Rigoni-Stern meant single (marriageable) and 'celibate' may have meant, simply, unmarried (Kiernan, 1988, 1989). Both have connotations of sexual activity today that they may have lacked then. Some may disagree with Farr's observation that 'the family is the social unit; and it is founded in its perfect state by marriage' or, as he said elsewhere, that the marriage rate is 'a barometer of national prosperity' (Haskey, 1987), but the social scientific observations made were seminal.

The divorced are mentioned by neither Farr nor Rigoni-Stern because they were so few. Table 11.1 shows the changing marital status composition of the England and Wales population over time, in particular the changing numbers of

the divorced. They had no separate existence in the census of England and Wales until 1921. It was only in 1857 that an Act made civil divorce possible without the necessity of introducing a private Act of Parliament (Haskey, 1987), before which only the very rich had access to divorce (see Figure 6.16). The health of the divorced is now of particular concern (McAllister, 1995).

Several strong themes of research about living arrangements and health have emerged (Macintyre, 1992; 1994).

1. Marital status (with or without cohabitation) is correlated with health, partly through the prevalence of risky health behaviours (Blaxter, 1990; Wyke and Ford, 1992; Joung *et al.*, 1995 a, 1996), partly through selection for marriage (divorce) and remarriage, and partly due to the potential benefit of a partnership. The health of single parents and their children, and the divorced in particular, may generally be poorer than that of others (Popay and Jones, 1990; Coombs, 1991; McAllister, 1995; Judge and Benzeval, 1993). The loss of a spouse or partner through death may have a real impact on the remaining partner, which then probably lessens with the passage of time (Martikainen and Volkonen, 1996).

2. Within marriage and cohabiting partnerships, the competing demands of employment, domestic and parenting responsibilities may create 'role-strain', but the effects of this on aspects of health are unclear. The effects may be greater for women, but disentangling the ways in which these different roles may create (or reduce) health problems is immensely complicated (Gove, 1974; Gove and Geerken, 1977; Glenn, 1975; Renne, 1971; Verbrugge, 1979; Verbrugge and Madans, 1985; Kandel *et al.*, 1985).

3. Social networks (contacts with neighbours, church and other social organisations, extended family, work contacts, etc.) appear to be important for good health. In recent decades the importance of social networks from a variety of different settings, social structures and contexts starting with the Alameda County Study has been confirmed (Berkman and Syme, 1979; Kawachi *et al.*, 1996; House *et al.*, 1988). A recent review has estimated the impact of social networks on cardiovascular mortality in middle-aged Danish men and found it to be comparable in size with that of traditional cardiovascular risk factors (Olsen, 1993). The nature of the problem makes it very difficult to address using routinely available data. We do not pursue it here further, but note it as an area of current research interest.

4. Geographical variations at the macro and micro level appear to be persistent (Britton, 1990). For instance, for many and complex reasons, the health of those living in inner city areas in England and Wales is poorer than that of those living in rural areas. This is one example of the way in which geography appears to be related to health independently of other socio-economic influences that

Table 11.1

Population and marital condition distribution (percentages), by sex and age at various censuses, England and Wales, 1851, 1921 and 1991

		1851		1921		1991	
		Males	**Females**	**Males**	**Females**	**Males**	**Females**
15–19	Single	100	97	100	98	99	98
	Married	0	3	0	2	0	2
	Widowed	0	0	0	0	0	0
	Divorced			0	0	0	0
	Total number	873,236	883,953	1,727,823	1,775,231	1,636,124	1,569,340
20–24	Single	80	69	82	73	88	76
	Married	20	31	18	27	11	23
	Widowed	0	0	0	0	0	0
	Divorced			0	0	1	2
	Total number	795,455	871,152	1,448,385	1,703,067	1,844,532	1,886,843
25–34	Single	36	33	34	34	42	29
	Married	63	64	65	63	53	63
	Widowed	2	3	1	3	0	0
	Divorced			0	0	5	8
	Total number	1,317,234	1,429,367	2,621,280	3,139,939	3,758,504	3,835,113
35–44	Single	16	16	15	19	14	8
	Married	79	76	83	75	76	79
	Widowed	4	8	2	6	0	1
	Divorced			0	0	9	12
	Total number	1,006,891	1,050,287	2,496,375	2,850,034	3,469,743	3,500,554
45–54	Single	11	12	12	16	9	5
	Married	80	72	83	72	81	80
	Widowed	8	16	5	11	1	4
	Divorced			0	0	9	11
	Total number	738,986	768,804	2,133,179	2,287,098	2,898,231	2,895,249
55–64	Single	10	11	10	15	8	6
	Married	75	59	78	60	81	72
	Widowed	15	30	11	25	4	14
	Divorced			0	0	7	7
	Total number	482,132	525,465	1,382,843	1,529,885	2,510,602	2,614,972
65–74	Single	9	11	9	14	8	7
	Married	63	40	65	39	78	54
	Widowed	29	49	25	47	11	35
	Divorced			0	0	4	4
	Total number	266,370	311,311	729,854	913,019	2,022,992	2,481,918
75–79	Single	8	11	7	13	6	9
	Married	49	24	50	21	70	33
	Widowed	43	65	42	65	21	56
	Divorced			0	0	2	3
	Total number	65,016	81,086	158,540	234,038	651,394	1,011,946
80 and over	Single	7	11	7	13	6	12
	Married	36	13	36	11	54	16
	Widowed	57	76	57	76	38	71
	Divorced			0	0	2	1
	Total number	44,929	62,112	91,836	163,818	563,173	1,312,660

Notes: *The divorced were not separately identified until the 1921 Census. Before that time no provision was made in the schedules for the return of divorced persons, and they were included in the other categories according to their census returns.*

Sources: *1851 Census, population tables II, volume I, p. cci.*
1921 Census, general tables, pp127–128, 138.
1991 Census.

can be easily measured (Dalgard, 1980). Disentangling relationships between material features of areas, and general levels of socio-economic status, is difficult, even today (Sawchuk, 1993; Mackenbach, 1993; Macintyre *et al.*, 1993). There is a long tradition of area-based analyses of mortality in particular, and the difficulties of analysing urban-rural differences over time are many (Fox and Goldblatt, 1982). Routine statistics allow areas to be characterised at different geographical levels, and by census–based indices of deprivation (Drever and Whitehead, 1995; Charlton, 1996; Eames *et al.*, 1993), but the importance of investigating the characteristics of individuals and the neighbourhoods in which they live is increasingly recognised (Sloggett and Joshi, 1994; Mcintyre *et al.*, 1993). This is an area of considerable current research interest, involving multi-level modelling, but is not covered in any detail in this chapter (Shouls *et al.*, 1996).

11.2 Changes in the social fabric

Britain was the first country in the world to experience mass urbanisation (see Chapter 6). In 1800, three quarters of the population of England and Wales lived in villages of 50–500 people, but by the end of the nineteenth century about three quarters lived in urban areas, a much higher proportion than in any other country. Urbanisation was also extremely rapid, and many of the problems of inner city areas today are related to the way in which cities developed in the nineteenth century (Allnutt and Gelardi, 1980). Our understanding of the social support offered by the rural communities left behind, and those joined and created in towns and cities, is fragmentary.

Figure 11.1

Household composition and crowding, 1801–1981

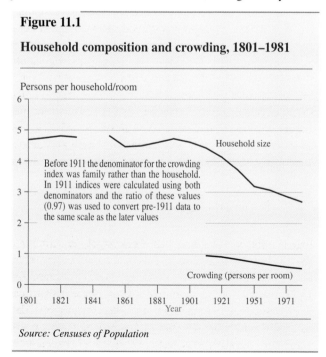

Source: Censuses of Population

By 1841, the start of the period covered by this book, towns and cities were massively overcrowded, social and housing conditions were abominable, and the poor, rural areas were denuded. The dead competed with the living for space to rest,

with 50,000 corpses interred in London each year (Healing *et al.*, 1995). Population density within buildings and in buildings per land unit increased and new meanings to neighbourhood and household must have emerged. Figure 11.1 shows one dimension of the problem, crowding within dwellings over time, as measured at successive censuses. Population density and concentrations have also changed over time (Craig, 1975; Dorling and Atkins, 1995).

In the last part of the nineteenth century, the growth of municipal and voluntary sector housing of a high standard alleviated the situation. The introduction of cheap public transport (see Figures 6.8 and 6.9) allowed the boundaries of cities and suburbs to expand. Movement from the centre to the periphery has continued since, though many working-class families remained at the urban centre. The problems of the urban sprawl and inner city decay are both aspects of the decentralisation that has taken place. New towns and cities, estates and high-rise buildings are largely postwar features of the scene, whereas slum clearance has been a continuous process (see Chapter 10), entailing displacement and disruption of previously well established neighbourhoods and communities.

It seems likely that the accompanying social changes over this period must have had an impact on health. We are hampered by a lack of detailed information for much of the period, but present what data there are on living arrangements and health, and review the evidence that they are related.

11.3 Changes in attitudes and 'connectedness'

While the physical living environment changed, different features of the changing social connections within this environmental context may have played a part in sustaining health and creating disease. Most people married, though the ages by which they had done so varied depending on circumstances. At the outset of marriage registration (in 1837) the minimum legal age for marriage was considerably lower than required today – 14 for boys and 12 for girls. But in fact fewer married at young ages then than now, probably because they could not afford to marry and leave the family home, and average age at marriage fluctuated around the mid-twenties throughout the period (Haskey, 1987) (see Figure 6.2). One of the biggest changes has been the marital status of those marrying. Widows and widowers have contributed a diminishing proportion from 1845 (apart from effects of wars), and recently there have been increases in divorced people remarrying. Reconstituted ('second') families have, therefore, been an enduring feature of society throughout the period.

When Farr observed that 'marriage is a healthy estate' he was careful to discuss several reasons for this observation, but he was expressing a current (if sentimental) view of the 'companionate' marriage. But it has been suggested that this was then a relatively recent perception of how individuals in such relationships might be expected to feel and behave towards one another. It had emerged over several hundreds of years, mirroring many changes in social organisation, including the prioritisation of the nuclear family as a feature of the more general growth of 'affective individualism' (Stone, 1990). While we may today, guardedly, have some affinity for this view of partnerships, it is not clear that even in the mid-nineteenth century it was shared among all classes equally, nor are all partnerships beneficial to health (Smith *et al., 1992)*. Even today, there are allegedly different cultural attitudes to children (manifest in attitudes to their survival), and these vary with the child's sex. The compromised attachment to children (and adults) where the risks of premature death were enormous and well known may have influenced the emotional quality of relationships in the nineteenth century.

Similar issues are raised in terms of attitudes to privacy; for the mass of people in the nineteenth century 'personal space' would have been virtually nonexistent by today's standards and perceived requirements. Would this have been a material factor affecting the quality of relationships, stress and mental health then as now? Certainly there seems little doubt that population density materially affected the risks of transmission of the major infectious diseases of the time, because of sheer crowding and proximity. The age-structure of households, with substantially greater numbers at young ages until the start of the twentieth century, may also have played a part (Reves, 1985; Knodel and Hermalin, 1984; Woods *et al.*, 1988, 1989) (see Figure 6.1). Living conditions may also have contributed directly to the development of some chronic diseases. Domestic pollution from cooking and heating with coal fires, and the increased risk of chronic obstructive pulmonary disease (COPD) have been referred to elsewhere in this book (see Chapters 9, 10, 12 and 20), as has the possible relation between overcrowding and social conditions in childhood generally, transmission of *Helicobacter pylori* infection and subsequent peptic ulcer (and perhaps gastric cancer) (see Chapters 9, 17 and 22). Indirectly, family size may protect women through hormonal mechanisms against breast, ovarian and endometrial cancers, but the combination of marriage by the early twenties with short life-spans probably meant really large average family sizes were only generally experienced in the nineteenth century.

A recently observed phenomenon is the increased risk of childhood leukaemia in populations formed by the rapid mixing of rural and urban groups, for instance in the new towns and among evacuees during the Second World War (Kinlen and John, 1994), which may suggest an infection as a cause of this rare disease. Urban-rural mixing was probably involved in the spread of many infectious diseases in the nineteenth century, as was possibly the Irish immigration (Mercer, 1990) (see Figure 6.3). No doubt there are other examples of the way in which changing aspects of the material living environment may have affected health over a century and a half.

Broader changes in the social composition of living arrangements that may have had an impact on health have also been apparent, particularly in the twentieth century.

Although in the mid-nineteenth century children may have contributed significantly, through their labour, to the household income, and functioned as 'little adults' in many respects, they are generally regarded as dependants today. Likewise with people over retirement age, although they may play an important part in the wider household economy (see Chapter 26 and Figure 6.5). Both groups arguably require more health care. The important role of family and neighbours in self-care and health maintenance, as well as indirectly supporting the health services (e.g. through allowing early discharge), has long been recognised. The break up of tightly knit neighbourhoods and communities may have prejudiced such informal support (Graham, 1991). Changes in family formation and retention patterns have altered the pattern of household composition. Three-generation households are even less common, and, with the growth of the elderly population, an increasing proportion live alone. The numbers of households headed by a lone adult have increased, particularly in recent years (see Figure 6.20), as have those households with no children. Changes in age at first cohabitation and at childbirth, with or without subsequent marriage, have also altered the pattern of relative ages of household members. Lone adults (whether single or married) continuing to live with parents may do so for health reasons, particularly as community care is promoted. Accompanying these household and family changes is the massive increase in divorce rates until the most recent period. About 4 in 10 marriages would end in divorce in England and Wales if divorce rates were to remain at recent levels, the highest rates in Europe. There has been a secular increase over the century, and rapid acceleration during the 1960s and early 1970s (England and Wales) and late 1970s (Scotland), with the introduction of major changes to divorce laws (see Figure 6.16). Divorce law reform has tended to have only a temporary effect on the underlying upward trends. Remarriage patterns and cohabitation influence the number of reconstituted (second) families and part-time parenting arrangements. Cohabitation and births outside marriage (currently 1 in 3) reinforce the complexity of living arrangements. Unemployment and changing employment patterns for men and women (see Figures 6.10, 6.11 and 6.19) will have had an impact on the morale and numbers of those available to undertake essential domestic tasks in households.

11.4 Data limitations

Examination of these issues has been largely undertaken in the postwar period, though Farr's pronouncement about marital status indicates the enduring interest in examining social statistics, about mortality at least. Some insights can be obtained using routine data from ONS, though special data collection studies are necessary to make real headway with unravelling the intricacies of the relationships between social position and health. In the following analyses we restrict attention to those under 75 because, for mortality data at least, marital status is apparently recorded with decreasing accuracy above that age. Also, the survey data used are usually based on private households and are thus more representative of people aged under 75 (see Chapter 26). Census and mortality data cover the whole population, general practice data cover those registered with GPs (nearly all), hospitalisation data cover people who use NHS hospitals and the GHS covers only residents in private households. Assessing the health of the whole population involves knowledge of the status of those within as well as outside institutions, and there have been major changes in institutional populations over the period considered (see Figure 6.6). Finally, detailed adjustment for age is necessary when comparing the experience of marital status/household groups because their age-structures differ in important ways. Adjustment for the confounding effects of more general socio-economic determinants of health would be desirable but is seldom possible.

11.5 Mortality data

Data about all-cause mortality in England and Wales by sex, age and marital status are available from 1911 (women) and 1938 (men) to 1973 in the Registrar General's annual reviews and from ONS (series DH1 volumes) for 1974 onwards. Population estimates by age, sex and marital status are available from 1981 to 1993, and for earlier years from the censuses. They were published from 1931 onwards in the Registrar General's Annual Reports. In most cases they were based on the previous decennial census, but were less reliable between 1930 and 1950 – the Registrar General's reports at the time describe the particular difficulties surrounding the creation of these estimates around the war years and before the introduction of the Population Statistics Act in 1938. The divorced were first enumerated separately at census in 1921, but it is only since 1961 that the widowed have been shown separately from the divorced in the mid-year population estimates. Mortality data about both are available from 1961 for men and 1959 for women. For the year 1981, when there was an industrial dispute involving local Registrars, data on marital status at death were considered unusable. For all other years, marital status at death was generally well recorded ('not

stated' were less than 1 per cent for women throughout the period, but only after 1961 were they about 1 per cent for men). For Scotland, similar population estimates were only published from 1958 onwards, and these show widowed and divorced separately only from 1968 (Registrar General's Annual Reports); we have used these published figures. Scottish mortality by marital status was available for both sexes since 1911, and marital status was unstated in a tiny proportion of deaths throughout the period. Using these data we calculated, for males and females separately, all-cause standardised mortality ratios (SMRs) for the single, married, widowed and divorced, for ages 15–74. Sex-specific rates in 5-year age-groups for the period 1971–75 in England and Wales were used as the standard in each case.

Figures 11.2–11.5 show that the married did better than all other groups throughout. The relative positions of single, widowed and divorced varied, but there were cyclical fluctuations between censuses in the accuracy of population estimates. There are also inaccuracies of statements about marital status at death compared with census enumeration (numerator-denominator bias). When numerator-denominator bias is allowed for the data still imply protection of the married for both sexes (Murphy, 1996). Moreover, men may be more protected by marriage than women (Riessman and Gerstel, 1985). This is irrespective of whether an additive or multiplicative excess risk is implied, when comparing the married with the non-married of each sex separately, and is apparent with both direct and indirect standardisation (not shown). Such all-cause mortality patterns are frequently observed, and are apparent for most individual causes of death (Hu and Goldman, 1990; Joung, 1996). The graphs that simply compare the mortality of the married with that of all others combined eliminate much of the numerator-denominator bias visually, though misclassification between married and 'other' remains. The data suggest a widening gap between the married and 'other' over time. This might be related to changing levels of bias, but is more likely to be real. Data from the Netherlands (Joung et al., 1996) and Hungary (Hajdu et al., 1995), though

Figure 11.2

All-cause mortality at ages 15–74 by sex and marital status, England and Wales, 1938–93

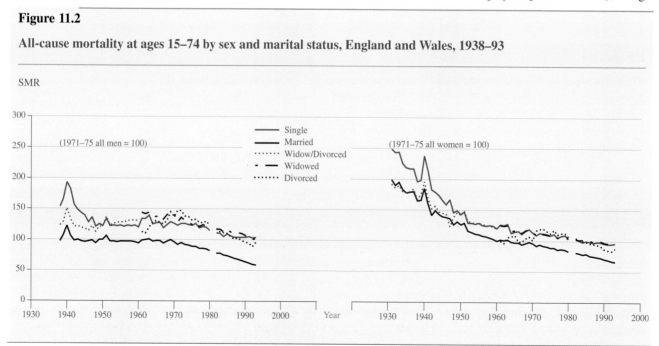

Figure 11.3

All-cause mortality at ages 15–74, by sex and whether married or not, England and Wales, 1938–93

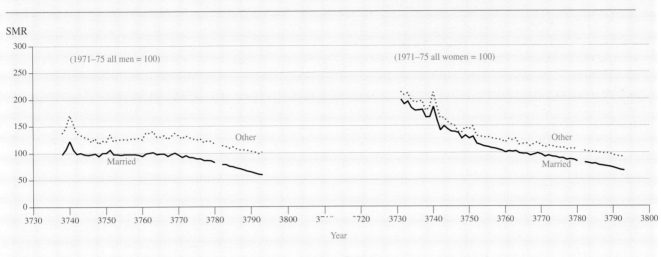

Figure 11.4

All-cause mortality at ages 15–74, by sex and marital status, Scotland, 1958–93

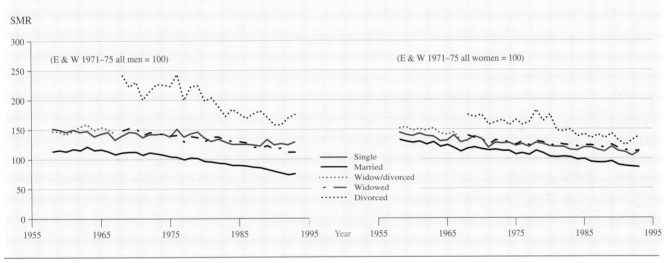

Figure 11.5

All-cause mortality at ages 15–74, by sex and whether married or not, Scotland, 1958–93

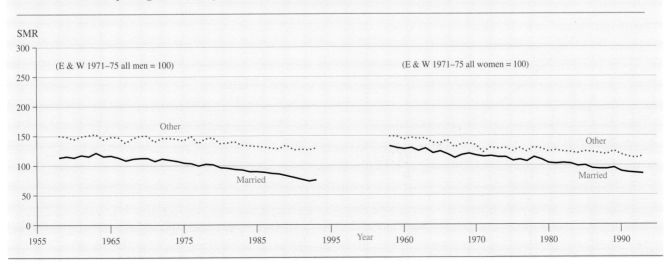

Table 11.2:

Observed deaths and standardised mortality ratios (SMR) at age 16–64 by sex and marital status in 1971 and 1981, based on all deaths in the period 1981–89

Marital status in 1981

Marital status in 1971		Single	First marriage (all)	First marriage (absent spouse)	Remarried (all)	Remarried (absent spouse)	Widowed	Divorced
Males								
Single	observed	1,447	190	20	12	1	24	31
	SMR	132	83	123	85	167	154	153
Married	observed	138	10,546	259	1,121	25	1,068	357
	SMR	161	94	116	96	97	127	140
Widowed	observed	21	5	1	78	4	366	4
	SMR	132	96	91	94	93	123	121
Divorced	observed	21	6	2	54	2	5	150
	SMR	184	128	133	116	167	106	132
Females								
Single	observed	1,126	111	5	4	1	19	11
	SMR	114	100	75	89	250	133	162
Married	observed	17	5,552	167	591	22	1,955	213
	SMR	108	92	103	112	130	106	114
Widowed	observed	8	6	9	53	0	1,455	7
	SMR	131	109	145	89	0	111	108
Divorced	observed	3	6	3	27	1	22	155
	SMR	81	200	273	97	48	105	107

Source: ONS Longitudinal Study

Table 11.3

Standardised mortality ratios (SMRs) by sex and marital status in 1971 and 1981 based on all deaths in the period 1981–89, ages 16–64 (England and Wales = 100 derived from data in Table 11.2)

Marital status in 1981

Marital status in 1971	All	Single	First subsequently married (spouse present)	First subsequently married (spouse absent)	Widowed	Divorced
Males						
Single	124	132	83	125	154	153
Married	98	161	94	114	127	140
Widowed	117	132	94	93	123	121
Divorced	131	184	117	148	106	132
Females						
Single	113	114	99	85	133	162
Married	97	108	94	105	106	114
Widowed	110	131	90	95	111	108
Divorced	106	81	107	125	105	107

Source: ONS Longitudinal Study

not explicitly presented in this way, provide the same picture. There has been considerable research into whether widowhood (and divorce) specifically trigger early death in the remaining partner (Susser, 1981). Whether these transitions also affect survival from cancer, perhaps by delaying detection or reducing host resistance, is also debated, but the results are inconclusive (Ben-Shlomo *et al.*, 1993; Neale *et al.*, 1986; Kvikstad *et al.*, 1995; Ader *et al.*, 1995).

The ONS Longitudinal Study (LS) has overcome some of the problems of cross-sectional data usage. It reports a true protective effect of marriage for both sexes, with some evidence of selection playing a part (Fox and Goldblatt, 1982). Tables 11.2 and 11.3 show, for men and women in the LS at age 16–64 in 1971, subsequent death rates between 1981 and 1989. This is cross-tabulated by the marital status of individuals in 1971 and again in 1981 (marital status was obtained from the linked census records). Small numbers preclude a detailed interpretation, though the data might suggest a protective effect of remarriage and the attenuation of this depending on whether the married subjects live alone or in a partnership. The LS was one of the first prospective studies of the complex relationships between family/household characteristics and mortality (Fox and Goldblatt, 1982). It has also been used to examine the relation between household characteristics that might imply role strain and mortality (Fox and Goldblatt, 1982; Mercer *et al.*, 1989; Mercer, 1991; Weatherall *et al.*, 1994). However, the results with mortality as the outcome were usually suggestive but inconclusive, save that important interactions with more general socio-economic determinants were apparent.

11.6 Hospital admission data

Hospital admission data for England and Wales are available by age and marital status from HIPE, HAA and HES. They are readily available from 1968 to the financial year 1993/94. Scottish hospital in-patient data in the same form are continuously available from 1961 to 1993, in the SHIPS dataset. Figures 11.6 and 11.7 show age-adjusted admission ratios by marital status at age 15–74 in England and Wales 1968–93, and Scotland 1961–93, using all admissions in Scotland in 1984 as standard; different pictures emerge for each country and in each sex. Numerous problems of interpretation affect these data as measures of health by marital status category. Data collection systems have changed and in part account for a varying proportion of the admitted population where marital status was unknown. The proportions with unknown marital status are sometimes large enough to distort potentially the patterns for the widowed, divorced and even the single at these ages. Numerator-denominator bias between admission and population estimate data is unquantified. These data also relate to episodes rather than people, though Scottish record linkage data indicates that, when episodes are converted to individuals admitted once or more within a year, by marital status for 1984–90, it makes little difference to the Scottish pattern. Another data source is the Oxford Record Linkage Study (ORLS) which provides a detailed picture of admissions around the time of the 1981

Census. The ORLS allows estimates of episodes of admission/persons admitted by marital status from 1979 to 1983. Age-adjusted rates at ages 16–64 show that for all discharges, the married and divorced men had the lowest rates and the single and widowed the highest. For women, the single and married had the lowest rates and the widowed and divorced the highest.

Two studies (Butler and Morgan, 1977; Morgan, 1980) have examined hospital use by marital status in England and Wales. Butler and Morgan used 1973 HIPE data and the ORLS in a detailed examination of the higher admission rates of the non-married compared with the married. This included the role of multiple admissions and transfers in determining the higher rates. Morgan also used census data about patients in non-psychiatric hospitals in England and Wales on census night in 1971 to examine differences in bed occupancy by marital status and found higher rates among single, widowed and divorced. Such data are not easily available from the 1981 and 1991 Censuses. Direct age-standardisation to the European population, using these census data for 1971, shows that for men at age 15–74 or at 25–74, the lowest rates are indeed for the married, followed by the divorced, then widowed, with the single having the highest rates. For women aged 15–74 the lowest rates were seen in the widowed, then divorced, then married, then the single. Among women aged 25–74, the married had the lowest rates, then the widowed, then the divorced, then the single. The change when using different age-groups in women may be due to obstetric admissions at younger ages in the married. We extracted equivalent data for Scotland also, and found broadly the same pattern.

11.7 The General Household Survey – NHS utilisation rates

Data available from the GHS about self-reported NHS utilisation rates between 1984 and 1994 are shown in Table 11.4. From 1986 onwards, anyone reporting themselves as cohabiting is included with the married, but otherwise the categories relate to legal marital status; attention has been confined to the more stable rates at ages 25–74. For men, the single, married and widowed reported the lowest hospitalisation rates in the previous year, with the separated and divorced reporting the highest rates. For women, the separated and divorced also had the highest rates and the single and widowed had the lowest.

The 1971 GHS report published out-patient department (OPD) attendance rates in the previous 3-month period. In every age-group, the rates were lowest for single people, intermediate for the married, and highest for the widowed, divorced and separated. Among men aged 25–74 in 1984–94, the married consulted less than the single, who in turn consulted less than the separated, widowed and divorced. For women, the married consulted less often than the widowed, who consulted less than single, who consulted less than the separated and divorced (see Table 11.4). Morgan (1980) discussed the conflicting evidence from several special studies about OPD attendance by marital status.

Figure 11.6

Age-standardised hospital discharge ratios for ages 15–74 by sex and marital status, England and Wales, 1968–93

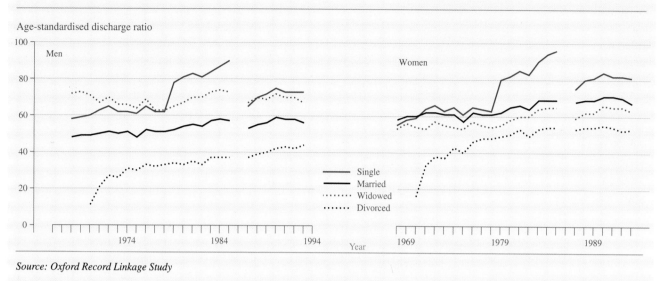

Source: Oxford Record Linkage Study

Figure 11.7

Age-standardised hospital discharge ratios by sex and marital status, Scotland, 1961–93

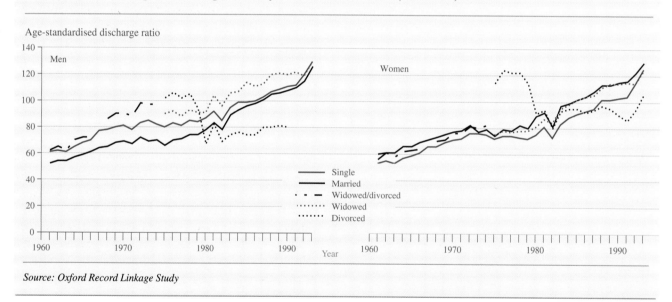

Source: Oxford Record Linkage Study

One study using GHS data for 1983 and 1984, described OPD and in-patient admissions of single mothers compared with other mothers (Beatson-Hind *et al.*, 1989) at age 16–64. OPD attendance was lower among single compared with the married, with higher rates for the widowed, divorced and separated. Ages of dependent children separately influenced rates of attendance, with the likelihood of OPD attendance decreasing with young age of children (in the opposite direction to GP consultations). For hospital admissions (excluding maternity admissions), the widowed had the lowest rates, then the married, then the single, and then the separated and divorced, after adjustment for confounders. This picture is very different from that presented by the crude rates in the same dataset.

A study in the Netherlands examined specialist (OPD) consultations and hospital admissions by marital status and living arrangements (Joung *et al.*, 1995b). Access to care in the Dutch system should be as good as that in England and Wales. After adjustment for socio-demographic influences and health status, the initial high rates of OPD attendance among the widowed and divorced resembled the low rates associated with the never-married by comparison with baseline rates of the married. Health status influences the attendance of the widowed and divorced, but the single have low rates for other reasons. After controlling further for living arrangements and presence of a partner, the single rates, as well as the divorced and widowed OPD rates, more closely resembled those of the married. In-patient admissions were low for the never-married compared with the married, and high for the widowed and divorced. This pattern persisted after control for socio-demographic confounders, health status measures and partnership/living arrangements, suggesting different determinants of in-patient admission and OPD visits.

The picture of OPD and in-patient stays cannot easily be summarised because different data sources from closely similar countries show conflicting results. Effective age-adjustment is essential and the level of non-statement of marital status makes definition of the rates difficult. Differences in definition also intrude and comparisons are being made between point prevalence and period prevalence rates. It is not certain who has the lowest and highest rates of admission or OPD attendance.

Table 11.4

NHS utilisation rates, 1984–94, by marital status Directly standardised rates per 1,000, to European standard population

	GP consultations in 2 weeks	OPD visits in 3 months	Hospital in-patient in 1 year
Age 25–74			
Males			
Single	6	338	101
Married	1	297	99
(Married inc. separated)	2	298	99
Separated	33	354	138
Widowed	100	362	92
Divorced	16	465	145
Females			
Single	9	384	116
Married	1	311	152
(Married inc. separated)	2	315	153
Separated	28	412	195
Widowed	31	363	136
Divorced	10	488	192
Age 15-74			
Males			
Single	5	323	95
Married	6	278	96
(Married inc. separated)	6	279	96
Separated	35	321	123
Widowed	176	293	94
Divorced	21	385	122
Females			
Single	7	357	115
Married	2	296	201
(Married inc. separated)	4	299	201
Separated	42	376	231
Widowed	120	294	110
Divorced	107	423	188

Source: GHS

11.8 GP morbidity data

Data about patterns of patient consultations in primary care are an indirect measure of morbidity. The number of contacts with GPs are available from the General Household Survey (but not the reason for the contact). More detailed information on marital status and living arrangements is available from the Second, Third and Fourth studies of Morbidity in General Practice. The proportion of patients consulting within a year (rather than the number of consultations) has been used as a measure of the prevalence of morbidity.

The Second Morbidity Study (RCGP *et al.*, 1974, 1979, 1982) covering 1970/71 demonstrated (after age-adjustment in broad age-groups between 15–64 or 15–74) that single men and women were least likely to consult. For men, there was little difference between the ever-married, but for women the divorced were more likely to consult than the married and widowed groups. There were variations depending on the condition consulted for, but this basic pattern was generally present with high rates for widowed and divorced, particularly for mental disorders, accidents, and injury and poisoning.

The third study (RCGP *et al.*, 1986, 1990) covering 1981/82 again found that generally among those aged 16 and over the single were least likely to consult, and the widowed and divorced group (not split for the analysis) most likely. Again there was variation, by severity of condition (serious, intermediate, trivial) and diagnostic type, but broadly similar patterns to those seen in 1970–71 were observed. The study also looked at consultation patterns by household type. Three types of household were defined – young people aged 16–24 living alone in private households, people aged 65 and over living alone in private households (neither institutional nor supported directly by others in the household, hence presumably healthier), and children under 16 living with a lone adult (presumably the children of single parents). When compared with other people of the same age, living in all other household types combined, no important differences emerged for any of these three groups.

The fourth, most recent and largest survey (McCormick *et al.*, 1995), covered the year 1991/92. Age-adjusted rates of patients consulting for ages 16–64 indicated only a small difference between the single (who were least likely to consult) and the married. (The one exception was for mental disorders, where the single were more likely to consult.) There were considerably higher rates among the widowed and divorced across most severity and condition types, including the conditions highlighted from the earlier surveys. Among those aged 65 and over, the higher rates among the widowed and divorced were not so pronounced as for younger people. Single men of this age, and to a lesser extent women, were more likely to consult for mental disorders than married people, though still less than the widowed and divorced group.

The fourth survey also presented more detailed analyses of the probability of consulting in terms of living arrangements, including cohabiting status. It categorised subjects as single (not cohabiting), married and cohabiting, or widowed/divorced/separated (not cohabiting). The picture was similar to consultation patterns by legal marital status, but more pronounced . At ages 16–64, the excess consultation rate among those widowed/divorced/separated (not cohabiting) was uniformly high for different categories of consultation relative to the married/cohabiting, for both males and females. The single (not cohabiting) were significantly less likely to consult than the married/cohabiting, except, once again, for mental disorders (where in particular single males and females without children had raised rates). Above age 65, the differences were less marked, but the same rank ordering persisted generally.

The fourth survey also used multivariate analysis to control for confounding factors when interpreting the impact of living arrangements on consultation rates. Not all possible combinations of age, marital status, cohabitation, presence of children, etc., were modelled, but principal household types were included. Broadly speaking, the results of the univariate analysis were confirmed. Thus, girls in single parent households generally consulted more, while boys consulted more only for mental disorders. At ages 16–64, widowed/divorced/separated adults of both sexes with and without dependent children generally had raised rates (compared with married/cohabiting people with dependent children), as did married/cohabiting people aged 45–64 without dependent children, but to a lesser degree. Single people without dependent children generally had low rates (apart from mental disorders), whereas single people aged 45–64 (both sexes) with dependent children had somewhat higher rates. At age 65 and over, single people consulted less (apart from mental disorders) whether they lived alone or shared with another adult, compared with those married/cohabiting. Separated, widowed and divorced women, whether sharing or not, were generally more likely to consult; for men this applied for mental disorders.

The morbidity surveys are the most important source of primary care consultation data. The General Household Survey is another source of data. It has collected and published data at various times between 1971 and 1994 on consultations in the previous 2 weeks with a general practitioner. Bearing in mind the sample size and the presentation of the data, it seems reasonably clear that, after age-adjustment, for both sexes, the widowed/divorced/separated consult the most. Table 11.4 shows age-adjusted rates of consultation for the single, married, separated, widowed and divorced for 1984–94 combined. From 1986, those reporting themselves as cohabiting were included with the married in the GHS tables presented here. Previously, there was no question on cohabiting. This change had little effect on the distribution of marital status. The higher consultation rates of the widowed, divorced and separated appear to be confirmed. The differences between the single and married (whether the separated are included or not) are less clear, with the suggestion that the single consult most frequently.

The health and health service use of single mothers aged 16–64 in Britain has been analysed using GHS data for 1983 and 1984 (Beatson-Hind et al.,1989). Legal marital status of mothers with children had little impact on their GP consultations, in contrast to levels of self–reported illness, and other aspects of health service use. In two related studies from the Netherlands (Joung et al., 1994, 1995a) it was found that legal marital status and living arrangements made separate contributions to the degree of self–reported morbidity. GP consultations (among other health care utilisation) were greatest among the widowed and divorced and least amongst the single. These differences persisted after controlling for differences in health status, socio-economic factors and separately for partnerships/living arrangement, though the fact of a partnership/cohabitation brought consultation rates for the single and widowed/divorced closer to the intermediate group of the married.

In summary, legal marital status seems to have the biggest effect on consultation rates, for both men and women, with single people consulting least and widowed/divorced/separated people consulting most. These differences are, however, attenuated to some extent by cohabitation.

11.9 Self-reported health

The OPCS surveys of psychiatric morbidity among adults living in private households found that, after adjusting for age and other confounding factors, couples had the lowest rates of neurotic symptoms, and single adult households (with or without children) the highest (Meltzer et al., 1995). Single adult households were also at greater risk of depressive episodes, mixed anxiety/depression, alcohol dependence and, for single adults without children, drug dependence. Adults living with parents were at greater risk of drug and alcohol dependence.

The GHS has included questions about long-standing illness, limiting long-standing illness, acute sickness and restricted days due to acute sickness, practically since its inception. Data on limiting long-standing illness covering the entire population were also available for the first time in the 1991 Census. There are differences in the wording of the limiting long-term illness question in the two sources, which affect interpretation (Charlton et al., 1994).

Tables 11.5 and 11.6 are based on data from the 2 per cent sample of anonymised 1991 Census records (Marsh and Teague, 1992), and show rates for men and women living in various types of household, by their marital status. For both sexes, married people were least likely to report limiting long-term illness, whether in their first marriage or not. The widowed reported the most, with single and divorced occupying an intermediate position. Remarried males, however, reported quite high rates. When the same data are considered by household type, no clear pattern emerges in relation to the presence of children. Lone parents appear to report higher rates of limiting long-term illness, with higher rates among those with non-dependent children than those with dependent children.

Table 11.5

Prevalence of limiting long-term illness, by marital status and family type
Age adjusted rates per 100 individuals aged 15–74 (using 5–year age-groups, to European standard population)

Marital status	Single	Married	Remarried	Divorced	Widowed	All
Males (living in household of:)						
Cohabiting couple, no children	13.6	8.4	9.0	10.0	11.2	10.7
Cohabiting couple, non-dependent children	15.8	12.0	0.0	6.9	7.7	10.6
Cohabiting couple, dependent children	12.7	10.5	5.4	10.3	11.4	10.4
Lone parent, non-dependent children	18.1	16.6	13.4	11.4	15.3	16.7
Lone parent, dependent children	6.1	9.8	12.8	9.3	15.3	13.2
Married couple, no children	—	11.1	15.9	—	—	11.3
Married couple, non-dependent children	17.7	22.1	10.9	—	—	12.8
Married couple, dependent children	5.8	10.3	12.8	—	—	10.1
N/A	17.0	12.2	22.3	17.3	25.6	16.3
All	16.8	10.9	17.2	15.1	21.8	
Females (living in household of:)						
Cohabiting couple, no children	11.4	11.2	4.1	10.8	10.1	11.0
Cohabiting couple, non-dependent children	16.5	5.2	0.0	7.7	13.9	12.6
Cohabiting couple, dependent children	4.5	4.4	9.6	3.5	9.7	5.2
Lone parent, non-dependent children	19.1	11.9	12.1	17.2	11.3	16.8
Lone parent, dependent children	7.1	18.4	15.8	11.0	11.8	12.6
Married couple, no children	—	10.3	12.9	—	—	10.6
Married couple, non-dependent children	16.5	15.5	10.7	—	—	11.5
Married couple, dependent children	7.6	8.7	8.6	—	—	8.6
N/A	15.1	12.4	14.8	18.8	20.2	15.3
All	15.5	9.5	11.3	15.4	16.3	

Source: Sample of anonymised records (SARs) from the 1991 Census

Table 11.6

Prevalence of limiting long-term illness by family type
Derived from Table 11.5 to summarise the marginal totals

	No children	Dependent children	Non-dependent children	N/A
Males				
Married couple	11.3	10.1	12.8	
Cohabiting couple	10.7	10.4	10.6	16.3
Lone parent	—	13.2	16.7	
Females				
Married couple	10.6	8.6	11.5	
Cohabiting couple	11.0	5.2	12.6	15.3
Lone parent	—	12.6	16.8	

	Single	Married	Remarried	Divorced	Widowed
Males	16.8	10.9	17.2	15.1	21.8
Females	15.5	9.5	11.3	15.4	16.3

Figures 11.8–11.12 show GHS data on self-reported health from 1975 to 1994. Marital status is based on legal marital status for the years 1975–85. From 1986 onwards, however, any respondent (irrespective of legal marital status) who reported that they were cohabiting, has been included with the married. Once again, for both sexes, for (limiting) long-standing illness it appears the married do best, but there is some overlap between the remaining groups. Self-reporting of health as 'good' or 'not good', and the proportions cutting down on activities due to health, show somewhat clearer pictures; the married and single apparently fare better compared with the widowed, separated and divorced.

Figure 11.8

Percentage with limiting long-standing illness at ages 25–74, 1975–94

Per cent with limiting long-standing illness

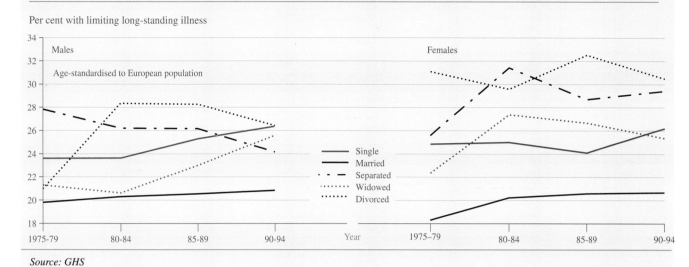

Source: GHS

Figure 11.9

Percentage with long-standing illness at ages 25–74, 1975–94

Per cent with long-standing illness

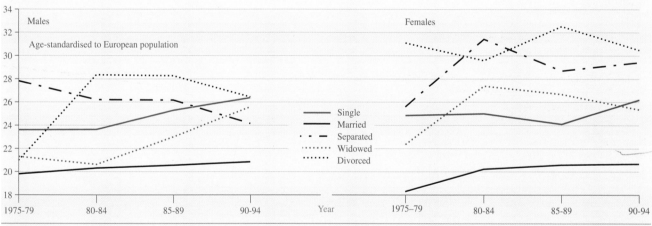

Source: GHS

Figure 11.10

Percentage cutting down on activities due to health at ages 25–74, 1975–94

Per cent who cut down activities

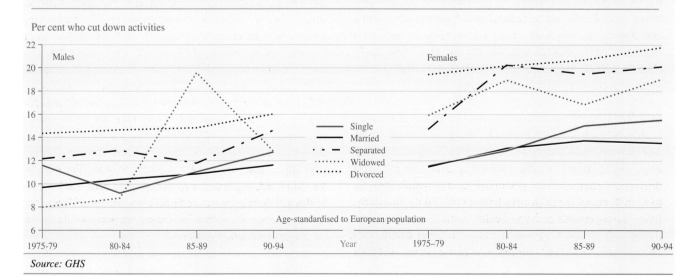

Source: GHS

Figure 11.11

Percentage of people rating their health as 'not good' at ages 25–74, 1975–94

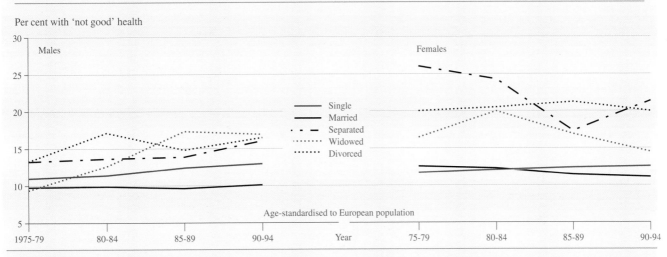

Source: GHS

Figure 11.12

Percentage of people rating their health as 'good' at ages 25-74, 1975-94

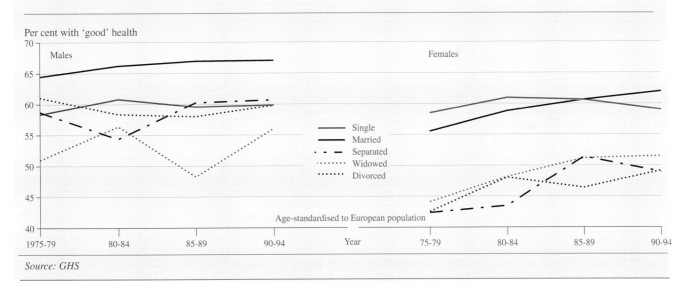

Source: GHS

A study of the health of single mothers aged 16–64 (compared with all other mothers) suggested that the never-married have lower rates of self-reported acute illness than married mothers, and the widowed/separated/divorced have higher rates. With regard to self-reported chronic illness the same study (Beatson-Hind *et al.*, 1989) indicated higher rates for all groups by comparison with the married.

In a Dutch study, perceived general health and subjective health complaints were found to be worse among the single and divorced than among the married and widowed (Joung *et al.*, 1994). After controlling for living arrangements, these differences attenuated for perceived general health but only to a small extent for subjective health complaints. Similarly, living arrangements affected health, with partnerships and living with parents being associated with better health. Any excess risks of morbidity for the non-married decreased after

controlling for living arrangements, but both marital status and living arrangements affected health. However, a further study (Anson, 1989) found no separate effect of living arrangements in addition to marital status on perceived health, in a study of women aged 18–55, and found never-married women to have better perceived health than married. A further study of limiting long-term illness among ages 20–59, using GHS data for 1985 and 1986, attempted to control for social class, paid employment and family roles by multi variate adjustment (Arber, 1991). Marital status and parental status did not appear to be importantly associated with mens' health after adjustment for a variety of other variables. For women, the widowed, separated and divorced experienced poorer health and there appeared to be a significant protective effect of the presence of children, but the picture was complex given the range of variables modelled.

In summary, different measurements of self-reported health may have different associations with the marital status and household characteristics that are being examined in these studies. It is known from comparison of the responses to the 1991 Census and GHS questions about limiting long-standing illness, that even small changes to a question about the same aspect of perceived health may elicit substantial variation in response. It seems likely that married people resemble cohabiting unmarried people with regard to their perception of their health, but that those whose marriages have terminated, for whatever reason, perceive their health to be worse. The perceived health of the intentionally never-married is not yet clearly established.

11.10 Conclusions

The evidence seems to be strong that marital status and presence of a partner independently affect a number of measures of health. These findings alone suggest that both the selection of the healthy (and deselection of the less healthy) for entry to various marital status categories is important, as well as the social support offered by occupying different social positions (through the shock of separation or bereavement, reduction of risky behaviours or encouraging healthy ones, or other forms of social support). Where studies made it possible, these effects appear to be separate from more general socio-economic or more material wealth influences. How health is affected by other features of household life, such as the employment status of one or both partners in a relationship, and the presence or absence of children of certain ages in the household (due to natural cycles of leaving home, intentional family restrictions or involuntary sub-fertility), or even the presence of other adults beyond the partner in the household, is not yet clear.

ONS data, particularly the GHS and LS data, can be used to provide some insights into the association between health and social relationships. The proper disentanglement of these connections from closely associated geographical and socio-economic features must, however, await further detailed studies. It will be very surprising if the effects of human contact and social support are ever explained away by the intervention of other intermediate factors.

Acknowledgements

Figure 11.1 was compiled by the authors Burney and Marks, as part of their chapter on respiratory diseases.

Chapter 12

Air pollution, climate and health: short-term effects and long-term prospects

By
Alison Macfarlane, Andy Haines,
Stéphanie Goubet, Ross Anderson,
Antonio Ponce de Leon and
Elizabeth Limb

Summary

- Over the past 130 years, the mean annual temperature in the United Kingdom has risen by about 0.5 degrees Centigrade. Recent discussion of the impact of global warming has renewed interest in links between climate and health, but this goes back many centuries.

- In addition to long-term and seasonal changes, short-term changes in weather can have an impact on health. In England and Wales, mortality can rise on unusually hot days in summer and during exceptionally cold periods in winter.

- Pollution from the burning of coal was recognised as a health hazard in London as long ago as the thirteenth century and was much discussed by seventeenth-century writers. Analyses of data for the nineteenth and twentieth centuries show that on numerous occasions up to the mid-1960s, severe fogs, with high concentrations of smoke and sulphur dioxide, were accompanied by very obvious peaks in mortality.

- Changes since the 1940s in the type of fuel burned in the United Kingdom have led to a decline in emissions of smoke and sulphur dioxide. As a result, severe fogs have not occurred since the mid-1960s. On the other hand, the increasing volume of road traffic has increased the concentrations of other air pollutants, notably nitrogen dioxide and carbon monoxide.

- The average concentration of ozone has not risen in recent years, but it is thought to have increased over the previous century. Less is known about trends in concentrations of fine particles, but there is concern about the possibility that they can affect health.

- The associations between these pollutants and ill health as measured by mortality and use of health services are difficult to assess. This is partly because high concentrations of air pollution tend to coincide with periods of exceptionally hot or cold weather. In addition, it is difficult to measure individual people's exposure to the pollutants. Nevertheless, the more powerful statistical techniques that have been developed in recent years suggest that raised concentrations of ozone and fine particles may affect health in the short term, but it is unclear whether this is also the case for nitrogen and sulphur dioxide.

'Any investigation of the laws of health and sickness, life and death in connexion with meteorological phenomena, which is confined in its scope to mean temperatures, must be imperfect and can hardly be expected to be crowned with any important results. ... The temperature, weight, humidity, of the atmosphere, and other physical forces should not be masked under mean values, but laboriously traced throughout their course from day to day, and if it were possible, from morning to night and from night to morning, and observed in connexion with the contemporaneous facts that relate to human life, as these are also successively recorded, if the sway which they exercise is to be appreciated in its full significance'.

William Farr, 1865

12.1 Introduction

The recognition that climate in general, and seasonal and short-term variations in weather conditions in particular, can affect health goes back at least to the ancient Greeks and appears in theories set out by Hippocrates and Galen (Adams, 1849; Greenwood, 1921). Nearer our own era, data from the 'bills of mortality', which were compiled in London and some other large cities, were compared with meteorological observations in analyses published from the middle of the eighteenth century onwards.

The introduction of death registration in England and Wales in 1838 gave added impetus to this activity, and nineteenth-century annual reports of the Registrar General contained commentaries on the weather during the year. William Farr commented on associations between exceptionally cold weather and higher than average mortality in the second and third annual reports of the Registrar General (Farr, 1840, 1841). He continued this theme on a number of subsequent occasions (Farr, 1885).

In 1843, William Guy, Professor of Forensic Medicine at King's College Hospital, read a paper entitled 'An attempt to determine the influence of the seasons and weather on sickness and mortality' to the Statistical Society, of which he was a leading member (Guy, 1843). He returned to the subject nearly 40 years later with a paper 'On temperature and its relation to mortality: an illustration of the application of the numerical method to the discovery of the truth' (Guy, 1881).

This time, instead of dividing the year into the conventional four quarters, he divided it into three periods of 4 months each, 'The four hottest months being June, July, August and September; the four coldest, December, January, February and March; and the four temperate, April, May, October and November'. This is similar to the approach Michael Curwen has used in his work on seasonal variations in mortality, which is described in the next chapter.

Meanwhile, the association between weather and disease continued to be of interest in the nineteenth century to both doctors and meteorologists (Haviland, 1855; MacDowall, 1895). Analyses in the first half of the twentieth century also found associations between low temperature and mortality (Young, 1924; Woods, 1927; Wright and Wright, 1945).

Pollution from coal burning has long been seen as a problem in this country (Brimblecombe, 1987). As early as the thirteenth century, complaints were made about the effects of smoke from the burning of 'sea coal', that is, coal brought by sea to London. A commission was set up in 1285 to investigate it and propose solutions. In the seventeenth century, the diarist John Evelyn still had cause to complain about the effects of sea coal in a number of publications, including his classic 'Fumifugium', published in 1661. In his satirical tract 'A character of England', he wrote that London was cloaked in 'such a cloud of sea coal, as if there be a resemblance of hell upon earth, it is in this volcano in a foggy day; this pestilent smoak, which corrodes the very yron, and spoils all the moveables, leaving a soot on all things that it lights: and so fatally seizing on the lungs of the inhabitants, that cough and consumption can spare no man' (Evelyn, 1659). His contemporary, John Graunt, attempted to draw some conclusion about associations between London's high mortality compared with rural areas, which he found in his analyses of the bills of mortality and the City's 'stinks and airs' (Graunt, 1662). In the same period, Sir William Petty went to considerable lengths to collect data about coal consumption.

In the mid-nineteenth century, William Farr recognised that London fogs were harmful to health, but did not find evidence that they increased mortality (Farr, 1843). These were the fogs that pervaded Charles Dickens's novels *Bleak House* and *The Old Curiosity Shop*. Further industrial growth and the expansion of cities made the problem grow, and severe fogs became more common later on in the century (Brodie, 1891). They cast a blanket over the criminal activities in Arthur Conan Doyle's novels and featured in Claude Monet's paintings of London. The most severe fogs, in 1873, 1880, 1882, 1891 and 1892, were accompanied by rises in mortality, particularly from bronchitis, and also by low temperatures (Ministry of Health, 1954). Analyses done in the 1920s of fog episodes in Islington and St Pancras at this period suggested that fog on its own did not have an effect but when it was accompanied by low temperature, mortality rose (Russell, 1924, 1926).

A 'London fog inquiry', undertaken jointly by the London County Council and the Meteorological Office during the winters of 1901–02 and 1902–03, appears to have been followed by a period of relative decline in the number and intensity of fogs (Brodie, 1905). The extent to which this resulted from the activities of the Coal Smoke Abatement Society, founded in 1899, the introduction of gas and electric light, central heating in public buildings, or a change in the prevailing weather, is unclear (Bernstein, 1975).

Nevertheless, fog carrying smoke and sulphur dioxide pollution was prevalent in the 1920s and 1930s. Fogs in many industrial areas during November 1921 and in London in December 1924 were not accompanied by exceptionally low temperatures or increases in mortality. Other severe fogs occurred in Glasgow in November 1925, and in London in February 1929 and December 1935 (Ministry of Health, 1954). In 1920, the composition and concentration of atmospheric pollution was described in a Medical Research Council report (MRC, 1920) and a government committee was set up to examine its effects. The renamed National Smoke Abatement Society was actively concerned throughout the 1930s with the association between pollution and levels of bronchitis and heart disease (Wadsworth, 1995).

At the outbreak of the Second World War, a number of initiatives were set up to encourage more efficient and therefore less polluting uses of coal to preserve coal stocks. These moves were temporarily halted by a demand for industrial smoke to screen important targets from German bombers, but shortages of fuel in 1941 prompted a return to the wartime drive for fuel efficiency (Hartley, 1962).

Nevertheless, fogs continued to occur in the post-war era. A fog which was considered to be the worst for a number of years occurred at the end of November 1948. It was accompanied by an increase in mortality similar in size to those observed during the fogs at the end of the nineteenth century (Logan, 1949; Ministry of Health, 1954).

In this chapter, we describe changes in the patterns of climate and air pollution which have been taking place in the latter half of the twentieth century and attempts to assess the impact of short-term changes in weather and air pollution on health and mortality. The effects of the longer-term changes which are taking place in climate and air pollution are largely unknown so far, but we briefly discuss the possible impact of climate change resulting from the accumulation of greenhouse gases in the atmosphere.

12.2 Air pollution

Most air pollution arises either directly or indirectly from the burning of fossil fuels. The effects of air pollution are complex and wide-ranging and are not restricted to humans. Pollutants in the air can also affect soil, insects, fish, vegetation, buildings and the climate. They may be carried for hundreds or thousands of miles from their source.

In the United Kingdom, air pollution is monitored via a network of urban and rural sites. The monitoring was coordinated by the Warren Spring Laboratory until it closed in 1994, when the work was transferred to AEA Technology at Harwell. A range of air pollutants is monitored, including ozone, particles, sulphur dioxide, oxides of nitrogen and carbon monoxide. In London, some local monitoring is coordinated by the London Air Quality Network, which is based at the South East Institute of Public Health.

12.2.1 Present levels and composition of outdoor air pollution

The sources and ambient concentrations of air pollutants have changed markedly since the 1950s. Emissions of sulphur dioxide have declined (Quality of Urban Air Review Group, 1993a). This decrease is commonly attributed to the Clean Air Acts of 1956 and 1968, under which local authorities were empowered to enforce smokeless zones and give people grants to convert their home heating from coal to smokeless fuel, gas or electricity. In many places, however, the decrease in emissions was simply a continuation of trends which were already apparent before the Acts were passed (Auliciems and Burton, 1973; Wadsworth, 1995). There has also been a change to less sulphurous coal. Belfast, where coal and solid fuel is still burnt in domestic grates, is the remaining major city in the United Kingdom which experiences high sulphur dioxide levels. High levels also occur in some parts of Northern England, where domestic consumption of coal is still high.

The decreases seen elsewhere in the United Kingdom have been helped by the fact that emissions from non-nuclear power stations now tend to be away from concentrations of population. This has been reinforced more recently by the move away from coal and oil and towards natural gas for electricity generation. On the other hand, high stack emission with efficient dispersion has led to a widespread exposure to low levels of sulphur dioxide.

Emissions of smoke also declined between the 1960s and the 1990s (Quality of Urban Air Review Group, 1993a). This was due to the reduction of coal burning in domestic grates and the increased combustion efficiency of power and industrial sources. Again, the impact of the Clean Air Acts is unclear. In 1971, a report from Warren Spring Laboratory commented on the reasons for the decrease in smoke emissions: 'it is impossible to decide from the data to what extent the Clean Air Act of 1956 has been responsible or to what extent it has been due to modernisation of habits of living' (Craxford et al., 1971).

There has been a further decline in emissions of black smoke since 1980. This downward trend in particulate emissions has now ceased because of the increased contribution from road traffic, mainly diesel engines, which emit small carbon-rich particles (Quality of Urban Air Review Group, 1993a, 1993b). Early monitoring of pollution in London showed particles to be very small and acidic (Lawther et al., 1968). Particulate air pollution was measured by drawing air through a filter paper and measuring the intensity of the black stain as an estimate of the concentration of black smoke (Lee et al., 1972; Bailey and Clayton, 1982).

With the change in patterns of air pollution and greater diversity of sources, attention is now focused on the smaller particles from sources other than coal. Particles which are less than 10 microns (PM10) are of major interest in studies of pollution and health as they are small enough to reach the smallest airways of people's lungs. The number of particles inhaled is also important and this is highest for smaller particles, in particular those smaller than 2.5 microns. Increasing attention is being given to the effects of 'fine' and 'ultra-fine' particles (Department of Health Committee on the Medical Effects of Air Pollutants, 1995b).

Measures of concentrations of black smoke in the air made using the traditional smoke stain method are now at historically low levels. The particle fraction also contains chemicals such as sulphuric acid aerosols and sulphates, but these are not measured by this method because they do not stain black. A newer gravimetric method has been developed to measure particles whose size is less than PM10 but it has not been in use long enough in the United Kingdom to generate data which can be used to determine trends (Department of Health Committee on Medical Effects of Air Pollutants, 1995b).

Oxides of nitrogen, NO_x are produced in high combustion conditions such as petrol and diesel engines. Emissions have increased, with an increasing proportion coming from mobile sources. Trends in emissions are projected to stabilise as a result of the introduction of three-way catalytic converters but to rise again as traffic volume increases. At the time they leave a vehicle's tail pipe, only about 10 per cent of oxides of nitrogen consist of nitrogen dioxide, NO_2. The rest are mainly nitric oxide, NO, which is not thought to be a danger to health. Once in the ambient air, nitric oxide is oxidised to nitrogen dioxide, which is regarded as potentially harmful to health (Department of Health Advisory Group on the Medical Aspects of Air Pollution Episodes, 1993).

Exposure to nitrogen dioxide is related to traffic density. In the country as a whole, nitrogen dioxide concentrations increased by 35 per cent between 1986 and 1991. Despite this, there has been no upward trend in the annual ambient concentrations of nitrogen dioxide in Central London over the past 20 years, but this may be explained by traffic saturation. An exception occurred in December 1991, during a period of stagnant winter weather, when London experienced historically high levels of nitrogen dioxide which exceeded WHO guidelines by a factor of two. Other areas, such as Manchester and Birmingham, have also experienced similar episodes. Personal exposures to nitrogen dioxide can also be influenced by indoor sources, such as gas cookers.

Ground level tropospheric ozone is formed mainly as a 'secondary' pollutant by the action of sunlight on nitrogen dioxide and oxygen in the presence of volatile organic compounds and hydrocarbons, which act as catalysts. Volatile organic compounds, such as benzene, are also emitted by combustion sources such as motor vehicles and from a wide range of industrial processes. Emissions of these compounds, particularly those from road transport, have increased slightly over the past 20 years. Concentrations of ozone tend to be lower near to sources of emission of oxides of nitrogen

because nitric oxide reacts with ozone to form nitrogen dioxide. In certain weather conditions in the summer, large parts of the population may be exposed to higher than usual levels of ozone.

Background levels of ozone at ground level have risen gradually but markedly over the past century, with a doubling of the base-line long-term average level. Nevertheless, since the 1970s there has been little evidence of a systematic increase in annual average levels (Bower et al., 1995). High concentrations are more frequently observed in the south than in the north of the country and are particularly likely to occur under anticyclonic conditions (Department of the Environment, 1992; Photochemical Oxidants Review Group, 1993). Sporadic episodes, such as those occurring in 1976 and to a lesser extent in 1990 in Southern England, tend to reflect the variable nature of English summer weather rather than an upward trend.

Carbon monoxide emissions have also increased since 1980, also as a consequence of the increasing volume of motor vehicle traffic. Unfortunately, technical problems make it difficult to monitor trends since the early 1980s in the concentrations actually present (Bower et al., 1995).

In 1990, the Department of Health set up the Advisory Group on the Medical Aspects of Air Pollution Episodes to evaluate the effects on health of air pollution (Department of Health Advisory Group on the Medical Effects of Air Pollution Episodes, 1991; Cameron and Maynard, 1992). In 1991, the Group reported on ozone. This was followed by reports on the effects of sulphur dioxide, acid aerosols and particulates, on oxides of nitrogen and on mixtures (Department of Health Advisory Group on Medical Aspects of Air Pollution Episodes, 1992, 1993, 1995a, b). The Department of Health's Committee on Medical Effects of Air Pollutants, which was set up in 1992, has produced reports on non-biological particles and health and on air pollution and asthma (Department of Health Committee on Medical Aspects of Air Pollutants, 1995a, b).

In people with chronic lung disease there may be interactions between the effects of their exposures to different pollutants. For instance, in experimental studies where people with asthma have been exposed to ozone, it is possible to detect a response in their airways to concentrations of sulphur dioxide at levels which are lower than those to which they would otherwise be sensitive. On the other hand, if they are first exposed to nitric acid or water vapour fog, this may attenuate the reductions in their lung function which arise from exposure to ozone (Hazucha et al., 1989; Aris et al., 1991). Experimental studies also suggest that low ambient concentrations of ozone may increase the response to inhaled allergens in people with seasonal symptoms of asthma and positive skin tests for ragweed or grass (Molfino et al., 1991). In general, though, ozone does not appear to affect asthmatics to a greater degree than non-asthmatics. Thus it differs from sulphur dioxide, to which people with asthma are known to be more sensitive.

12.3 Changes in climate

Although the subject of climate change has only relatively recently reached its current high public profile, it has been recognised for many years (Gribbin, 1978). Changes have been taking place for very much longer. Over the past 130 years, the mean annual temperature in the United Kingdom has increased by around 0.5°C. The increase seems to be particularly marked in the winter half of the year. As our climate is strongly affected by the surrounding ocean it is possible that temperatures in the United Kingdom may increase by a lesser degree than those on the continent of Europe, but prediction is difficult.

In the world as a whole, the mean surface air temperature has increased by 0.3 to 0.6°C over the past century (Houghton *et al.*, 1990). The magnitude of this increase is compatible with predictions of climate models based on the growing concentrations of greenhouse gases, including carbon monoxide and methane. The balance of scientific evidence now suggests a discernable human influence on the world's climate (Houghton *et al.*, 1996). Recent years have been among the warmest since 1860, with 1995 being the warmest so far.

In the northern hemisphere, the rise in mean temperature appears to be due principally to an increase in daily minimum temperatures. This means that there is a reduction in the daily range of temperatures. In contrast, in Australia and New Zealand, there has been no decline in the mean daily temperature range. It is possible that in the northern hemisphere, sulphate aerosols, which are produced by fossil fuel combustion and block sunlight, might have led to relative cooling of the air during day time hours and so reduced the daily range of temperatures.

The Intergovernmental Panel on Climate Change (IPPC) suggested that, based on the range of sensitivities of climate to increases in concentrations of greenhouse gases and plausible ranges of emissions, the global mean surface temperature is likely to rise by between 1.0 and 3.5°C by the year 2100 (Watson *et al.*, 1996). In this, its second report, the IPPC went on to review the possible impact of these changes on health.

As well as the direct effects of temperature which are discussed later, the rise in temperature can affect health indirectly in a number of ways (Haines and Fuchs, 1991). These include reductions in food supply, particularly in developing countries, thus increasing the numbers of people at risk from hunger (Haines and Parry, 1993; Parry and Rosenzweig, 1993; Rosenzweig *et al.*, 1993). There are also likely to be changes in the distribution of vector-borne and parasitic diseases (Shope, 1991; Cook, 1992).

The complex interactions of possible effects on human health pose a challenge to epidemiology, as it is conventionally concerned with the relationship between specific exposures, usually to individual agents, and the risk of disease or death

(McMichael, 1993). Nevertheless, after many years of inactivity, there is now a considerable volume of research taking place and the people involved can draw both on the experience of the past and the much more powerful statistical techniques available today.

Human physiology is geared to an optimum body temperature of 37°C. Elderly people and pre-term newborn babies are more vulnerable to changes in environmental temperature than adults or older children (Curwen, 1990). As Michael Curwen describes in the next chapter, there is considerable seasonal variation in mortality in the United Kingdom, with a preponderance of deaths in the coldest four months from December to March.

12.4 Methods of assessing the effects on health of short-term changes in weather conditions and air pollution concentrations

Assessing the effects of pollutants on health is beset by many problems. Only in rare instances, for example, asbestos, are the diseases caused by chemical and physical agents distinguishable from other diseases. Otherwise, the mechanisms by which environmental factors cause disease are often complex and still poorly understood. There are serious methodological problems which make it difficult to understand or quantify the relationships. Exposure to pollutants is often difficult to measure. Populations are exposed to low concentrations of a range of both synthetic and naturally occurring chemicals and these may interact in unknown ways. There are a number of ways in which exposure may be related to response. These include:

1. A dose-dependent relationship above a threshold, below which no adverse effects are discernible.

2. A dose-dependent relationship without a 'safe' threshold, as happens with ionising radiation and certain carcinogenic chemicals.

3. Hypersensitivity reactions for which prior exposure is necessary. Once this has occurred, allergic reactions result from exposure even to low doses, although, for a given person, the intensity of the allergic reaction is dose-related.

People can vary in their susceptibility to environmental factors. Differences may depend on age, sex, previous disease, nutritional status and genetic influences. There may also be synergistic interactions between environmental exposure and lifestyle, as happens between exposure to asbestos and smoking. It is possible that there is a period of latency between exposure and effect. This latent period can last for many years, as in the case of cancers arising from exposure to radiation, and may further complicate investigations of causal relationships.

The simplest method of assessing the effects of high pollution or extreme weather is to compare measures of adverse health effects during the episode with data for the periods immediately preceding or following the episode and corresponding periods in other years. In the past, the data available were often already aggregated into weekly totals. Episode studies are difficult to interpret because it is not possible to control adequately for confounding due to temperature or coincidental influences such as epidemics of influenza and other respiratory diseases.

These limitations led to the development of methods of studying daily variation in health indicators. This approach was first used in England in the investigation of the 1866 cholera epidemic (General Register Office, 1868) and has been used in studies of air pollution since the 1950s (Macfarlane, 1976). It gives the potential to control for possible confounders and to separate the effects of different pollutants. This is because multiple rather than single days are analysed and the various factors which might influence health rarely co-vary completely. Initially the analyses took the form of calculating deviations from 7 and 15 day moving averages (Martin, 1961; Gore and Shaddick, 1958; Waller et al., 1969). In recent years, there has been a considerable advance in the statistical methods available with the development of new techniques which are sensitive to much smaller changes in pollution levels (Schwartz et al.,1996).

Even with these more powerful statistical techniques, the fact that high levels of air pollution tend to be accompanied by extremes of temperature makes it difficult to assess their relative effects on health (Katsouyanni et al., 1993). One approach which has been used to tackle this problem is synoptic evaluations. Days with similar meteorological characteristics are identified as a homogenous group, or 'synoptic type', which represents a distinctive type of air mass (Kalkstein, 1991a). If an air mass is associated with high levels of mortality or morbidity, it can be studied separately to assess which factors may be responsible. Another approach has been to identify separately in the regression analysis days with extreme weather conditions.

A further consideration is that extreme conditions may have a disproportionate effect on the most ill and thus most vulnerable members of the population, whose death may be accelerated by perhaps only a short time. This may lead to exceptionally low mortality in the immediate aftermath of an extreme event (Ministry of Health, 1954; Macfarlane, 1984; Kalkstein, 1993). This effect has been referred to as 'mortality displacement'.

Short-term variations in mortality take place against a backdrop of major seasonal variation in mortality, with death rates in England and Wales being higher in the winter than in the summer. Most winter periods include peaks in mortality of varying magnitudes, coinciding with influenza epidemics. In the chapter which follows, Michael Curwen describes one approach to quantifying these major swings and trends over time, but there are others. The majority of studies which focus on shorter-term variations construct statistical models which include terms to allow for seasonal variations and influenza

epidemics along with other systematic variations, notably the day of the week (Katsouyanni et al., 1996). These statistical models could equally be used to focus on seasonal variation and mortality during epidemic periods.

There are two main types of daily time series study. One type of study is based on individuals who may be either healthy or have pre-existing respiratory disease. Either they are asked to complete diaries to give their perceptions of their health each day (Lawther et al., 1970), or they are followed day by day with measurements of symptoms, lung function, or use of medication. These 'panel studies' have the advantage of analysing the data at an individual level. In a recent British panel study for which full results have been published, it was found that in a panel of adults with chronic obstructive lung disease, high ambient levels of ozone and sulphur dioxide were associated with lower lung function and more respiratory symptoms than on days with lower levels of ozone and sulphur dioxide (Higgins et al., 1995). Another recent study looked at daily variations in the lung function of Surrey primary school children during a recent summer period. It found a small but significant negative association with particles but no association with concentrations of nitrogen dioxide or ozone (Scarlett et al., 1996).

Most daily time series studies are of the second type. These use aggregated routinely collected data about mortality or health service usage in defined populations on each day. Unlike panel studies, the data can be analysed only at group level. Such studies can effectively control for 'stable' confounding factors, such as social class, smoking and occupational exposure, because these do not change measurably from day to day. On the other hand, without appropriate statistical analysis, they are prone to confounding by temporal factors, which may be related to both air pollution and health effects, the chief ones being seasonal factors, weather and epidemics of respiratory disease, notably influenza.

Measures of adverse health effects include daily mortality, hospital admissions and contacts with general practitioners. Daily death totals were compiled specially for studies of daily mortality in conurbations in England and Wales in the 1950s and 1960s (Martin, 1961; Waller et al., 1969). Since 1 April 1969, the date of deaths occurring in England and Wales has been coded routinely for analysis. Developments in computing power have increased the potential for extracting daily death totals for populations defined geographically, either in terms of people's usual place of residence or of their place of death.

In the nineteenth century, records of individual hospitals were used to analyse changes in admission rates. The studies of mortality in Greater London in the 1950s and 1960s used applications to the Emergency Bed Service as a measure of excess pressure for hospital admission (Abercrombie, 1953; Evans, 1985). Since the Hospital Episode System was set up in 1987, data about all consultant episodes in NHS hospitals or purchased by the NHS in England should be available at national level. These are being used in studies of short-term associations with measures of air pollution and climate.

The Royal College of General Practitioners uses a weekly returns service from general practices to obtain information about variations in disease incidence. It covered an average weekly population of 239,984 over the period 1980–89 (Fleming *et al.*, 1991), but now covers a larger population. To look for potential impacts of air pollution which may be transient, disaggregation of weekly returns into half-weekly or even daily records would be necessary. Nevertheless, in its present format, useful data have been produced, including, for instance, data on the annual and seasonal variation in the incidence of common diseases. It showed, for example, the rise in the mean weekly incidence of asthma in the 1980s compared with the late 1970s, which is discussed by Marks and Burney in Chapter 20.

The development of large computerised general practice databases has made it increasingly possible to collect consultation data on a daily basis in large numbers of practices. By 1990, 63 per cent of practices used computers, although not necessarily for recording consultations (Gray, 1992). The General Practice Research Database was set up by the VAMP software company in May 1987. Its intention was to recruit sufficient practices to build up a database containing information about 4 million people, who would be representative of the national population. By 1990, it had become the largest commercial supplier and about 30 per cent of general practices used its systems. In May 1994 this database was transferred to OPCS to manage on behalf of the Department of Health. Originally it was obligatory for practices contributing data to the VAMP research bank to record a diagnosis when a prescription was issued, but not for consultations where no prescription was given. Increasingly, all consultations are being recorded. The data it contains are now being used for a variety of studies, many related to prescribing, but also for other purposes. This includes studying the possible effects of air pollution episodes through studies of associations between consultations with general practitioners and daily variations in air pollution and temperature.

12.5 Studies of the effects of air pollution on health

In the next two sections, we describe how mortality, hospital and general practice data have been used in such studies and focus in depth on two episodes of air pollution, one in the summer and one in the winter.

12.5.1 Episodes of fog and low temperature in winter

The 1952 London fog
The best known air pollution episode in the United Kingdom, with the highest concentrations of black smoke and sulphur dioxide measured in the latter half of the twentieth century,

occurred in London from 5–8 December 1952. Unusually calm weather conditions led to a temperature inversion and a persistent dense fog covered the Greater London area (Ministry of Health, 1954; Brimblecombe, 1987). The weak December sun was insufficient to penetrate the air mass, which remained cold and immobile. The smog consisted of soot,

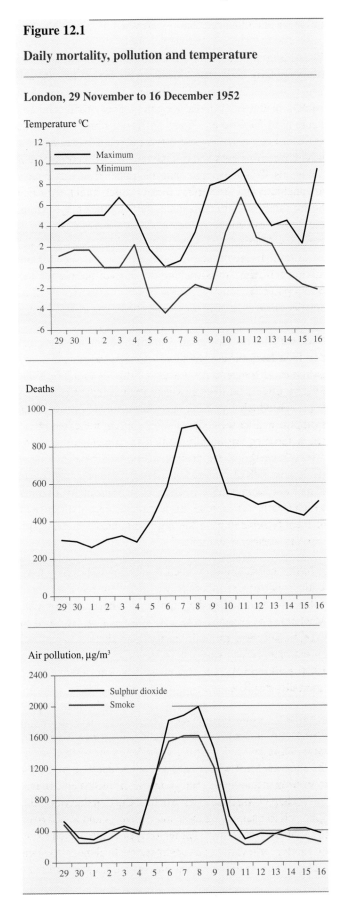

Figure 12.1

Daily mortality, pollution and temperature

London, 29 November to 16 December 1952

sticky particles of tar and sulphur dioxide, and dilute sulphuric acid was created by reactions, leading to an intense form of acid rain. The concentration of smoke recorded reached a maximum of 4460 μg/m³.

Immediate press attention focused on the economic impact of the fog rather than the health effects, which became apparent slightly later. The Ministry of Health's enquiry, published in 1954, concentrated on the fatalities. It concluded that 'The number of deaths in excess of those which would normally have been expected during the first three weeks of December was between 3,500 and 4,000'. The death rate increased shortly after the fog commenced and fell rapidly again as it dispersed, although it remained at a somewhat higher level than before the fog for several days, as Figure 12.1 shows. The rise in mortality was most marked for deaths attributed to respiratory causes. The deaths were largely concentrated among elderly people, but the death rate among young children doubled during the week of the smog. Although the fog was accompanied by low temperatures, it was clear that the fog was the major hazard. Only small rises in mortality were observed in other parts of Britain, which also experienced cold weather but not an increase in air pollution levels. The Ministry's report concluded that 'The fog was, in fact, a precipitating agent operating on a susceptible group of patients whose life expectation, judging from their pre-existing diseases must, even in the absence of fog, have been short' (Ministry of Health, 1954).

The fog was also accompanied by a major peak in applications to the Emergency Bed Service (Abercrombie, 1953). John Fry, a general practitioner in Beckenham, Kent, described the increase on his workload on the third and fourth days of the fog in an article in the *Lancet* (Fry, 1953). He found that the majority were elderly people with severe respiratory illness, but commented that 'although there are quite a number of asthmatic children in the practice, none of them was affected;' Some of the cattle at the Smithfield show, which was held during the fog, were affected, so much so that one died and 12 had to be slaughtered (Ministry of Health, 1954).

Fogs in London in subsequent winters
Severe fogs continued to occur during winters in the 1950s and early 1960s. Daily readings of smoke and sulphur dioxide were compared with daily mortality data, using deviations from moving averages in an attempt to adjust for seasonal variation. These analyses showed peaks in daily mortality and in applications for admission to hospital under the Emergency Bed Service during periods when air pollution levels were high (Logan, 1956; Bradley *et al.*, 1958; Gore and Shaddick, 1958; Martin and Bradley, 1960; Martin, 1961, 1964; Waller *et al.*, 1969; Macfarlane, 1977).

During the exceptionally cold winter of 1962–63, a particularly severe fog formed in London on the anniversary of the 1952 fog. Although sulphur dioxide concentrations reached a peak of 3500 μg/m³ similar to those in 1962, there was less black smoke and the marked peak in mortality was not as high as in 1952. While the higher peaks in air pollution were accompanied by peaks in daily mortality, it was difficult

to quantify the extent of the statistical association. This is because the fogs were accompanied by low temperatures resulting from the temperature inversions and sometimes coincided with influenza epidemics, which often appeared to be preceded by spells of low temperature (Macfarlane, 1977).

As overall levels of smoke and sulphur dioxide declined during the latter part of the 1960s, fogs became rarer and much less severe, and the easily identifiable peaks in mortality disappeared. A review at the end of the 1970s concluded that 'In the absence of the previous very high concentrations which occurred in acute episodes such as the 1952 London smog, any short term effects on mortality are not in any way outstanding in comparison with those brought about by extreme temperatures, both hot and cold' (Holland *et al.*, 1979). It reached a similar conclusion about morbidity.

A return to the use of coal rather than nuclear power for electricity generation in the United States in the early 1980s and a search for air quality standards prompted a number of reanalyses of the London data for the 14 winters 1958–72. Two analyses suggested that daily mortality in London was significantly associated with aerosol acidity, smoke and sulphur dioxide in winter months, even at levels of pollution which were low compared with those seen in the 1950s and early 1960s (Thurston *et al.*, 1989; Mazumdar *et al.*, 1982). An attempt to find a threshold below which no effects were observable failed to find one (Ostro, 1984). A more recent study using autoregressive models found that during winters in London, levels of sulphur dioxide as well as smoke were strongly correlated with mortality and that these associations were still detectable as late as 1972 (Schwartz and Marcus, 1990).

A number of more recent studies in the United States have shown that changes in concentrations of smoke, measured as total suspended particulates were strongly associated with short-term changes in mortality (Schwartz and Dockery, 1992a, b; Pope *et al.*, 1992; Dockery and Pope, 1994; Schwartz, 1994a). In a study in Philadelphia, the association was stronger among elderly than in younger people and for respiratory than for total mortality. The relationship appears to be non-linear, but, as in the London data, no threshold has been detected. The exposure response curve appears steeper at lower air pollution levels (Schwartz and Dockery, 1992a). A number of other studies have shown non-linear relationships between smoke concentrations and mortality (Schwartz, 1992, 1994d; Thurston *et al.*, 1994; Waller, 1984).

Taking a cross-sectional approach, a geographical study compared concentrations of air pollution and mortality rates in six US cities. It concluded that although the effects of other, unmeasured risk factors cannot be excluded with certainty, it is likely that fine particulate air pollution or a more complex pollution mixture associated with fine particulate matter contributed to excess mortality (Dockery *et al.*, 1993).

Other studies from North America show associations between levels of air pollution which are regularly encountered in Britain and are usually well within WHO guidelines and raised levels of daily mortality, hospital admissions, attendances at accident and emergency departments, lung function and symptoms in people with asthma (Dockery and Pope, 1994; Schwartz, 1991a, b, 1994a b, c, e; Burnett *et al.*, 1994,1995; Cody *et al.*, 1992; Delfino *et al.*, 1994; Pope *et al.*, 1991; Roener *et al.*, 1993; Schwartz *et al.*, 1993). In addition, several studies have indicated an increase in adverse health events associated with air pollution episodes on a scale which still occur in Britain (Department of Health Advisory Group on the Medical Aspects of Air Pollution Episodes, 1995a).

In response to renewed concern about the health effects of air pollution, there has been a return to research on the subject in the United Kingdom and air pollution episodes are now being investigated more fully, as the example which follows shows.

Health effects of an air pollution episode in London in December 1991

From 12–15 December 1991, London experienced a historic air pollution episode during which levels of nitrogen dioxide reached their highest level ever and remained above WHO guidelines for four successive days, as Figure 12.2 shows. The episode occurred because, at that time, anticyclonic weather created the stagnant and cold conditions which have historically pre-disposed the London basin to winter air pollution episodes. Emissions from motor vehicles and, to a lesser extent, central heating could not disperse and levels of nitrogen dioxide reached an hourly average concentration of 423 parts per billion at Victoria (Bower *et al.*, 1994). This was well above the WHO guideline of 210 ppb.

Figure 12.2

Daily concentration of nitrogen dioxide, black smoke and sulphur dioxide and daily temperature in London, December 1991

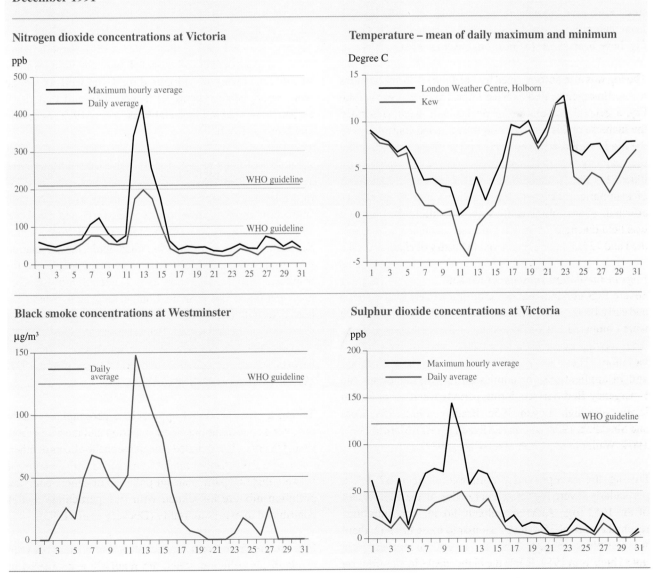

Particulate concentrations were also raised. The mean level of black smoke recorded by 11 stations on 12 December was 80 µg/m³ above the monthly mean of 30 µg/m³, but individual stations varied considerably. The highest level of black smoke, recorded at Ilford, was 228 µg/m³, well above the European Union guide value of 85–128 µg/m³. The highest level of sulphur dioxide, recorded in the City of London, was 144 µg/m³ compared with the European Union guide value of 100–150 µg/m³. In general, levels of sulphur dioxide did not increase to the same extent as those of nitrogen dioxide and black smoke. An official health warning was released and the episode received widespread publicity. London was the only city in the United Kingdom to experience an air pollution episode at this time.

A study was commissioned by the Department of Health for England to investigate whether the air pollution episode in London was associated with increases in numbers of deaths, hospital admissions or general practitioner consultations (Anderson *et al.*, 1995a, b). The hypothesis concerned both deaths and the use of health services for respiratory and cardiovascular diseases and for all causes combined. A second aim, assuming an increase was to be observed, was to investigate the causal role of air pollution.

The method adopted was to compare numbers of deaths and hospital admissions in the episode week, beginning on 12 December, with those predicted on the basis of events occurring in the previous week, and the corresponding weeks during December 1987, 1988, 1989 and 1990. The statistical technique was that of log-linear modelling. This was used to test whether the numbers of adverse health events in London in the episode week differed from those predicted from data for the control weeks and years, and to estimate the relative risks. The death registration and Hospital Episode System data were obtained through the OPCS. General practitioner consultations for 1990–92 were obtained from VAMP Research for a sample of London practices covering about 300,000 patients and these were analysed in a similar way.

The risks in London were also compared with those calculated in exactly the same way for three control areas where there were similar, if not more extreme, weather conditions but no air pollution episode. These were the rest of England, the rest of the South East, and Manchester, which was selected as a similar conurbation.

Analysis of the London data in Figure 12.3 showed that during the episode week, all cause mortality was 10 per cent higher than would have been expected; in other words, a relative risk of 1.10, which was statistically significant at the 5 per cent level. Increases of 14 per cent in cardiovascular mortality and 18 per cent in ischaemic heart disease mortality were observed. Deaths attributed to all respiratory diseases were 22 per cent higher, deaths attributed to respiratory infections 23 per cent higher and those attributed to obstructive lung diseases 23 per cent higher than in the comparison weeks; but these differences were within the limits of chance. When the control areas were included in the analysis, the relative

risks of death in London during the episode remained elevated but were no longer significant.

Analysis of the London hospital episode data in Figure 12.4 showed that the numbers of in-patient episodes for obstructive lung disease, which includes asthma, rose significantly by 14 per cent during the episode. Among people over 65, the numbers of in-patient episodes rose by 19 per cent for all respiratory diseases, 43 per cent for obstructive lung disease and 97 per cent for asthma. No significant difference was detected for ischaemic heart disease. When London was compared with the control areas, to take account of weather conditions, the relative risks tended to be smaller. Though

Figure 12.3

Relative risks for mortality in London during the episode week, by underlying cause of death

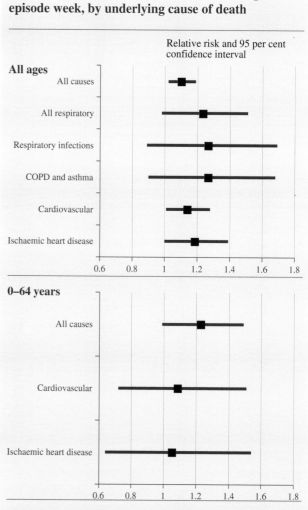

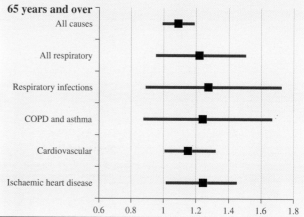

Figure 12.4

Relative risks for hospital admission in London during the episode week, by principal diagnosis

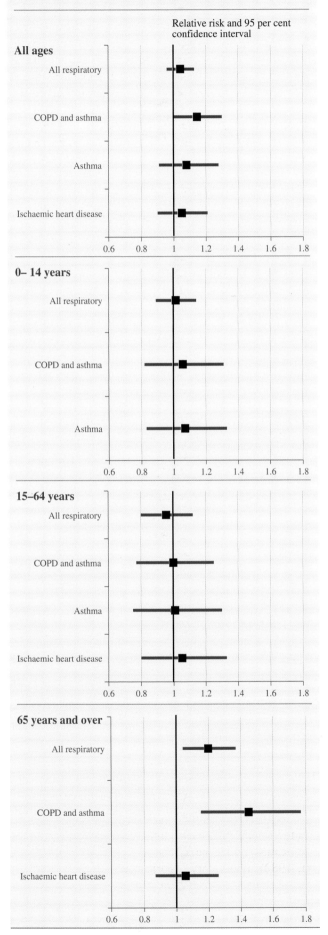

Figure 12.5

Relative risks for GP consultation in London during the episode week, in December 1991, by diagnosis and age

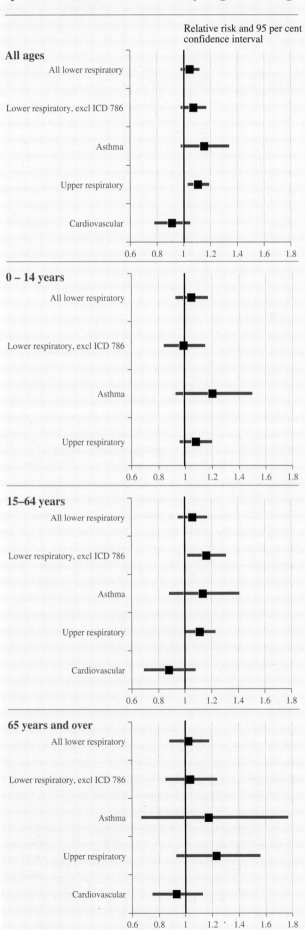

generally above 1.0, they were not statistically significant. The exception was a 55 per cent relative excess in admissions for obstructive lung diseases among people aged 75 and over.

Numbers of general practitioner consultations in London, shown in Figure 12.5, rose by 10 per cent for upper respiratory conditions but only 4 per cent for lower respiratory conditions. The rise of 14 per cent in consultations for asthma was not statistically significant.

Broadly, the results indicated that mortality and morbidity increased during the episode to a greater extent than would have been predicted and that the greatest rise was in respiratory diseases and among the older age-groups. This is unlikely to have occurred by chance alone because although only a few relative risks were statistically significant, the great majority of relative risks were greater than 1.0. Depending on which control area is chosen, the excess numbers of adverse health events during the episode were estimated conservatively as lying between 100 and 180 deaths from all causes and between 30 and 90 hospital in-patient episodes for respiratory conditions.

Various explanations for this excess mortality and morbidity were considered, including psychological factors, cold weather, a coincident epidemic of respiratory infection and air pollution itself. Publicity about the health effects of the episode could have inflated the numbers of adverse health events counted by increasing utilisation of services. Alternatively, it could have encouraged vulnerable individuals to take steps to protect themselves. Thus, publicity would have been more likely to affect admissions or general practice consultations, although it is not clear in which direction, and unlikely to have affected mortality. Cold weather increases mortality and possibly hospital admissions, but this seemed an unlikely explanation because it was just as cold, if not colder, elsewhere in the country. The excess of adverse health events in London was relatively greater than in the control areas. A coincident epidemic of respiratory infection could not be excluded although it was known that influenza was not occurring at the time. This factor would only explain a relative excess in London if the epidemic was affecting London more than the rest of the country but other available evidence suggests that this is unlikely.

It was concluded that the air pollution episode in December 1991 was associated with a rise in mortality and morbidity and that air pollution was a plausible explanation for at least some of this increase. The mixture involved was characterised by a high level of nitrogen dioxide and moderate levels of black smoke and sulphur dioxide. It is likely that this mixture would be typical of winter pollution episode situations in many other urban areas with high traffic density in conditions of stagnant weather. The detection of adverse health effects using the relatively insensitive approach of episode analysis is consistent with effects occurring at lower concentrations.

The only other recent episode study to be reported from Britain concerned an episode in Birmingham, which occurred from 17–27 December 1992. The level of sulphur dioxide rose to

130 ppb or 345 μg/m^3, nitrogen dioxide to 207 ppb and fine particulates measured as PM10 to 231 μg/m^3. This resembled the composition and scale of the episode in London in 1991. Diary data from 10 adults with 'mild' asthma and 14 with 'brittle' asthma living near the monitors were analysed to examine possible effects of the episode (Walters et al., 1993). The mild group showed no significant changes but the 'brittle' group showed evidence of adverse effects during the episode, indicated by reductions in peak flow, and increased use of medication.

Recent studies of winter daily mortality and hospital admissions in British cities

Analysis of the association between daily measures of air pollution and adverse health events enables more effective control of confounding factors, such as weather conditions, than is possible when looking at a single episode. Poisson regression analysis of daily counts of deaths (with adjustment for effects of secular trend, seasonal and other cyclical factors, day of the week, holidays, influenza epidemic, temperature and humidity) and auto-correlation were used to look at the association with air pollution in London during the period 1987 to 1992 (Anderson et al., 1996). In the cool period of the year, from October to March, a significant positive association was found between daily all cause mortality and black smoke on the previous day. There was no such association for nitrogen dioxide, sulphur dioxide or ozone.

The observed statistical distribution of each pollutant was used to derive its tenth and ninetieth centile. Then the numbers of deaths associated with exposure to each of these two concentrations were estimated and compared by calculating relative risks. A rise in concentration of black smoke from its tenth to its ninetieth centile, that is, from 9 to 26 μg/m^3, was associated with a rise by 1.6 per cent in numbers of daily deaths.

The same techniques were used to examine associations between air pollution and daily numbers of hospital admissions for respiratory disease over the same time period (Ponce de Leon et al., 1996). The only significant association found was with admissions of men aged 15–64 for respiratory conditions. A 3.9 per cent rise in these was associated with an increase in 24-hour sulphur dioxide levels from the tenth to the ninetieth centile, from 18 to 49 μg/m^3. An association between sulphur dioxide and daily admissions to hospital was also found in Birmingham during the winters of 1989 and 1990 (Walters et al., 1994).

These recent English studies of daily mortality and hospital admissions suggest that even at the historically low levels of winter air pollution which now exist, adverse health effects may still be detectable.

12.5.2 Heat waves and air pollution

It has been recognised since the 1930s that heat waves can lead to increases in mortality rates in the United States. An analysis by the United States Public Health Service of weekly mortality rates for 86 cities during summers in the 1920s and 1930s showed positive associations between deviations from normal weekly death rates and deviations from normal weekly mean temperatures for the preceding week (Gover, 1938). These increases were more closely related to the rise in temperature than to the absolute temperature, and applied mainly to the first heat wave of each summer. Excess mortality during a second heat wave in any one year was relatively slight (Gover, 1938; Kalkstein and Davis, 1989). Only about a quarter of the excess deaths were attributed to 'excessive heat', with the balance being attributed to 'diseases of the heart, cerebral haemorrhage, nephritis and pneumonia, (Gover, 1938). More recent studies have also shown direct effects of temperature on health include rises in numbers of deaths from cardiovascular and cerebrovascular diseases following hot spells (Kalkstein, 1991a).

Similar effects were found during many studies of heat waves in the United States in the 1950s and 1960s and in retrospective analyses of data for heat waves in the early years of the century. These were summarised in an extensive review by Surgeon Captain FP Ellis (Ellis, 1972), a Royal Navy doctor concerned about the effects of heat on the crews of naval ships, particularly submarines. He confined his attention to the United States at a time when similar increases had not been detected in the more temperate climate of the United Kingdom. As the increases are sudden and transient and much less marked than in the United States, daily mortality data are usually needed to detect them.

They were certainly needed for looking at the impact of a short but acute episode in July 1968. On 30 June, a so-called 'Sahara dust storm', resulting from movements of warm air in northern Africa, led to a warm night with a minimum temperature of 20.2°C. The next day, 1 July, was particularly hot, with a maximum temperature of 32.6°C and was followed by a further warm night. Death rates attributed to cardiovascular, respiratory and other causes rose sharply on 1 July and remained high on the following day. The increase was confined to people aged over 60. Only a very small peak was visible in weekly registration data, however (Macfarlane, 1976).

It has been suggested that a rise in night time temperatures could have a significant impact on health. This is because heat-related deaths appear more likely when a hot day is followed by a warm night which does not permit adequate cooling (Kalkstein, 1991b). The research on successive heat waves in the United States suggests that people become acclimatised to sharp increases in temperatures and that this could appreciably reduce their adverse effects on health.

In 1969, England and Wales experienced a hot spell during which temperatures built up gradually over a number of days. At this time, the highest mortality tended to follow the greatest increases in temperature, but was not invariably related to the highest temperature. There were also associations between increases in daily mortality and relatively hot weather in London, even when there was no exceptional heat wave (Macfarlane, 1978).

The summers of 1975 and 1976 were exceptionally hot. Heat waves occurred in late July to early August 1975 and in late June and early July 1976. They were accompanied by increases in mortality which were large enough to be apparent in weekly registration totals (Macfarlane and Waller, 1976). These heat waves occurred at a time when monitoring of ozone was just getting under way in the United Kingdom. No marked increase in ozone levels was observed during the 1975 heat wave, but a major increase was observed in 1976. This raises the question of the relative contribution of heat and air pollution to the rise in mortality.

High temperature and ozone during the summer of 1976
During the summer of 1976 levels as high as 248 ppb were observed at Harwell (Apling et al., 1977). Typically, levels of ozone are higher in rural areas than in conurbations, but levels of ozone did reach 212 ppb at the County Hall monitoring site in Central London.

Data for analysis of the episode were obtained from the Warren Spring Laboratory, the OPCS, and the Climatic Research Unit at the University of East Anglia. As well as overall daily deaths, subtotals were available for cardiovascular disease, (ICD 390-458) and respiratory disease, (ICD 466-519).

None of the six ozone monitoring sites in London had a continuous set of daily readings between May and September 1976. After checking that the six sites cross-correlated strongly, with greater variations at the peripheral sites at Teddington and Hainault, the log-transformed mean level of the six sites was used for analysis. The greater variation at peripheral sites and at the County Hall monitoring site is explained by their position. The Hainault and Teddington sites were adjacent to parklands and the measurements at the County Hall were made on a rooftop. Ozone at such sites is less likely to be broken down by compounds in car exhausts, and this explains the higher maxima (Bower et al., 1990).

Complete sets of levels of sulphur dioxide, acid aerosols and smoke were also available for analysis. Time series analysis was used to investigate the association of high temperatures and levels of pollutants with death rates in London (Goubet, 1993). A study in the Netherlands had shown that wind speeds and relative humidity have a different relationship with death rates on hot and cold days (Kunst et al., 1993). For this reason, interactions between wind speed, relative humidity and maximum temperature were entered in the regression models. Only the interaction between maximum temperature and relative humidity was found to be statistically significant. All results were adjusted for weather variables, including maximum temperature, relative humidity, wind speeds, interaction between maximum temperature and relative humidity. The temporal relationship between air pollution, maximum temperature, and vascular and respiratory deaths is shown in Figure 12.6.

Figure 12.6

Daily air pollution, temperature and mortality in Greater London, summer 1976

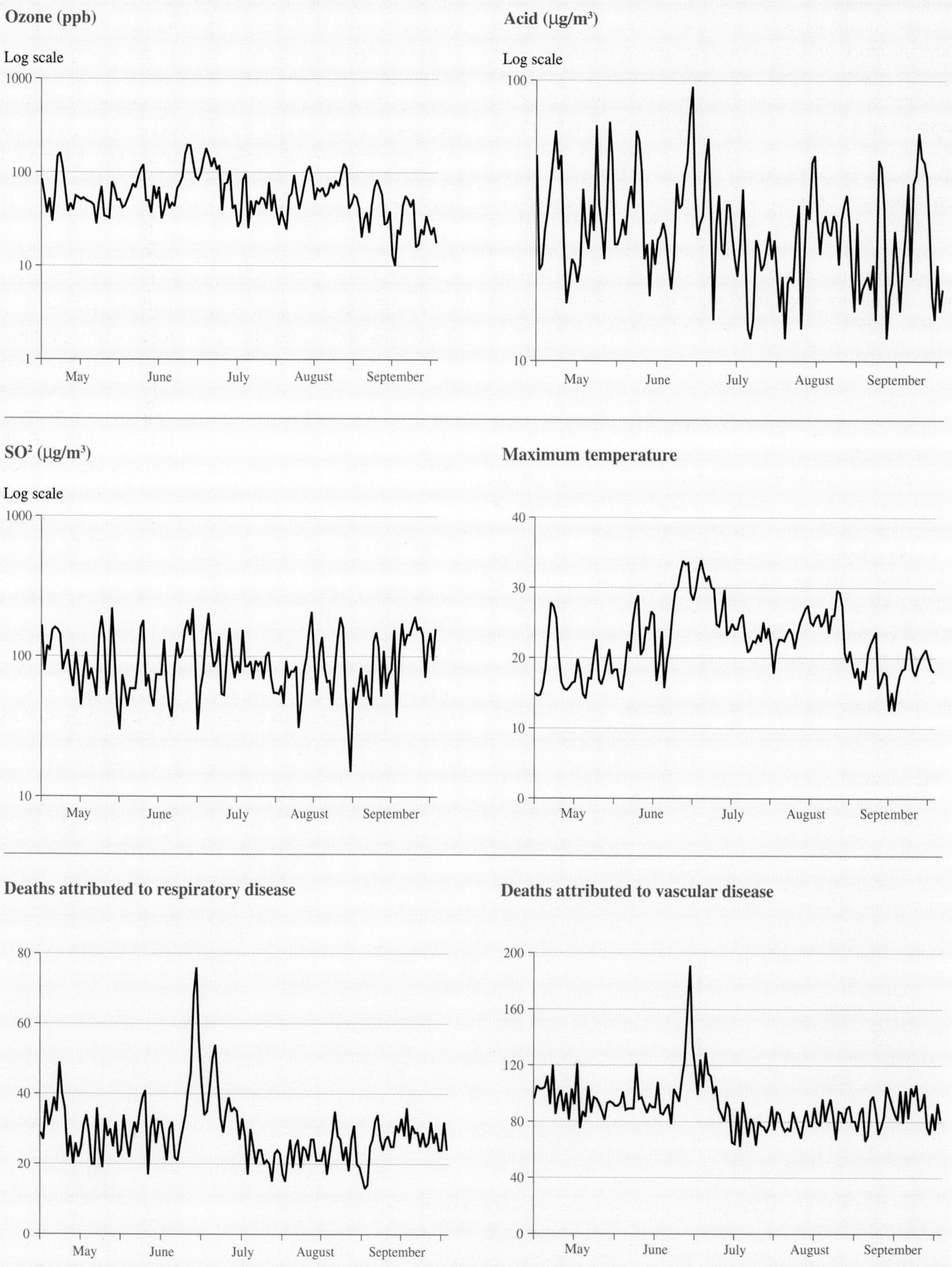

Ozone (ppb)

Acid (µg/m³)

SO² (µg/m³)

Maximum temperature

Deaths attributed to respiratory disease

Deaths attributed to vascular disease

There was no evidence of a day-of-the-week pattern in the numbers of deaths. Highest levels of pollutants and maximum temperature were observed on days when death rates rose above their ninetieth centile. Rises in levels of ozone, sulphuric acid and sulphur dioxide were associated with increases on the same day, and at 1 and 2 day lags, in deaths attributed to respiratory or vascular diseases. There was only a weak association between rises in levels of smoke and numbers of deaths attributed to respiratory disease, and no association was found for deaths attributed to heart disease.

The associations between levels of sulphur dioxide and smoke and numbers of deaths attributed to cardiovascular or respiratory disease disappeared after adjustment for levels of sulphuric acid. The association between ozone and numbers of deaths attributed to cardiovascular diseases was lower but was statistically significant, while there was no longer an association between numbers of deaths attributed to respiratory diseases.

The 153 days between May and September were divided in four climatic categories: sunny and cool, overcast and windy, rainy, and oppressive. This last category was defined by high day-time and night-time temperatures. Days within the oppressive cluster were examined more closely to determine which aspects of weather or pollution appeared to be most related to mortality. There were a few days when mortality and ozone concentrations were low, although the day and night -time temperatures were high. These were days of high wind speed, however. The wind can not only remove pollutants but can also alter people's perception of heat.

Over the whole period studied, deaths among people aged 65 and over accounted for 73 per cent of deaths from all causes. They made up 88 per cent of deaths attributed to respiratory causes and 80 per cent of deaths attributed to cardiovascular causes. It is likely that some of these people were already quite ill. There was a fall in numbers of deaths in the month following the heat wave, as Figure 12.6 shows. It could be that the high death rates during the heat wave left fewer susceptible people to die subsequently. An alternative hypothesis is that people had become acclimatised to oppressive weather and high levels of pollution. It was estimated that between 40 per cent and 60 per cent of the overall numbers of deaths during the period between 22 June and 9 July 1976 were due to the oppressive and polluted conditions.

The missing data and local geographical differences in ozone levels made examination of a dose-response relationship difficult. It was hard to distinguish between effects of pollutants and climate because ozone is formed during periods of hot, anticyclonic weather, and sulphur dioxide and acid concentrations were also high at this time. Statistical analysis suggested independent associations between pollution, in terms of 3 day average concentrations of acid and ozone and 2 day average concentrations of sulphur dioxide and smoke, and death rates attributed to both respiratory and cardiovascular diseases, taking into account the climatic conditions.

Air pollution, hot weather and adverse health events during recent summers

The analysis of daily mortality in London from 1987 to 1992, which was described earlier, also included time series analyses which attempted to identify independent associations with

Figure 12.7

Relative risks of daily mortality from all causes in London during the 'warm' months, April–September, 1987–92

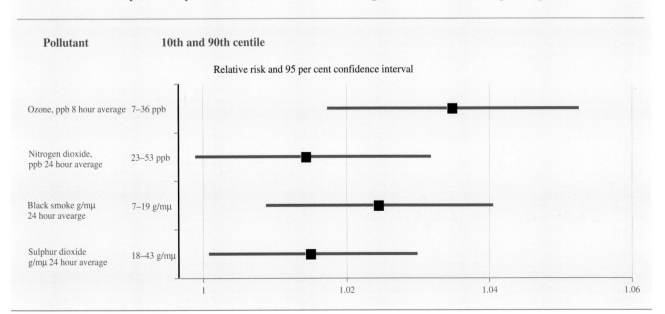

summer air pollution and temperature during the 'warm' months from April to September (Anderson *et al.*, 1996). The results, shown in Figure 12.7, are again expressed as relative risks associated with an increase in the concentration of each air pollutant from its tenth to its ninetieth centile. Significant associations were observed between all cause mortality and ozone on the same day, and sulphur dioxide and black smoke on the previous day. The strongest association was with ozone, with increases of 3.5 per cent in all cause mortality and 5.4 per cent in mortality attributed to respiratory causes associated with an increase in pollution levels from the tenth to the ninetieth centile. The association between mortality and black smoke was stronger in the summer than that in the winter described earlier. The associations with ozone and black smoke were independent of each other. They were similar in size to those observed in some North American cities (Schwartz, 1996).

Over the same period, summer air pollution in London was also associated with hospital admissions for respiratory disease (Ponce de Leon *et al.*, 1996). As Figure 12.8 shows, significant associations were observed between admission of people of all ages and ozone concentrations on the previous day and nitrogen dioxide concentrations two days earlier, but not with concentrations of black smoke or sulphur dioxide. Ozone was more important in the adult age-group, with a 6 to 8 per cent increase in admissions being associated with a rise in concentration of ozone from the tenth to the ninetieth centile. In the 0–14 age-group nitrogen dioxide appeared to have a greater impact. It was associated with a 4 per cent increase in admissions. For ozone, there was evidence for a threshold at about 50 ppb, below which no association could be detected. Similar associations with ozone have been found in North America (Schwartz, 1996), but the association with nitrogen dioxide is unusual.

This study forms part of the APHEA project in which data from 15 large European cities have been analysed according to an agreed protocol (Katsouyanni, 1996; Katsouyanni *et al.*, 1996) before being combined in pooled analyses. The findings for the individual cities are broadly consistent with analyses for cities in North America.

Reports from the United States, notably from Chicago, described increases in mortality associated with a heat wave from 12–16 July 1995, when temperatures ranged from 33.9°C to 40.0°C (Mortality and Morbidity Weekly Report, 1995). This was also a hot summer in the United Kingdom, although temperatures did not reach the levels experienced in Chicago. Figure 12.9 shows total deaths in England and Wales over the months of May to September, together with the maximum and minimum 'Central England' temperatures. Data for this period are being analysed in much greater detail by the Office for National Statistics in collaboration with the London School of Hygiene and Tropical Medicine, but a number of features are apparent in Figure 12.9. The period with the highest temperatures did not occur until August, and the peak in mortality associated with it was small compared with that for 1976 as shown in Figure 12.6. This may be a reflection of other differences. The 1976 data in Figure 12.6 relate to a major city with an 'urban heat island' effect and are restricted to deaths attributed to cardiovascular and respiratory causes. In addition, the 1976 heat wave occurred earlier in the summer, compared with that in 1995, which was preceded by a number of relatively hot periods. During these, some highly vulnerable people may have died while others may have become acclimatised to higher than average temperatures. The analysis referred to above should allow these possibilities to be explored.

Figure 12.8

Relative risk of daily hospital admission in London for respiratory conditions during the 'warm' months, April–September, 1987–92

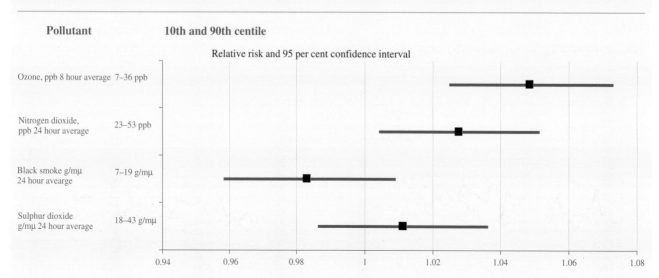

Figure 12.9

Daily mortality and temperature, England and Wales, May to September 1995

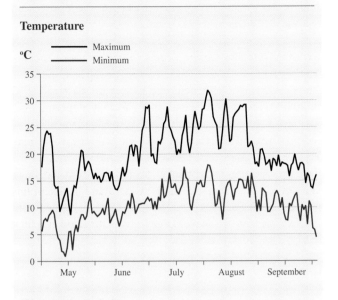

Temperature

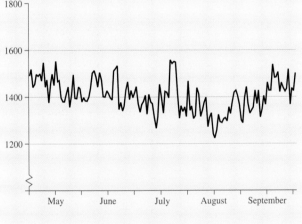

Total deaths each day

12.6 Asthma and thunderstorms

Episodes of asthma have been reported during and after thunderstorms in Birmingham in July 1983 (Packe and Ayres, 1985) and in the south of England in June 1994 (Murray *et al.*, 1994; Campbell-Hewson *et al.*, 1994). Similar episodes have occurred in Melbourne, Australia (Bellomo *et al.*, 1992). Levels of ozone and nitrogen dioxide were not high at the time of the June 1994 outbreak. It was considered that the surge in attendances at accident and emergency departments was more likely to be associated with increases in concentrations of aeroallergens, particularly grass pollen. These may be inhaled at times of high humidity, such as those that occur during thunderstorms (Celenza *et al.*, 1996).

12.7 Global warming and the depletion of stratospheric ozone

Concerted attempts to assess the impact of global warming on health are relatively recent (Watson *et al.*, 1996). This means that until the research currently being done has progressed further, there are rather more hypotheses than results. It has been suggested, for example, that there might be a 'trade-off' between decreasing mortality associated with warming in winter months and the impact of heat waves on mortality (Langford and Bentham, 1995). Others have suggested that this is unlikely, as the excess of mortality in winter is actually smaller in a number of countries with colder winters than in the United Kingdom, and much of the excess may be related to communicable diseases (Kalkstein, 1991a). This may be associated with the extent to which people can be protected from extremes of temperature by controlling their indoor environment.

The overall effect remains to be determined and will probably vary as global warming progresses. To determine the vulnerability of the United Kingdom population to extreme

Figure 12.10

Malignant melanoma death rates, England and Wales, 1950 - 1994

Males   Females

Death rate per million population (standardised to European population)

temperatures and to rises in night-time relative to daytime temperatures in the summer months, it will be necessary to monitor daily deaths, particularly among elderly people who are the most likely to be susceptible to extreme weather conditions. This could also lead to better information about the potential for acclimatisation to high temperatures. Further work is also needed on the relative importance of weather and pollutants in causing morbidity and mortality and on other possible long-term consequences of climate change, including rises in sea levels, disturbances of ecosystems and weather-related disasters.

The same consideration also applies to the possible longer-term consequences of the depletion of stratospheric ozone, which leads to increases in levels of ultra-violet radiation, which can lead to melanoma, non-melanoma skin cancer and cataracts. The relation between malignant melanomas and ultraviolet radiation is not simple, as melanomas can occur on non-irradiated parts of the body and may be related to exposure in childhood. A number of factors are likely to have contributed to the rise in mortality from melanoma, as shown in Figure 12.10 (Streetly and Markowe, 1995). These include in particular the changing patterns of exposure of people usually working indoors to outdoor recreational activities. More recently, mortality rates have declined among younger women, while remaining level for men.

12.8 Discussion and conclusions

The studies of daily mortality and morbidity are prone to confounding by factors which are related to both air pollution and the adverse health outcomes, and to other statistical problems. The statistical methods have developed rapidly over the past decade (Schwartz *et al.*, 1996). Despite the possibility of residual confounding, the results are generally accepted as indicating a causal relationship.

It is clear that seasonal variation in mortality is associated with raised mortality in winter and that mortality is higher than usual during periods of exceptionally low temperature. Hot spells in summer are also associated with peaks in mortality, especially among elderly people. Because periods of high concentrations of pollution tend to coincide with extremes of temperature it is difficult to assess their relative contribution to observed increases in mortality. Some studies have restricted their focus to weather (Ramlow and Kuller, 1990; Kalkstein, 1991a; Biersteker and Evendijk, 1976).

Studies which have included data about weather and air pollution have started by adjusting for weather variables, but have still detected associations with air pollution. The main indicator pollutants to be associated with short-term health effects are particles and ozone. The effects of nitrogen dioxide and sulphur dioxide are much less certain (Department of Health Advisory Group on the Medical Aspects of Air Pollution Episodes, 1991, 1992, 1993, 1995a, b). These associations remain after allowing for association with extremes of temperature.

The consistency of the evidence across different studies in different places in the United States, Europe and elsewhere, and in different climates is striking. Biological plausibility has been demonstrated to some extent in the case of ozone, using human chamber studies, but to a lesser extent in the case of particles, which are difficult to study in chamber conditions. The mechanism by which daily health events are caused is thought to be by effects on the airways of individuals who are already very vulnerable as a result of existing respiratory or cardiac diseases. The degree to which death is brought forward is unclear. Thus, it is not possible to extrapolate from these studies to estimate effects on longer-term mortality or on the development of chronic disease. For this, studies of a different type are required (Dockery *et al.*, 1993).

The monitoring of the potential impacts of global climate change needs to be undertaken on a worldwide basis, looking for both direct and indirect effects (Haines *et al.*, 1993; McMichael *et al.*, 1996). In the United Kingdom, daily death totals from death registrations could be used to monitor deaths from heat waves and to determine the magnitude of any acclimatisation effects. Changes in the balance between winter and summer mortality may occur and their impact should be monitored. Computerised general practice datasets offer the potential for studying morbidity in relation to temperature and air pollution. To collect fuller data, surveillance should be undertaken in a more systematic fashion, linking environmental and health indicators. Monitoring systems for air pollution should be linked with potential sources of data on mortality and morbidity.

Meanwhile, evidence from other countries, supported by recent research from the United Kingdom, indicates that current levels of air pollution have small but detectable short-term effects on health. This applies both to winter pollution characterised by particles and nitrogen dioxide and summer pollution characterised by ozone. It is not known to what extent these short-term effects represent a significant shortening of life, nor is it known whether air pollution at levels current in Britain is likely to have long-term effects on the health of the population.

Chapter 13

Excess winter mortality in England and Wales with special reference to the effects of temperature and influenza

By
Michael Curwen

Summary

- Mortality rates in England and Wales are higher in winter than the rest of the year.

- Excess winter mortality (EWM) was brought into prominence in recent years by: a) the recognition that hypothermia is a distinct cause of death and; b) the finding that EWM is considerably higher in Britain than in neighbouring countries.

- Hypothermia is not a major cause of EWM in England and Wales – recent analyses have shown that EWM in any one year is strongly affected by the mean national average winter temperature and the number of registered influenza deaths. In 1949–85, 88 per cent of the variation in EWM was associated with variations in temperature, influenza and a year-on- year decrease in EWM.

- These findings are confirmed by a more detailed analysis for 1970–71, where, disregarding influenza, in each of the seven months September–March there is a significant correlation between EWM and temperature.

- A parallel analysis using RCGP sickness figures confirmed the validity of influenza mortality as a measure of influenza prevalence.

- The 1949–85 analysis showed that on average each death attributed to influenza was associated with 2.6 excess deaths attributed to other causes. These are referred to as "hidden" influenza deaths, and 2.6 as the "hidden" factor.

- Subsequent analyses have suggested that the hidden factor is rising. Values as high as 20–30 for some age groups were recorded for the years 1976–88.

- The importance of hidden influenza deaths came into prominence during the epidemic of 1989–90, which was responsible, over a 12-week period, for about 25,000 excess deaths in England and Wales compared with 2,500 registered influenza deaths, giving a hidden factor of about 9.

- EWM takes its greatest toll among the elderly, but it is by no means confined to these groups. In particular the temperature effect is applicable at all ages. However, there is less association between EWM and social class than might be expected.

- The immediate causes of EWM are much the same as of all adult mortality – respiratory and cardiovascular disease.

- It has been suggested that the deficit of deaths following a major influenza epidemic is simply the result of the deaths of vulnerable people being "brought forward" by a few weeks. The present analysis casts doubt on this .

- An explanation of the marked difference between the British experience of EWM and that of other European countries will require a major effort and a multi-disciplinary approach.

13.1 Introduction

It has long been known that mortality rates in England and Wales are higher in winter than in the rest of the year. In the Registrar General's Third Annual Report Farr devoted several pages to the effect of low temperature on mortality in London during the years 1838–41 (GRO, 1841). Since at least 1850 the Annual Report has included a table showing how the national crude quarterly death rate varies from the annual rate. Taking the whole year as 100, the index for the January–March quarter increased from an average of 110 for the period 1841–50 to 128 for 1921–30 (McDowell, 1981). One cause of the increase was the gradual elimination of various causes of specifically summer mortality – particularly among children. Since 1930 the index has been falling steadily and has reached 111 for the years 1986–90.

The causes of Excess Winter Mortality (EWM) seem to have been taken for granted. Was it not obvious that cold weather 'carried off' frail, old or poor people? But Farr, for one, did not consider the problem insoluble. At the end of a cold spell in December 1874 it was presumably he who wrote (GRO, 1874):

> *But it must not therefore be assumed that the mortality (caused by this cold spell) is beyond control. The cold is most effectively combated by exercise, which excites the heating energy of the system, and warmth is sustained by nutritious food, by artificial heat, by warm woollen or fur clothing and by the respirator which returns the heat exhaled by respiration [!] The aged poor in this cold season of pressure require all these helps and have claim not only upon their kindred, but upon their wealthier Christian brethren.*

The cold winter of 1963 stimulated much interest in the subject of EWM. Hypothermia was recognised as a distinct and presumably preventable cause of death (RCP, 1966), but one which, to judge from current figures, plays only a small part in EWM as a whole. The quarterly index of 111 implies some extra 34,000 deaths in the March quarter. Since 1975, when special records were first kept, there have never been more than 600 annual deaths in England and Wales with hypothermia mentioned on the death certificate. In a wide-ranging review Alderson dealt with many aspects of seasonal mortality some of which are discussed throughout this chapter (Alderson, 1985).

Another factor that has brought the problem of EWM into prominence has been the wide range of international mortality statistics now available (UN, 1987). From these it appears that EWM is considerably higher in Britain than in neighbouring parts of Western Europe and in Scandinavia (OPCS,1987). Table 13.1 compares the latest available values of the Excess Winter Death Index (EWDI), as defined in a footnote to the table, for selected countries throughout the world.

In a similar international comparison (McKee, 1989) it was concluded that 60 per cent of the variation in EWM in 18 European countries could be accounted for by variations in minimum average monthly temperature and per capita GNP. The fact that this is only a part of the story is emphasized by comparing the UK with two of its closest neighbours, Holland and Belgium, where the EWM is around half that in the United Kingdom in spite of slightly colder winters and only slightly higher GNP. It should be pointed out that there is an error in McKee's Table 1; the EWM percentage for Belgium should read 7.2 instead of 13.9.

No attempt is made here to throw any light, except perhaps indirectly, on these international comparisons. The purpose is to explore, mainly by means of OPCS mortality statistics, the variations of EWM within England and Wales, analysed over time and by means of the usual axes such as age, sex and cause of death, using simple methods. Most of the material has already been published (OPCS, 1987; Curwen and Devis, 1988; Curwen *et al..* 1990; Curwen, 1991), but the opportunity has been taken of presenting some new material relating to monthly mortality and corresponding sickness data derived from the Weekly Returns Service of the Royal College of General Practitioners (RCGP). The finding of a relationship between temperature and mortality is of course not new. Since at least 1970 there have been studies, many from America, specifically linking low temperatures with deaths from many causes (Bull and Morton, 1978; Larsen, 1990; Keatinge *et al.,* 1989; Mannino and Washburn, 1989; Vuori, 1987; McKee, 1990). Some of these have taken into account the confounding effects of influenza.

There are many different approaches to exploring such variations. The aim of this chapter is to show that the relationship between temperature, influenza and mortality can be demonstrated and to a certain extent quantified over a long period of time using only published sources and the simplest of statistical methods.

13.2 Trends in excess winter mortality

Seasonal mortality may be studied on the basis of quarterly, monthly, weekly or even daily statistics; each method has advantages and disadvantages. The use of the four traditional quarters of the year, which divides December from the rest of the winter, has little to recommend it except for historical purposes. Weekly data have long been used, for example in the monitoring of epidemics, but are difficult to handle in the analysis of longer periods; not least among the difficulties is the fact that published weekly mortality is not analysed by age and sex, and is based on registrations rather than occurrences – a distinction which is important, for example, during holiday periods such as Christmas and the New Year. For recent years true weekly or daily mortality figures may be directly derived from the computer files.

This leaves the month as a unit for analysis. The fact that the months are of unequal length is a small disadvantage compared with the fact that the numbers of monthly occurrences of death, routinely analysed by age, sex and cause of death, have been published in England and Wales since at least 1945. In the following analysis the year is divided into three, almost exactly equal, four–month periods, December–March (winter), April–July (summer) and August–November (autumn). This is the method used, with appropriate modifications, in the international comparisons of Table 13.1. In any one year the number of Excess Winter Deaths (EWD) is defined as the number of winter deaths less the average of the numbers in the preceding autumn and the following summer.

13.2.1 Variations in EWM 1949–1991

When the numbers of deaths in England and Wales are plotted over these 42 winters (Figure 13.1) the striking feature is the erratic year-to-year variation in the numbers of winter deaths compared with steady trends (increasing with the age of the population) in the other two seasons. This contrast provides good justification for the use of the four-month division of the year in any preliminary study of seasonal mortality. A more detailed analysis, based on separate months, appears later.

Table 13.1

Mean excess winter deaths index for selected countries, 1976–84.

British Isles		Eastern Europe	
England and Wales	21	Austria	11
Scotland	20	Bulgaria (a, b)	19
Northern Ireland (5) (a, b)	18	East Germany (a, b)	10
Irish Republic (7) (a)	24	Czechoslovakia (a, b)	9
Scandinavia		**Other countries**	
Denmark	9	Canada (7)	7
Finland	8	USA (4)	9
Norway	9	Israel (7)	26
Sweden	10	Japan	17
		Australia (c)	20
Western Europe		New Zealand (c)	25
Belgium	11		
France (3)	11		
West Germany	8		
Italy (4)	19		
Netherlands	9		
Portugal (7)	26		
Spain (3)	19		
Switzerland (6)	10		

The Excess Winter Death Index (EWDI) is defined as the percentage excess of deaths in the four winter months of highest mortality (December–March unless otherwise specified) compared with the average of the numbers in the preceding and following four-monthly periods. The figures given are the mean EWDI for the eight winters 1976–84, except where the number of winters are shown in brackets.

(a) Based on registrations not occurrences.

(b) January–April.

(c) June–September.

Source: UN Demographic Yearbook, 1985

Figure 13.1

Seasonal mortality 1949–91: number of deaths in England and Wales, four-monthly periods

The numbers of expected winter deaths are based on the 1949–88 regression analysis)

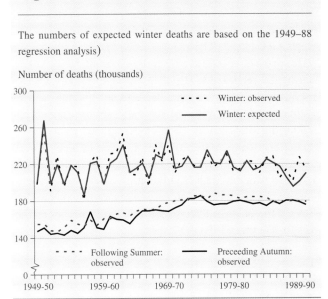

It has been shown by means of Pearsonian regression analysis (OPCS, 1987) that about 88 per cent of the variation in the numbers of EWD in the years 1949–85 could be accounted for by three variables – temperature, influenza and time. The figure shows how well the predicted model fits the original data. The analysis may be summarized as follows:

(1) Each degree Celsius by which the national mean winter temperature varied from year to year was associated with some 8,000 more or fewer EWD.

(2) Each registered influenza death was associated with between three and four EWD.

(3) Holding the other two factors constant there were, on average, 500 fewer EWD per year.

Two examples may be used to illustrate the relationship. In the winter of 1975/76, which was slightly warmer than average, the severe influenza epidemic, with 6,100 registered influenza deaths, was responsible, on this model, for about 21,000 of the observed 58,000 EWD. Three years later a particularly cold winter (but minimal influenza) apparently led to 14,000 out of the total 48,000 EWD.

It must be emphasized that the two main independent variables are no more than proxies, one for all the climatic features which may be linked with temperature and another for national influenza incidence. The analysis does nothing to explain the underlying excess winter mortality in this country, that is to say, the number of EWD that might be expected in a 'normal' winter without any influenza. Still less does it throw any light on the contrast between British experience and that of most of the rest of Europe. The underlying downward trend of EWM is discussed later.

13.3 The effects of temperature on mortality

The measure of temperature used here is a single figure for each winter – the average temperature measured during the four winter months at a number of weather stations throughout England and Wales (see Table 13.3). That being so it is perhaps remarkable that it should evidently be so effective as an indicator. It does not distinguish between day and night temperature (is a habit of sleeping with the window open particular to this country?). It does not attempt to measure sudden changes in temperature, still less the chill factor (wind speed plus coldness) or humidity – all factors which, on a common-sense view, characterize the English winter ('damp and treacherous') .

Another factor possibly related to temperature is atmospheric pollution. The extensive literature on the relation between mortality and various forms of atmospheric pollution is discussed in Chapter 12. For example, the London fog of 1952 stimulated a number of studies using daily deaths in Greater London in an attempt to disentangle the effects on mortality of atmospheric pollution, low temperatures and influenza (often associated in time with one another) (MOH, 1954; MacFarlane, 1976, 1977, 1984). It would be impracticable to apply these methods to the longer-term national trends discussed in this chapter.

13.3.1 A new monthly analysis

In order to throw more light on the temperature effect a new analysis has been undertaken based on the 12 months taken separately – rather than on the average for the four winter months. The period August 1970–July 1991 was chosen for this analysis, the year 1970 being something of a watershed, with fewer severe influenza deaths epidemics since then.

To separate the effects of temperature and influenza, regression analysis has again been used – with one refinement. In order to reduce the distorting effect of major epidemics, months in which the numbers of registered influenza deaths exceeded an entirely arbitrary figure of 500 have been omitted. In the absence of an epidemic there are seldom more than a few hundred such deaths per month, while in epidemic years it may even reach 3,000. Details of the nine excluded months are shown in Table 13.2.

Table 13.2

Months with more than 500 registered influenza deaths during the period August 1970 to July 1991, England and Wales

Year	Month	No of influenza deaths
1972	January	905
	February	614
	December	1,522
1973	January	2,214
1976	February	3,075
	March	2,755
1977	April	528
1978	February	502
1989	December	2,142

Source: RCGP Weekly Returns Service

The model for the new regression analysis is as follows:

Excess deaths in month = B1 * excess temperature in same month + B2 * excess temperature in previous month + B3 * excess influenza deaths in same month

In each case the 'excess' is measured from the mean of the appropriate non-excluded months. All calculations are performed within months of the same name; thus their differing lengths does not effect the analysis. Deaths are for all ages. Table 13.3 gives the estimated values of the regression coefficients for temperature. Discussion of B3, the influenza coefficient, appears in the next section. A model taking account of influenza deaths in the previous month did not prove useful and was discarded.

Table 13.3

Monthly deaths related to temperature, August 1970 – July 1991, England and Wales

	Number of months	Average deaths ('00)	Number of excess deaths (all causes) per degree colder	
			In current month	In previous month
	(a)	(b)	B1	B2
August	21	416	(50)	430
September	21	427	**640**	(160)
October	21	454	**920**	(-50)
November	21	479	**1,120**	(80)
December	19	529	**1,060**	(310)
January	19	561	**1,050**	620
February	18	542	**1,360**	(630)
March	20	528	820	(380)
April	20	489	(250)	(530)
May	21	458	(350)	(70)
June	21	441	(-60)	(600)
July	21	428	(130)	(-50)

(a) Excluding months in which the number of registered influenza deaths exceeded 500.

(b) Average number of deaths, all causes, adjusted for unequal length of months.

Significance (two-tailed):	**bold**	=	*1%*
	normal	=	*5%*
	(brackets)	=	*not significant.*

Source: Author's unpublished data

The analysis confirms the earlier one – that in much of the year total mortality is independently related to temperature and influenza. (In fact there is virtually no correlation between temperature and influenza mortality except in January, where there is a just significant positive correlation coefficient, i.e. more influenza in warmer Januaries.) In each of the seven months September–March there is a significant relationship between temperature and mortality, the regression coefficient (measuring excess deaths per degree of temperature) rising from 640 in September to 1,360 in February and falling back to 820 in March.

The significant figure for September is perhaps surprising. It is well known that this is the time when mortality begins to rise after the August minimum, but to judge from the total numbers of deaths shown in Table 13.3, the increase between August and September is quite small; what has been demonstrated here is that any such increase seems to be specifically related to temperature. This finding is perhaps foreshadowed by the analysis of daily deaths in England and Wales in the two years 1970–71 which concluded that mortality from most causes of death was correlated with temperature throughout the year (Bull and Morton, 1978).

The coefficient B2 indicates how, after allowing for the effect of the current month's temperature, mortality is related to temperature in the previous month. It can be seen that all but two of the values of B2 were in the expected direction, but only in January and (curiously enough) August can the coefficient be regarded as significant. This is obviously a crude model making no distinction between potential time-lags ranging from a few days to eight weeks. However, the general conclusion to be drawn from the low values of B2 is that the average time-lag of any association between temperature and mortality is a relatively short one – perhaps no more than a week or two. This again confirms the finding of time-lags ranging from one to six days (Bull and Morton, 1978).

Another finding which should be noted is the apparent 'fading' of the temperature effect during, or after, March, in spite of the fact that March is on average colder and has a higher mortality than October and April than September. By the spring it is presumably the cumulative effects of the winter's bad weather that are taking their toll, thus blurring the picture. Also it is not usually until February that influenza begins to play a more important part than temperature. But it would be naive to suppose that a simple regression analysis could distinguish between the associations of mortality with temperature and influenza – which in any case vary from year to year.

13.4 The effect of influenza

The original regression analysis covering the years 1949–1985 suggested that each death registered as being due to influenza was associated with 3.6 EWD, that is to say, with 2.6 deaths registered as due to causes other than influenza. It is convenient to refer to these as 'hidden influenza deaths' and the figure 2.6 as the 'hidden factor'.

A systematic analysis in the Netherlands of mortality covering the 22 years 1967–89 yielded the identical figure of 2.6 for the number of hidden influenza deaths for every registered influenza death (Sprenger et al., 1993). This analysis took no account of temperature, nor was there any suggestion of any change in the hidden factor over the period. The same authors cite Farr, writing 150 years ago, as having arrived at the figure of 3.5 as this hidden factor (Langmuir, 1976).

In recent years it has appeared that the fit of the 1949–85 model was not as close as it had been previously. It seemed possible that a model, largely based on a period with frequent severe epidemics, was no longer applicable to the low levels of influenza between 1976 and 1989. A fresh analysis was carried out for the 12 winters 1976–88 using a more sophisticated model, based on five separate age-sex groups (Curwen and Devis, 1988). The surprising feature of this was that not only did influenza continue to be an important contributor to EWM, but that as measured by the hidden factor, its importance was greatly enhanced. Instead of two or three hidden influenza deaths for every one registered, there were, when the age-groups were taken separately, perhaps as many as 20 to 30 (Table 13.4). Another confirmation of raised levels of hidden influenza deaths derives from a study of regional mortality discussed in the next section.

Table 13.4

Estimates of hidden influenza deaths, England and Wales

			Average no. of registered influenza deaths	Hidden factor (a) (with 95% confidence limits)
Regression method: 4-month winter				
1949–85	all ages		2600	2.6 (1.8–3.4)
1976–88 (b)	ages 45–64	M + F	33	20 (8–32)
	ages 65–74	M	36	35 (24–46)
		F	32	24 (7–41)
	ages 75+	M	105	22 (9–35)
		F	246	14 (5–23)
Regression method: individual months				
1970–91 all ages (c)	December		68	17 (2–32)
	January		154	10 (2–18)
	February		122	11 (3–19)
	March		150	15 (9–21)
	April		84	6 (0–14)
	May		30	14 (3–25)
Weekly analysis of epidemics: all ages (d)				
			Actual no. of deaths	
1969–70	(wks 49–6)		9510	1.8
1972–73	(wks 47–6)		3440	4.6
1975–76	(wks 5–17)		5220	2.3
1989–90	(wks 46–5)		2510	8.9

(a) The hidden factor is the number of excess deaths associated with influenza, but not registered as such, to the number registered as due to influenza.
(b) A period with no major epidemics.
(c) Omitting months with more than 500 influenza deaths.
(d) Excess deaths calculated by comparison with corresponding weekly deaths in previous winter.

Source: GRO and ONS

The importance of hidden influenza deaths came into prominence at the time of the epidemic of 1989/90 – the first of such magnitude since that of 1975/76. This epidemic seems to have been responsible, over a period of 12 weeks, for about 25,000 excess deaths in England and Wales compared with 2,500 registered influenza deaths, thus giving a hidden factor of about 9 compared with 2.3 for 1975/76. Excess deaths were calculated by comparison with the corresponding weeks of the previous winter (Curwen et al.,1990).

These latter estimates of hidden influenza deaths were based on a detailed study of weekly mortality figures, comparing them with three measures of influenza incidence: laboratory reports, general practitioner returns and the number of registered influenza deaths, all of which, generally speaking, concurred in the dates when the epidemics began, peaked and ended. Here we have much stronger evidence of the reality of the hidden influenza death phenomenon than can be gained from regression analysis. It is difficult to escape the conclusion that the same agent, labelled as 'influenza' by pathologists, general practitioners and some certifiers was, directly or indirectly, responsible for a great many deaths which did not bear this label. What in fact did cause these excess deaths is discussed later.

Table 13.4 gives the various estimates of the hidden factor derived from all these sources, including the monthly regressions. The fact that the factor tends to be lower during well publicized epidemics than in low-influenza periods is presumably due to certifiers being then more likely to be alerted to the possibility of influenza as the cause of death.

The literature on the association of mortality with influenza is probably as extensive as that with temperature. In the United Kingdom the most important recent work has been that from the Public Health Laboratory Service (Clifford *et al.*, 1977; Tillett and Spencer, 1982; Tillett *et al.*, 1983), who are careful to distinguish the effects of temperature and influenza. One finding was that the effects of cold weather and influenza were multiplicative rather than additive. This is in spite of the finding reported here that cold weather and influenza are not usually associated with each other. The present work has confirmed the PHLS evidence of excess deaths associated with influenza in non-epidemic years.

13.5 The effect of age

Since at least the time of Farr it has been recognized that it is the elderly who are particularly at risk during cold weather. From Table 13.5 it will be seen that there is a marked age-gradient in the EWDI (which measures excess winter mortality as a percentage of non-winter mortality), the index for all causes of death in the years 1976–83 being more than twice as high at ages of 75 and over, compared with those of 45–64. By the years 1986–91 the gap between these two age-groups had widened as a result partly of the 1989–90 influenza epidemic and partly the increasing average age of those in the oldest group.

Below the age of 45 the measurement of EWM is complicated by the excess summer mortality largely due to accidents in young adults, particularly males, thus giving negative values of the index. For the sake of completeness the following values of the EWDI for the years 1986–91 are recorded here; ages 1–14, Male: 5, Female: 8; ages 15–34, Male: -5, Female: -1; ages 35–44, Male: 6, Female: 2. The question of seasonal infant and childhood mortality is outside the scope of the present analysis.

It is apparent that EWM is by no means confined to the elderly. For example, the cold winter of 1984/85 was evidently responsible for the deaths of about 4,500 men and women in the 45–64 age-group – comparable for example to the annual toll of genito urinary cancer at those ages.

Table 13.5

Mean excess winter death index by age, sex and cause of death 1976–83, 1987–91, England and Wales

		Age-group		
		45–64	65–74	75+
1976-83				
Ischaemic heart disease	M	16	20	27
	F	18	20	25
Cerebrovascular disease	M	16	20	30
	F	16	19	27
Other circulatory disease	M	20	24	34
	F	22	28	31
Respiratory disease	M	53	53	53
	F	54	57	58
Accidents and violence	M	8	15	36
	F	12	20	38
All other causes	M	3	5	11
	F	3	5	9
ALL CAUSES	M	13	18	27
	F	11	18	27
1987–91				
ALL CAUSES	M, F	11	14	24

Source: GRO and ONS

The effect of temperature and influenza on monthly mortality over the period 1970–91 has been analysed separately for three broad age-bands. Broadly speaking, the results are similar to those described above for all ages. The temperature effect may be summarised by looking at the average number of extra deaths in each of the six winter months October–March associated with each degree Celsius below average, and showing these as percentages of the corresponding averages of all deaths in these months.

The figures are as follows:

	Below 65	65–74	75+
Average extra deaths	140	260	680
per month per degree	(1.2%)	(1.9%)	(2.5%)

These figures may be compared with those of Larsen (Larsen, 1990), who showed that in parts of the United States of America the cumulative effect of low temperatures in each of the months December–February was an increase between 1 per cent and 2 per cent of the crude death rate per degree Fahrenheit. (There were only slight increases in September.)

13.6 Cause of death

In the period 1976–83 circulatory disease caused 55 per cent and respiratory disease (including influenza) 33 per cent of all excess winter deaths among adults aged 45 or more. For non-winter deaths the corresponding proportions were 52 per cent and 16 per cent. It follows that, as might be expected, it is in respiratory mortality that winter has the greatest proportional effect.

Table 13.5 gives the EWDI by age and sex for men and women aged 45 or more in six main cause-groups. It is seen that winter increases the chance of dying from respiratory disease by more than 50 per cent, the risk varying little with age. For the three main types of circulatory disease identified in the table – ischaemic heart disease, cerebrovascular disease and 'other'– the increased risks are lower, but the age-gradients are steeper. For example, the male ischaemic EWDIs range from 16 at ages 45–64 to 27 at over 75. There is no real evidence from these figures distinguishing any one of the three categories of circulatory disease.

The gradient is particularly steep in the category of 'injury and poisoning'. Roughly half the excess winter deaths classified thus were associated in some way with hypothermia. Numerically speaking these are not, however, an important source of mortality. Taking out these five cause-groups leaves a residual group where the EWDIs are mostly well below 10 – indicating that the main sources of EWM have been identified.

The foregoing special analysis was based on the years 1976–83, a period relatively free from influenza. During influenza epidemics there is, as will be seen, a steep age-gradient in respiratory disease. Interpretation of these figures, particularly for the elderly, is made difficult by a blurring of the distinction between respiratory and circulatory causes of death as recorded on death certificates – a problem only partly solved by the change in the rules for selecting the underlying cause made in 1984. (Monthly mortality is not routinely tabulated by age and cause of death together.)

These findings accord with those of many other studies cited above, in which increased mortality due to ischaemic heart disease, strokes and pneumonia is specifically associated with low temperatures. Seasonal variation in plasma fibrinogen concentration is among the mechanisms that have been suggested as a cause of increased circulatory mortality (Stout and Crawford, 1991). The same range of diseases, with predictably more emphasis on respiratory conditions, are associated with influenza (Tillett et al., 1983; Ashley, et al., 1991). Other diseases whose mortality is claimed to be associated with influenza include diabetes mellitus and musculo-skeletal disease (Tillett et al., 1983; Diepersloot, et al., 1990).

13.7 Social class

As with other forms of mortality and other health statistics it is pertinent to ask whether the extra risk of dying in winter is related to socio-economic circumstances. The most recent evidence on this matter is derived from the Longitudinal Study (Fox and Goldblatt, 1982) which uses, among others, two socio-economic markers: housing tenure – distinguishing mainly between people with owner-occupied and those with rented accommodation; and car-access – distinguishing those who have access to a car within the family. Taking two contrasting groups classified in 1971 and followed up until 1985 the following EWDIs have been calculated:

	Males	Females
Owner-occupation with car-access	18	18
Rented accommodation without car-access	22	25

These differences are perhaps less than might be expected, although it should be pointed out that the analysis excludes those in institutions – and that in any case car access is less relevant for the very old.

13.8 Geographical region

In view of the international variations in the level of EWM, variations within England and Wales might have been expected. But an analysis covering the eleven winters 1976–87 (during which there was no influenza epidemic) showed that, on average, there was remarkably little variation in EWM between the standard regions. A slight North to South gradient may perhaps be detected, although a high figure for Greater London – regarded as a separate region – suggests an effect of urbanization (Curwen, 1991).

Although there was little suggestion that EWM varied on average between the regions, there were considerable year-to-year variations which can be attributed to differing geographical patterns of regional influenza incidence – as measured by crude influenza death rates (and often on extremely small numbers of influenza deaths). This pattern is not in any way related to temperature, for which the regional ranking order is virtually unchanged from year to year. Taking each winter separately, the regional EWDIs were positively correlated with the local influenza death rates in nine out of the 11 winters (five of the correlation coefficients being significant at 5 per cent).

13.9 Measures of influenza sickness

At the time when the methods of analysis described here were first undertaken it seemed that the only appropriate measure of influenza incidence was that of the number of deaths registered as due to influenza. To use these as an 'independent' measure when studying variations in all deaths (of which influenza deaths are a subset) may be criticised as involving a logical circularity.

Since 1967 information about episodes of many common illnesses have been collected from a sample of ('sentinel') general practitioners throughout England and Wales (Fleming and Crombie, 1985). In the 1970s the sample of patients on these doctors' lists represented about 3.3 per thousand of the population, a figure which was raised to 4.7 in the 1980s. In 1989 there were about 230 participating doctors – mainly self-selected. There is no claim that the sample of patients is random, but at least in such factors as age and sex it can be shown to be reasonably representative. Independent studies have validated many of the findings based on the returns (OPCS, 1975) and they are being increasingly used for epidemiological purposes.

Among the list of diseases reported are 'epidemic influenza' (EI) and 'influenza-like illness' (ILI), although it is recognised that there is bound to be overlapping not only between these labels but between either of them and those of other respiratory conditions, such as the common cold. The following figures show the relative importance of EI and ILI in comparison with other such conditions for the period 1973–91 (in terms of average annual episode rates per thousand population).

	Average	Range
Epidemic influenza (EI)	10	4–32
Influenza-like illness (ILI)	33	14–47
Other respiratory conditions (mainly common cold, acute tonsillitis, acute bronchitis)	267	234–317

The RCGP material is routinely published by ONS in the form of weekly population-based rates. Tillett and Spencer compared several indices in assessing the size, timing and duration of influenza outbreaks during the 12 winters 1968–80. They concluded that the following indices were in general agreement in their estimates of the magnitude of epidemics: RCGP rate for EI, total deaths (from all causes), total respiratory deaths, influenza deaths and sickness benefit claims (Tillett and Spencer, 1982). Laboratory reports, although for various reasons not suitable for statistical analysis, are clearly important in identifying the nature of

outbreaks. In France and the Netherlands, where similar systems are in operation, weekly rates based on ILI (combined with EI) are used for monitoring influenza epidemics (Dab *et al.*, 1991; Sprenger *et al.*, 1991).

A practical difficulty in the use of the RCGP figures for long-term studies, such as those reported here, is that all rates are calculated on a weekly basis. In a recent study of seasonality (Fleming *et al.*, 1991) these have been aggregated into rates for 13 lunar months – a method which has yielded interesting results, but which cannot easily be used in conjunction with those based on calendar months.

For the purposes of the present study calendar-month rates for EI and ILI have been calculated for the period August 1970 to July 1991 by assuming that episodes reported in weeks overlapping two months are proportionately distributed. For example, three sevenths of the episodes in a week beginning 29 March are allocated to that month and, four sevenths to April.

Figures 13.2 and 13.3 show how these rates compare with those calculated from registered influenza deaths. The first thing to notice is the similarity of the trends. Each of the yearly rates shows a general decline, those for influenza deaths and influenza illness being punctuated by three major epidemics. It can be seen that the peaks of influenza mortality are more pronounced than those of influenza illness (a finding which corroborates the suggestion made earlier of lower values of the hidden factor during epidemics). As might be expected the trend of ILI fluctuates less than those of the other two rates. Turning to the monthly pattern, there is again close similarity between the three trends – the ILI rate rising about fourfold from a summer base-line to a peak in February, while the other two rates are almost zero in the summer months.

Figure 13.2

Three measures of influenza: deaths, episodes of epidemic influenza (EI) and episodes of influenza-like illness(ILI), annual rates (August–July)

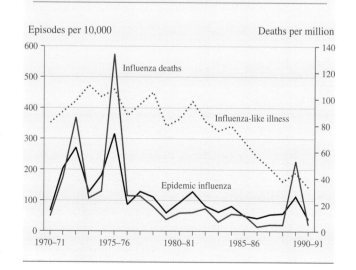

Figure 13.3

Three measures of influenza and temperature: average monthly rates (allowing for unequal month length.)

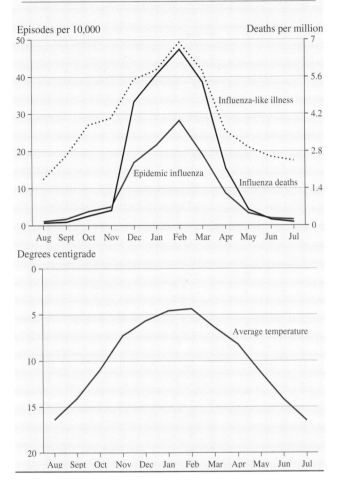

One result of this analysis has been to confirm the validity of using registered influenza deaths as a measure of influenza incidence. In fact the regressions of mortality with influenza and temperature are hardly altered if, instead of influenza deaths, we use either EI rates, or the sum of EI and ILI rates. It is only in the months of April and May where influenza sickness (including ILI) is an appreciably better predictor than influenza mortality.

Table 13.6

Correlation coefficients between the three measures of influenza, England and Wales

	Number of months (a)	Influenza deaths * EI episodes	Influenza deaths * ILI episodes	EI episodes * ILI episodes
August	21	(0.36)	(0.40)	**0.58**
September	21	0.52	**0.66**	0.46
October	21	**0.70**	**0.80**	**0.72**
November	21	0.46	**0.68**	0.54
December	19	**0.82**	**0.71**	**0.67**
January	19	**0.65**	(0.18)	**0.64**
February	18	**0.90**	**0.64**	**0.76**
March	20	**0.94**	**0.69**	**0.75**
April	20	**0.73**	0.54	**0.85**
May	21	0.52	0.50	**0.77**
June	21	(0.18)	0.46	**0.65**
July	21	(0.33)	**0.60**	0.50

(a)   *Excluding the nine months in which the number of registered influenza deaths exceeded 500.*

* *Indications of significance (two-tailed):*
         bold = *1%*
         normal = *5%*
         (brackets) = *not significant at 5%*

Before looking at the three monthly measures in detail it should be mentioned that the relationship of each with temperature has been examined in order to ensure that there is no general confounding between the effects of temperature and influenza on mortality. In fact there are as many positive as negative values amongst the 36 relevant correlation coefficients. Most of these are far from significant, the only exceptions being that, as already mentioned, influenza deaths are positively correlated with temperature in January (i.e. more deaths in warmer weather) while both EI and ILI are negatively correlated with temperature in October (when there is little influenza about).

Table 13.6 shows the correlation coefficients between the three measures of influenza for each of the 12 months (again omitting the epidemic months as previously defined). It will be seen that for all the eight months May to September there is a strong correlation between them. (The only exception, that between EI and ILI in January, is entirely due to an anomalous result in January 1990, which included the tail end of the recent epidemic although with not enough deaths to be excluded by the arbitrary criterion – and a marked reduction in the number of cases labelled ILI.) Even for the summer months, when there were sometimes no influenza deaths and only a handful of reported cases, there is evidence that the three indices are measuring aspects of the same phenomenon.

13.10 Age and influenza

During the period of this survey the proportion of older people in the population has increased, and consequently the age-distribution of deaths has changed. The proportion of persons aged 75 and over in the population rose from 4.8 per cent in 1971 to 7.1 per cent in 1991. This age-group accounted for 45 per cent of all deaths in 1971–75 and 56 per cent of all deaths in 1986–90.

The age-distribution of deaths registered as due to influenza has shown considerable fluctuation over the years – presumably as a result of changes in the immunity status of various sections of the population (OPCS, 1987). In the years 1971–75 the proportion of those over 75 amongst influenza deaths ranged between 49 per cent and 64 per cent, with an underlying upward trend to around 80 per cent in the years 1986–90. These changes are quite out of proportion to changes in general mortality, nor do they seem to relate to the severity of influenza epidemics.

For the two influenza epidemics of 1969–70 and 1989–90 the age-distribution of all (including 'hidden') influenza deaths has been estimated (Table 13.7). In the recent epidemic as many as 42 per cent of all such deaths were of people aged 85 and over (compared with 21 per cent for deaths due to all causes in a non-epidemic year). By contrast the contribution of the 45–64 age-group to the total of influenza-related deaths had almost disappeared by 1989–90. These findings are confirmed by the PHLS calculations (Tillett *et al.*, 1991), where they are related to the changing antigenic pattern of the circulating virus.

The use of the RCGP figures for cases of influenza and ILI makes it possible to calculate estimated fatality rates. Since the great majority of influenza deaths are of people aged 65 and over the calculation of such rates has been confined to this group. (The RCGP figures do not separate ages above 65.)

Omitting the epidemics of 1976 and 1989–90, the fatality rates, which again show considerable year-to-year fluctuation, have generally been declining. For the years 1975–78 the number of registered influenza deaths at ages of 65 and over ranged from 5 to 8 per thousand cases of influenza (EI plus ILI), falling to a range of 2 to 4 per thousand 10 years later. These rates are based on calendar years rather than winters.

The fatality rates at these ages for years with major epidemics were considerably higher – 24 per thousand in 1976 and 10 per thousand in 1989–90. It may be, of course, that these changes simply reflect changes in the perception of influenza as an underlying cause of death as the true prevalence of influenza varies.

Table 13.7

Percentage age-distribution of excess deaths during influenza epidemics, England and Wales

	All ages	65–74	75–84	85+
1969–70	100	47 (28)	21 (30)	7 (16)
1989–90	100	15 (24)	40 (35)	42 (21)

These figures are based on a comparison with the corresponding weeks in the previous year. The figures in brackets are the corresponding percentages for all annual deaths in the immediately following (non-influenza) year.

Source: GRO and ONS

13.11 Peaks and troughs of influenza epidemics: the question of deaths 'brought forward'

In a detailed analysis of the 1989/90 influenza epidemic (Ashley, *et al.*, 1991) it was suggested that in Great Britain the 29,000 'excess' deaths during the 56 days of the epidemic (17 November–11 January) were followed by a 'deficit' of about 11,000 deaths during the period up to 31 March, the explanation being that 'the influenza virus caused the death of people who might have died anyway in the next few months'.

A fresh analysis, presented here, casts considerable doubt on this finding. In the earlier analysis the expected mortality was based simply on the mortality recorded in the previous 4 years. A more reliable method of estimating the excess mortality takes account of the temperature. In fact the weather in the late winter and early spring of 1990 was exceptionally mild. For the months February–May the average temperature (in England and Wales) was more than 2°C higher than in the previous 4 years, and in February alone 4°C higher.

Figure 13.4 compares the two methods of calculation of the 'peak and trough'. The new calculation bases the expected deaths on the regression of total mortality with temperature for the months November–March, applying it to the actual temperatures in 1990. For the months December–March it also includes the regression with influenza mortality, applying it to an average non-epidemic year. For April and May the estimates of influenza sickness (EI plus ILI) – which, as described earlier, are better predictors – are used instead of mortality. It will be seen that the higher than average temperatures have led to larger estimates of the peak and considerably smaller estimates of the trough when compared with the 4-year method. Using monthly figures alone it is not, of course, possible to define the period of the epidemic with any precision but it seems that the proportion of deaths 'brought forward' by the epidemic was not more than 10 per cent of the total mortality. This figure compares with the previous estimate of 38 per cent. Such evidence as there is suggests that the troughs of mortality following the epidemics of 1972/73 and 1976 also represented slightly less than 10 per cent of the total mortality.

These findings may be compared with those of the PHLS analysis (Tillett *et al.*, 1991), where it is concluded that, although in previous epidemics there was no evidence of any

Figure 13.4

Excess and deficit of total monthly deaths, all causes, during and after influenza epidemic of 1989–90. Comparison of two methods of calculation

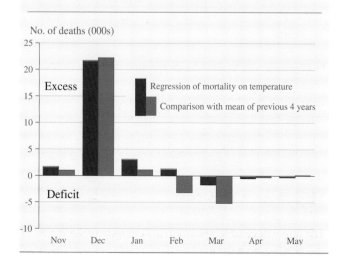

bringing forward of deaths likely to have occurred shortly afterwards, there was some evidence (not quantified) that such a phenomenon may have occurred in 1989–90. Data from the Netherlands also confirms the absence of reduced mortality following influenza epidemics (Mackenbach *et al.*, 1992).

A more general demonstration that there is no marked 'peak–trough' phenomenon in winter mortality derives from an analysis of EWD over the whole period 1950–1990; mortality in each of the four months April–July is, if anything, slightly positively correlated with total mortality in the preceding four months.

13.12   Long-term trends

The original analysis, based on the years 1949–85, showed that, allowing for changes in temperature and influenza, there were some 500 fewer excess winter deaths in England and Wales every year. This represented slightly less than 1 per cent of all excess winter deaths at the beginning of that period. This figure, however, was an underestimate of the true rate of decline, taking no account of the ageing of the population. The analysis of monthly mortality shows that in each of the three age–groups the underlying reduction in the annual excess mortality rates (again allowing for temperature and influenza) during the six months October–March was of the same order, about 1 per cent per year, during the period 1970–90 (see also Table 13.5).

In an exhaustive study of worldwide trends in seasonal mortality it was claimed that the increasing use of central heating had been a principal cause of the general reduction in seasonal swings ('deseasonality') throughout the present century (Sakamoto-Momiyama, 1977). If this, or any other, cause could be identified, we might have a clue to the problem of Britain's apparent lagging behind the rest of Europe. But neither she nor any subsequent writers seem to have found any firm evidence for this hypothesis. Indeed it is difficult to see how such evidence could effectively separate the effects of central heating from parallel socio-economic and environmental factors. A recent review suggested that the decline in EWM in the Netherlands was only partly due to decreases in influenza, that the role of central heating was minimal, and that 'a fundamental role is played by other factors closely related to socio-economic progress' (Kunst *et al.*, 1990).

In England and Wales the proportion of households with central heating rose from 13 per cent in 1964 to 82 per cent in 1991 (OPCS, 1994) and it has been argued, reasonably enough, that the absence of any corresponding decrease in arterial EWM suggests that outdoor exposures to cold weather may be chiefly to blame (Keatinge and Holmes, 1990).

13.13   Conclusions

The importance of temperature in determining the variations in EWM has been demonstrated in a number of ways, although nothing has emerged which throws any light on the way Britain differs from most of Europe. Even in Scandinavia, where the EWMI is about half of that in Britain, people are exposed to outdoor as well as indoor temperatures and to sudden changes of weather in the autumn. The relevant causative agent is presumably something that is related to temperature, but with the nature of the relationship differing in different places. Some such factors, including atmospheric pollution, have already been mentioned. It has indeed been suggested (Larsen, 1990) that variability in the weather has an even greater effect on mortality than temperature extremes. Since temperature fluctuations are generally greater during cold weather, it would be difficult to substantiate this idea, although it is a factor to be considered.

The relationship between mortality and influenza is a complicated and subtle one, not least because of the imprecision of the term 'influenza'. During major epidemics there is little problem: we have short periods where an identifiable virus (often isolated from children) is evidently causing a sudden increase in episodes of illness described as influenza by general practitioners; a sudden increase in deaths, mostly of old people, ascribed to influenza by certifying doctors; and a very much greater increase – also mainly in old people – apparently due to a whole variety of diseases other than influenza. But even in non-epidemic years – and during the summer – there is a ground-swell of something called 'influenza' which is associated with increased mortality.

Over the past 40 years there have been considerable changes in the virological pattern of influenza which presumably lie behind the reduced frequency and severity of epidemics and in the fluctuating – but generally increasing – age-structure of influenza mortality. It is against this background that the increasing level of what has been here called the 'hidden factor' must be judged. It may indeed be simply due to a changing perception among certifying doctors (often general practitioners) as to the role of influenza in the causation of death, which has been reflected in the apparently reduced fatality rates.

It has recently been suggested that respiratory syncytial virus (RSV) may be as important as influenza viruses in causing excess mortality among elderly people, and that it may be impossible to distinguish between the two causes by epidemiological studies alone (Fleming and Cross, 1993). It is even suggested that Britain's damper climate, compared with mainland Europe, may favour the spread of RSV. Perhaps the last word should go to McKee:

> *The continuing toll of premature death associated with cold weather deserves more attention than it has received in the past. There is now a need to explain why the UK has such a bad record. The answer is likely to require a multidisciplinary approach. The causes of death associated with the cold are now known. We need sociologists, economists and architects to tell us why elderly Britons seem to be exposed to the cold to a greater extent than their continental neighbours.*
> (McKee, 1991)

Acknowledgements

I wish to express my extreme gratitude to all those in ONS from Abe Adelstein onwards – too many to name separately – who have enabled and encouraged me to continue riding my hobbyhorse long into my retirement. I should also thank Donald Crombie and his staff at the Birmingham Research Unit of the Royal College of General Practitioners who have so freely given me the use of their morbidity data.

Chapter 14

Medical advances and iatrogenesis

By
John Charlton, Patricia Fraser and Mike Murphy

Summary

- Major advances in preventive medicine in the nineteenth century included vaccination against smallpox, the Pasteurisation process for milk and the introduction of antiseptics into surgery. Advances in medical technology, such as anaesthesia and antiseptics, made more complex surgery possible. Some specific indicators of medical advance between 1841 and 1950 were maternal mortality, infant mortality and tuberculosis.

- Since 1950, epidemiological studies, resulting in health education, have led to a reduction in smoking. Vaccine coverage has eradicated smallpox and greatly reduced the prevalence of diphtheria, pertussis, tetanus and poliomyelitis. Prevention has also played a role in reducing the number of accidents.

- Radiotherapy and cytotoxic chemotherapy have greatly improved the chances of survival for patients with cancers. Chemotherapeutic agents linked to monoclonal antibodies can now be used to attack cancer cells. Measures aimed at protecting body tissues from the side-effects of radiation and chemotherapy are also a recent development.

- Death rates from 'avoidable causes' showed a more rapid decline between 1950 and 1994 than death rates from 'non-avoidable causes'. Perinatal mortality rates and maternal mortality rates, both regarded as good indicators for antenatal and obstetric care, have fallen since 1950. Perinatal mortality rates have fallen by 80 per cent to 7.6 per 1,000, maternal mortality rates by 91 per cent.

- On the negative side, the unwanted effects of drugs have increased with their power and widespread use. Short-term unwanted effects of treatments, the effects of over-medication and malignancies following treatments such as chemotherapy are examples of these effects.

- It has been argued that the reduction of mortality has depended more on the control of the origins of disease than on knowledge of the mechanisms of disease. The health sector is still oriented towards therapeutic interventions rather than prevention. There is also a need for better evaluations of many medical treatments and surgical procedures.

14.1 Introduction

This chapter is concerned with the effects, positive and negative, that advances in medical knowledge and practice have had on the health of the British population. These are discussed using a few selected examples – a full review would require a book to itself.

Medical knowledge can have influences at various levels. At the individual level, a better understanding of hygiene and desirable health-related behaviour can reduce the risk of disease. At the level of society, medical knowledge can lead to legislation regulating food production and distribution, sanitation, air pollution, housing and employment. It may also lead governments to make provision for education (including health education), housing and social security benefits to those in need, and other measures to promote better health, such as those aimed at reducing the level of smoking. Finally, medical advance may lead to improvements in the treatments offered by doctors and associated professions.

Chapters 3 and 4 chart the considerable improvements that have occurred since 1841 in life expectation and mortality from various diseases. Similar increases in average life expectancy have occurred in other industrialised countries. The causes of increased longevity are many, including improvements in nutrition, housing, sanitation, occupational hazards, lifestyle (see Chapters 6 to 12) and medical care. There has been much controversy about the extent of the direct contribution made by the medical profession to the population's health over the past 150 years. Cochrane (1972), and McKeown (McKeown, 1976) have emphasised the need to evaluate properly the effects of new procedures and drugs (see below).

14.2 Medical advances 1841–1950

Infectious diseases were the major cause of death in the nineteenth century (see Chapters 4 and 15). The mechanisms were not at all understood, because for much of the nineteenth century these diseases were thought to arise from 'miasmas', malodorous poisons arising from unsanitary environments, rather than from microbes and viruses.

14.2.1 Prevention

Although Jenner introduced vaccination against smallpox, one of the world's most dreaded plagues, in 1796, it took some years for his evidence to be accepted by the medical profession and government. In 1853 smallpox vaccination was made compulsory for children within 4 months of birth, but this did not have an immediate effect (see Chapter 15) – there was a major outbreak in 1870 when 40,000 died, 10,000 in London. Vaccination was not always without problems, especially as the mechanism was ill-understood. Sometimes the vaccine contained the smallpox virus, and fatalities were not unknown. Smallpox was finally eradicated in 1977

through worldwide vaccination programmes promoted by the World Health Organisation (WHO).

In 1842 Chadwick wrote his *Report into the Sanitary Condition of the Labouring Population of Great Britain*. He was largely responsible for the Public Health Act of 1848, which, through a General Board of Health, furnished guidance and aid to local authorities. He was commissioner of the Board from 1848 to 1854. This had powers to establish local boards of health and investigate sanitary conditions in particular districts. The Act enabled local authorities to appoint Medical Officers of Health (MOHs) to oversee public health issues, but it was only with the introduction of the 1872 Act that they were required to do so. The nineteenth century approach to public health was for government to issue regulations (especially regarding buildings, nuisances and foods) and local authorities to implement the 'sanitary idea' (Lewis, 1991). Chadwick was succeeded by Simon (1855–76) who laid down principles that have become the foundations of public health. The success of his work owed much to the mortality statistics produced by Farr of the General Register Office (now ONS). Sanitation, the urban environment and Acts of Parliament to promote health are discussed in Chapter 6. Flinn (1965) has argued that the major contribution of doctors in Victorian Britain was in their promotion of an awareness of the association between dirt and disease.

Cross-infection was another mechanism contributing to iatrogenic mortality. In 1848, Semmelweis observed that the women who were delivered by doctors had puerperal fever mortality rates some two to three times higher than those delivered by midwives. He conducted one of the first clinical trials and established that if doctors washed their hands in chlorinated lime before each examination the maternal death rate dropped from 18.3 per cent to 1.3 per cent. His results were published in 1861. His superior and others in Austria would not accept his findings (although the Hungarians did) because the accepted wisdom was that miasmas were the cause of infection. He died in a mental hospital after a breakdown in 1865. Semmelweis's story provides a good example, too, of how the diffusion of medical knowledge can often take time.

A major breakthrough with infectious diseases occurred when Pasteur demonstrated the link between bacteria and disease in 1862. He invented the Pasteurisation process for milk, then a carrier of tuberculosis, brucellosis and other diseases. His discoveries led Lister to introduce antiseptics in surgery – from 1869 onwards he disinfected his hands and objects which came into contact with the wound before undertaking surgery, and covered the wound afterwards with gauze that had been dipped into a weak phenolic acid solution. Mortality in his patients fell from 6 per cent or more to less than 2 per cent within a few years, and wounds healed more quickly (Biraben, 1991). By 1871 his methods were widely used by other British surgeons, and a carbolic acid steam spray was in use in some operating theatres by 1875. Sterilisation techniques continued to be improved: surgical instruments were sterilised by dry heat by 1889, the same year that sterilised rubber gloves and operating tables were introduced. Between 1885 and 1895 knowledge and use of aseptic surgical procedures were widespread (Biraben, 1991). By 1895 they had caught the public's imagination as well, sometimes to excess – people hunted down flies, lice and midges, disinfected their bodies (sometimes causing dermatitis) and boiled food excessively so that it lost its vitamin C content, with the result that scurvy occurred among children in some well-off families (Biraben, 1991). Overall, however, the general awareness by 1895 of bacteria, asepsis and antisepsis brought positive results. In London the crude mortality rate fell by 19 per cent between 1861–70 and 1881–90, but by a further 25 per cent by 1901–05, an acceleration which Biraben (1991) attributes to knowledge of microbes. In Paris the corresponding figures were 7 and 32 per cent, the greater acceleration accounted for by the fact that antisepsis was introduced there earlier than in London. Lister paid tribute to Semmelweis: 'I think with the greatest admiration of him and his achievement and it fills me with joy that at last he is given the respect due to him'.

In 1880/81 Pasteur developed immunisation methods against two diseases caused by bacteria, rabies and anthrax. The tubercle bacillus was discovered and identified by the German physician Robert Koch as the main cause of tuberculosis in 1882. This disease had reached epidemic proportions in the rapidly urbanising towns and cities of the eighteenth and nineteenth centuries. In 1883 the diphtheria bacillus was discovered by Klebs and Loffler, and was followed shortly afterwards by production of an antitoxin by Behring and Kitasato that was efficacious in preventing death in those who already had the disease. However, parents were initially reluctant to accept this new treatment for their children (Morel, 1991). A toxin–antitoxin mixture was introduced in 1913 to immunise children, subsequently improved upon by Ramon in 1923. Mass immunisation of children was introduced in the United States and Canada in the late 1930s, and in Britain in the early 1940s, since when the disease has become practically non-existent, although it has recently begun to re-emerge. The BCG vaccine against tuberculosis was introduced in the early 1920s in Sweden, but only in the 1950s in Britain and the US. Serum effective against tetanus was prepared in 1890–92, but a vaccine only became available in the 1930s. Its use during the Second World War has demonstrated its high degree of protectiveness. In 1897 Beijerinck discovered viruses. Although effective vaccines have been developed against a number of important viruses, there are few effective drugs, even today (see section 14.3.2). Chapter 15 comments on the effects of immunisation on a number of infectious diseases.

14.2.2 Advances in medical technology

The stethoscope was invented in 1816, the hypodermic syringe in 1853 and the sphygmomanometer in 1896. X-rays were discovered in 1895 and anaesthesia was developed from 1844, which made more complex surgery possible. In 1891 Tuffier was successful in removing the apex of a tuberculous lung surgically using new techniques to prevent lung collapse, but such procedures were not generally carried out until much later.

A special issue of the *BMJ* celebrated medical progress over the period 1900 to 1950 (BMJ, 1950). In 1909 Ehrlich developed Salvarsan as a cure for syphilis, which was used successfully among soldiers during the First World War (see Chapter 16). Hopkins published a systematic investigation of vitamins in 1912, the 1920s were the 'golden decade' for the separation of different hormones and vitamins, and the 1930s witnessed the artificial synthesis of many of these (*BMJ*, 1950). Insulin was discovered in 1921 and used shortly afterwards with dramatic effects, particularly for early-onset diabetes (see Chapter 4). The average life expectancy of such newly diagnosed patients prior to the introduction of insulin was less than two years. Average life expectancy at birth for the juvenile diabetic has increased to more than 50 years, primarily as a result of the introduction of insulin and the effective management of the complications of diabetes (Bunker *et al.*, 1994).

Aspirin was discovered in 1897 as a valuable pain killer. Sulphonamide was discovered in 1932 and shown by Colebrook in 1936 in a controlled clinical trial to be effective against streptococcal septicaemia. Alexander Fleming discovered penicillin in 1928, but its manufacture took until 1939 to perfect. Wounded soldiers of the Second World War were among the first to benefit. These two drugs were shown to be effective for pneumonia, appendicitis, general infections especially in childbirth, syphilis, gonorrhoea, surgery and war wounds. Penicillin is not active against the tuberculosis bacillus, but in 1944 streptomycin was discovered and found to be effective in treating the disease. The bacteria become resistant to streptomycin, but fortunately other drugs which supplement its efficacy, para-aminosalicyclic acid (PAS) and isoniazid, were later discovered. The ABO blood grouping was discovered in 1901, and in 1914 sodium citrate was found to prevent clotting when added to blood. Blood was successfully transfused during the First World War, but only in small amounts directly between individuals. Modern drip methods were perfected in the 1930s, which made advanced surgery possible. Lithium treatment for manic depressives was introduced in the 1940s.

14.2.3 Some specific indicators of medical advance and iatrogenesis, 1841–1950

Maternal mortality
The number of deaths in England and Wales from puerperal fever did not decline until after 1880 (Chapter 15). Besides better hygiene, improved prenatal and other care were likely to have influenced maternal and infant mortality (Macfarlane and Mugford, 1984). Confidential enquiries into such deaths, which began in 1881, played a role. Initially the figures rose, probably as a result of more complete recording. Figure 14.1 shows that there was little improvement in overall maternal mortality until after 1890. Large improvements occurred from the early 1930s in Scotland and from the mid-1930s elsewhere in Britain, and have been attributed to the introduction of sulphonamide drugs for puerperal sepsis, the availability of penicillin and blood transfusions to women who haemorrhaged (Macfarlane and Mugford, 1984). By the time of the 1952–54 Confidential Enquiry, puerperal sepsis

accounted for only 3.8 per cent of maternal deaths, compared with more than half in 1848–72 (Macfarlane and Mugford, 1984; Logan, 1950). An interesting finding in the Registrar General's Supplement for 1930–32 was that maternal mortality rates were higher among wives of professional men than among wives of men in unskilled occupations, particularly for puerperal sepsis (General Register Office, 1938). Macfarlane and Mugford (1984) have suggested that this was because middle-class women were more likely to be able to afford to have their babies in nursing homes and other institutions, where they were at greater risk of acquiring infections than at home. Also, because of their ability to pay, they were more likely to receive unnecessary and sometimes inexpert medical interventions such as forceps delivery.

Figure 14.1

Maternal mortality, England and Wales, 1847–1994

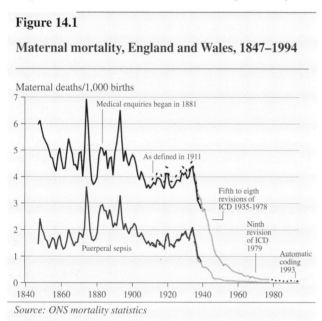

Source: ONS mortality statistics

Infant mortality

In the nineteenth century infant mortality was high and not falling (see Chapters 3 and 4). In 1848–72 the rate was 203 per thousand population for boys (167 for girls). The main causes were: infectious diseases (18 per cent) of which the most important three were non-respiratory tuberculosis, whooping cough and scarlet fever/diphtheria; 'infantile convulsions' (20 per cent); respiratory illnesses (15 per cent), mainly bronchitis and pneumonia; digestive diseases, mainly enteritis (10 per cent); and developmental and wasting diseases (27 per cent). In England and Wales the decline in the birth rate and stagnation of the death rate led, by about 1900, to an active infant-and-child-health movement (Dwork, 1987). Medical practitioners and health officials put pressure on the central and local authorities to provide infant milk depots and health visitors to visit the newborn. By 1901–10 mortality had fallen by 18 per cent. Notable falls were recorded for: typhus/typhoid (99 per cent); scarlet fever/ diphtheria (85 per cent); cholera (100 per cent); dysentery (93 per cent); non-respiratory tuberculosis (41 per cent); respiratory tuberculosis (78 per cent); and infantile convulsions (58 per cent) (see Table 4.2 of Chapter 4, which also shows the contribution each disease made to the overall fall in mortality). The pattern of disease decline suggests that the adoption of sanitary measures and health education of mothers over the period had some effect. The rapid decline

immediately after the Second World War may have been related to the introduction of antibiotics, mainly penicillin and sulphonamides. Other factors influencing recent declines are prenatal screening for congenital genetic defects (Harries and Rhine, 1993; Hey *et al.*, 1994), made more effective by new technologies such as ultrasound and biochemical tests.

Tuberculosis

Tuberculosis has been one of the most important diseases in the history of mankind, and continues to be one of the major fatal illnesses in the less well developed parts of the world. Most people infected with the bacillus do not suffer from the disease. Instead, it becomes trapped in body tissues, surrounded by defensive cells, and is finally sealed up in a hard calcified nodule called a tubercle. However, if the bacillus is not caught up in such a nodule it spreads in the lungs and into the bloodstream, from where it can reach almost any organ of the body. Most tuberculosis is of the pulmonary type, spread by droplets from infected persons. Overcrowding, poor hygiene (e.g. coughing and spitting) and poor housing standards are thus important factors in its transmission. The disease is most severe in malnourished people, but can afflict anyone.

Before curative drugs became available in the mid-1940s the disease was often fatal. The first hospital for its treatment was founded in 1841, The Brompton (Bishop, 1967). Cases were isolated to sanatoria to prevent the infection spreading, especially after Koch had established the infectious nature of tuberculosis in 1882. There, fresh air, rest and good food were prescribed. It was treated from 1894 by collapsing part or all of the lung to rest the affected part (Walton *et al.*, 1994), surgical removal of ribs, and later of the tuberculous tissue (introduced in 1891 but most widely used in the 1950s). The use of X-rays after 1895 led to more accurate and earlier diagnoses of the disease. Streptomycin, discovered in 1944, used in conjunction with PAS (1946) and isoniazid (1952), proved to be very effective at curing the disease. Mass screening for infected persons took place shortly after the Second World War.

As Chapter 4 showed, in the 1850s and 1860s respiratory tuberculosis accounted for more than 1 in 10 of all deaths, and other forms of tuberculosis (mainly derived through infected milk) for a further 4 per cent. Figure 14.2 shows the decline in tuberculosis mortality rates since 1851. Death rates fell at a fairly steady rate until the First World War. Between the two wars the decline was somewhat more rapid, but did not fall during the Second World War. Subsequently, rates declined at a much accelerated pace, with the rate of decline slowing down again in recent years. Notifications of tuberculosis have risen in Britain since 1987, with an increase in drug-resistant isolates. Recent developments in molecular fingerprinting, which enable the spread of individual strains to be tracked, represent an important new tool for surveillance and control of tuberculosis (Stoker, 1994) and other infections.

Similar patterns have been observed in Sweden for which there are reliable data over an even longer period (Puranen, 1991). Puranen found no evidence that the virulence of the bacillus has decreased, so this is unlikely to be a reason for

Figure 14.2

Tuberculosis mortality, 1851–1994 all ages, indirectly standardised (1950–52=100) rate per million population (log scale)

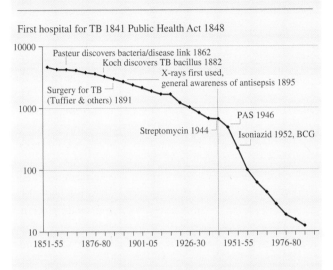

First hospital for TB 1841 Public Health Act 1848

Age-standardised rates per million (based on SMR for 1950–52=100)

	TB	All causes	% TB
1851–55	4,600	41,700	11
1856–60	4,200	39,900	11
1861–70	4,200	41,300	10
1866–70	4,100	40,800	10
1871–75	3,700	40,000	9
1876–80	3,600	38,400	9
1881–85	3,200	36,000	9
1886–90	2,900	35,100	8
1891–95	2,700	34,600	8
1896–1900	2,400	32,600	7
1901–05	2,100	29,100	7
1906–10	1,900	25,900	7
1911–15	1,700	24,000	7
1916–20	1,700	22,200	7
1921–25	1,200	18,400	7
1926–30	1,000	17,000	6
1931–35	800	15,700	5
1936–40	700	15,000	4
1941–45	700	13,100	5
1946–50	500	11,800	4
1951–55	200	11,300	2
1956–60	100	10,600	1
1961–65	60	10,500	1
1966–70	40	10,200	0
1971–75	30	9,900	0
1976–80	20	9,300	0
1981–85	20	8,900	0
1986–90	10	8,190	0

Source: OPCS DHI No 25 and OPCS Historic Deaths database

the decline. He argued that on the basis of evidence from developing countries, where tuberculosis is still common, acquired immunity is not particularly strong or long-lasting, so this too is unlikely to have been a major factor, and genetic and immunological factors are also unlikely, based on the available evidence (Puranen, 1991). Poor nutrition and poor housing are both important risk factors, and separating out their individual effects is difficult because the two usually occur together. A good diet is known to be protective (Marche and Grunelle, 1950; Leitch, 1945), and there is also an increased risk with high alcohol consumption, related to its effect on nutritional intake (Puranen, 1991). Alcohol consumption was high in Britain in the nineteenth century, and declined from the mid-1870s (see Chapter 8). Occupational exposure to high levels of certain dusts is also a risk factor (Puranen, 1991). Evidence from studies in Stockholm of data from 1749 to 1860 suggest that the environment, especially overcrowding, was the most important factor, far more important than nutrition. In Stockholm nutrition improved substantially but overcrowding did not, while tuberculosis mortality remained high, accounting for around half of all deaths (Puranen, 1991). Studies in Sweden between 1910 and 1920 found that improvements in housing produced considerable benefits (Puranen, 1991).

McKeown has argued that the fall in tuberculosis during the whole of the nineteenth century was due to a single factor, improved nutrition, and that medical treatment played little part because the decline occurred before effective treatment became available (McKeown and Record, 1962). Analyses by others over the past 30 years have shown that this conclusion was too simplistic. Swedish data collected over the course of 200 years show that exposure to the bacillus is strongly related to living conditions, especially standards of hygiene and population density, although occupation and location have also played an important role (Puranen, 1991). Public health measures taken to improve housing, new awareness of the risk of contagion and use of sanatoria are likely to have played an important role in reducing tuberculosis during the nineteenth century. Figure 14.2 also shows that although tuberculosis mortality was falling at a similar rate to all-cause mortality up to around 1865 (remaining at some 11 per cent of overall mortality), it subsequently declined faster than general mortality. This suggests that factors other than improvements in general standard of living were involved in more recent declines.

From the end of the nineteenth century onwards a number of new technological tools became available, including X-rays for better diagnosis, surgical techniques and, finally antibiotics. Surgical innovations do not appear to have accelerated the mortality decline from a particular date, but the diffusion of the new techniques is likely to have taken some time. The introduction of effective antibiotics in 1944, 1946 and 1952 had a major impact in reducing disease mortality to its now very small proportion of overall mortality. The efficacy of these treatments was proved by randomised controlled clinical trials before their general introduction.

14.3 Medical advances since 1950

14.3.1 Prevention

Cigarettes, the only available consumer product which kills people when used as intended, are still one of the greatest threats to health. Tobacco kills over 111,000 people in the United Kingdom each year – 1 in 4 smokers will die prematurely as a result of the habit. The number of smoking, related deaths is five times higher than that of accidents, murder, suicide, illegal drug use and AIDS combined (Walton *et al.*, 1994). In 1605 King James tried to eliminate smoking in Britain as an unhealthy habit, but the Royal College of Physicians (RCP) dismissed the King's views and the habit spread, gaining a reputation of having medicinal value (Walton *et al.*, 1994). With the invention of the cigarette, smoking became cheaper and easier, and by 1920 cigarette smoking was common among men, and among women some 30 years later. The adverse effects became evident in the 1950s when epidemiological research confirmed the hypothesis that cigarette smoking is a major cause of lung cancer. However, it was only in 1962 that the message was brought home to the layman, with the publication of the Royal College of Physicians' report *Smoking and Health*, which recommended restricting tobacco advertising, increasing taxation on cigarettes, restricting the sale of cigarettes and smoking in public places, and the display of information on the tar and nicotine content of cigarettes. Doll and Hill published their findings on smoking among doctors in the mid-1960s and again in the mid-1970s and 1990s, which showed that the risks were high, and that giving up smoking reduced the risk of lung cancer (Doll and Peto, 1976; Doll *et al.*, 1994). In 1971 the RCP set up a charity, ASH, to educate the public following its second report, *Smoking and Health Now*. Chapter 9 describes trends in smoking-related diseases, and Figure 9.2 shows how the campaigning by the Royal College of Physicians had an effect on smoking rates.

The eradication of smallpox and the current low prevalence of diphtheria, pertussis, tetanus and poliomyelitis are largely a consequence of the development of effective vaccines and of national immunisation programmes. Hitherto, these infectious diseases had had a devastating effect on the health of the population, particularly children. Vaccine coverage now exceeds 90 per cent for all antigens, and the incidence of diseases that can be prevented by immunisation is at an all time low (Begg and Nicoll, 1994). The 1994 national measles and rubella campaign, which aimed to vaccinate 95 per cent of schoolchildren within one month, was one of the most ambitious vaccination initiatives ever undertaken in Britain (Miller, 1994). Its purpose was to prevent a predicted measles epidemic in 1995, and the primary prevention of rubella embryopathy, and it seems to have been successful (CMOs update, 1995).

Accidents and cirrhosis of the liver are two other important causes of death where prevention can play a role. Rates for the former have fallen (see Chapters 4 and 24), but cirrhosis of the liver is on the increase, as is the case for several other alcohol-related diseases, particularly among young men (see Chapter 8).

14.3.2 Advances in medical technology

The isolation in 1967 of the penicillin nucleus made possible the synthesis of new antibiotics that were better absorbed (e.g. amoxycillin), or active against a broader spectrum of organisms (e.g. carbenicillin) than the earlier penicillins (Burdon, 1982). Cephalosporins, aminoglycosides and trimethoprim are among the large number of chemotherapeutic agents introduced in the last 20 years for their potency against clinically important organisms. Effective chemotherapy is now available against most bacteria, rickettsiae, mycoplasmae and chlamydiae. The challenge now is to choose rationally from the many available agents and to use them in such a way as to avoid the emergence of bacterial resistance. Bacteria are, however, becoming resistant to antibiotics, especially among the hospital-acquired infections, and development of new drugs to overcome resistant strains is becoming an increasingly important challenge (Emmerson *et al.*, 1996; Johnson *et al.*, 1996; Obaro *et al.*, 1996).

Betablockers (for reducing high blood pressure) and anti-depressants were developed during the 1950s. Around the same time Medawar studied the body's tolerance to transplanted organs and skin grafts, Watson and Crick discovered DNA structures, and Salk vaccine against polio was developed. Ultrasound was developed in the late 1950s for producing images of structures within the human body. During the 1960s benzodiazepine tranquillisers were developed, and the first heart transplant was undertaken. In the 1970s CAT scanners (computer aided tomography, providing enhanced detail in X-rays) were introduced, and monoclonal antibodies were developed. The first 'test-tube' baby was also born in this decade, and smallpox was finally eradicated. In the early 1980s AIDS was first recognised, and the responsible virus identified. While there have been dramatic advances in the treatment of bacterial infections, the number of effective antiviral agents remains small and the clinical conditions in which they are useful is limited (Richmond and Longson, 1982). Until the introduction of acyclovir in 1977, only modest progress had been made in treating herpes virus infections with interferon and topical idoxuridine. Acyclovir, unlike the earlier antiherpetic drugs, acts selectively on herpes simplex virus-infected cells and its toxicity is low enough for systemic use in immuno-compromised patients with AIDS and other immune deficiency states. For serious virus infections, such as hepatitis B, prevention by immunisation remains a far more effective means of controlling the virus than treatment of the established infection. As yet it has not proved possible to find an effective antiviral agent for the treatment of AIDS, nor to prevent the disease through the use of vaccines, although recent results with combinations of antivirals including protease inhibitors are promising.

Since about 1970, subcutaneous cardiac pacemakers have revolutionised the treatment of arrhythmias and bradycardia and thus played a major role in increasing life expectancy in patients with coronary heart disease. Cardiac bypass surgery offers improved vascularisation of the heart and usually good symptomatic benefit. Successful transplantation of organs, especially of kidneys, rapidly restores health, and rather more than 90 per cent return to their normal activities (Johnson, 1992). Fatality rates for kidney transplants of under 1 per cent are reported from the best centres. Since the introduction of renal transplantation in the 1960s, there has been a massive increase in demand for transplants of every organ. Cardiac transplantation, pioneered in the late 1960s, offers help to a minority of patients untreatable by other means. Surgical practice has also been influenced by the introduction of new drugs. For example, the availability of aprotinin in cardiac surgery has reduced the need for blood transfusions, the anaesthetic agent propofol has extended the use of day surgery, and usage patterns of H2 antagonists for the treatment of gastric and duodenal ulcers have reduced the need for surgical intervention altogether (Dhillon, 1993), as has antibiotic treatment of *Helicobacter pylori* (see Chapter 22).

While gynaecologists have been performing laparoscopy for several decades for diagnostic purposes and sterilisation, it is only in the last decade that the development of a reliable video-chip camera and new instrumentation have brought about a revolution in laparoscopic surgery (McCloy, 1992). Laparoscopic cholecystectomy was the first major abdominal operation to be undertaken on a nationwide basis using the new minimal access surgery (MAS) techniques, but other operations, such as oesophagectomy and colectomy, are now being carried out successfully using these methods (McCloy, 1992). Randomised trials have shown that patients undergoing MAS are likely to be discharged home earlier and experience substantially less post-operative morbidity and mortality (Barkun *et al.*, 1992; McMahon *et al.*, 1994; McGinn *et al.*, 1995), but more recently evidence has mounted casting doubt on the general success of these procedures, and the risk of serious complications during and after surgery is greater, especially in the hands of less experienced surgeons (Majeed *et al.*, 1996; Downs *et al.*, 1996).

Radiotherapy, used alone or in combination with other treatment modalities, has also greatly improved the chances of survival for patients with cancers. Testicular cancer, some childhood malignancies and Hodgkin's disease are notable examples. Since the 1930s, radiotherapy has proved effective in treating women with invasive cervical cancer. Initially, radium implants were inserted into the vagina and uterine cavity. These intra-cavitary devices were later supplemented by various types of external beam therapy. More recently, the introduction of mega-voltage radiation, improved tumour imaging and localisation, and more efficient focusing and dose fractionation, have enabled the side effects of radiotherapy to be reduced, while achieving greater tumour resolution. Successful treatment has been a major factor in the decline in mortality from cervical cancer among those diagnosed early enough.

Since the 1960s, cytotoxic chemotherapy has become standard treatment for a number of forms of cancer (Kaldor and Lasset, 1991). It has radically reduced mortality from acute lymphoblastic leukaemia in children, Wilms' tumour, retino-blastoma, testicular teratoma, choriocarcinoma and several types of non-Hodgkin's lymphoma. Given as adjuvant therapy following surgery for cancers of the breast and ovary, chemotherapy appears to improve survival. More recently tamoxifen treatment seems to have increased survival of women with breast cancer (Quinn and Allen, 1996).

In recent years, the pharmaceutical industry has focused on the need for more specific drugs targeted to sites of action. For example, chemotherapeutic agents linked to monoclonal antibodies targeted to specific antigens can be used to attack cancer cells. Monoclonal antibody drugs are also under test for the treatment of conditions as diverse as chronic renal failure, diabetes, hepatitis, multiple sclerosis and rheumatoid arthritis (Dhillon, 1993). Liposomes may also be used as carriers for certain drugs to minimise toxicity and enhance efficacy by delivering the drug to a target site. Liposomal amphotericin, effective in a wide range of life-threatening fungal infections in immunocompromised patients, is the first licensed liposomal product to become available in the United Kingdom (Dhillon, 1993).

New cancer therapy products aimed at protecting body tissues from the side effects of radiation and chemotherapy are also a recent development. For example, recombinant human granulocyte colony stimulating factor reduces the duration of neutropenia and thus the patient's susceptibility to life-threatening infections, while mesna is now used routinely to block the urotoxic side effects which were previously dose-limiting in patients treated with cyclophosphamide. Techniques to replace defective tumour suppressor genes with engineered wild-type gene or its protein product are being developed to augment existing treatment options for common invasive cancers (Brewster, 1994).

Many common diseases have genetic components, and some less common diseases, such as haemophilia, cystic fibrosis and sickle cell anaemia, are caused by single genes. For some time, human gene products have been used for treatment. These include anti-haemophilia factor, human growth hormone and insulin (Harries and Rhine, 1993). Gene therapy offers the possibility of treating or curing hereditary diseases by transferring normal genes. Therapy involves using viruses as convenient vectors to introduce new DNA into host cells, which results in the expression of a new protein. The first diseases to be tackled by gene therapists were severe combined immunodeficiency, particularly adenosine deaminase (ADA) deficiency in children, type III familial hypercholesterolaemia, and cystic fibrosis (CF). In the United States, clinical gene therapy trials started in 1990, the first aiming to treat a rare, lethal immunodeficiency disease and had encouraging results. Trials of gene therapy for ADA and CF are under way in the United Kingdom (Bolton, 1994).

14.3.3 Some specific examples

Two important causes of mortality where there is now some evidence that medical advances have been effective in reducing mortality are not covered in this chapter because they are dealt with in detail elsewhere (see Chapters 18 and 24). For ischaemic heart disease thrombolytic treatment immediately after a heart attack can reduce fatality rates by some 25 per cent, and public health activities aimed at accident prevention, and to a lesser extent improved treatment (blood transfusions, modern surgery, etc.), have reduced the risk of fatality from injury and poisoning (see Chapters 4 and 24). The examples below were chosen to reflect a number of different aspects of medical advance (and iatrogenesis).

Poliomyelitis

Polio is one of several viral diseases that have been largely eradicated in Britain and most other countries through vaccination and rehabilitation (Hull *et al.*, 1994) (see Chapter 15, Figure 15.9). Management of polio was greatly improved by muscle relaxation techniques introduced by Sister Kenny, whose patients were left less stiff, less deformed and had better circulation than those on orthodox regimes. The medical profession were for some time extremely sceptical of her methods, but by the late 1940s opinion polls showed her to be, with Eleanor Roosevelt, one of the two most admired women in the world (Smith, 1989). Polio is particularly interesting in that during the epidemics of the 1940s and 1950s it hit 'clean' households to a much greater extent than others, since better hygiene delayed exposure to the virus, leaving young adults exposed to a more severe form of the disease (Paul, 1971) (see Chapter 15). In a sense the epidemics were exacerbated by the sanitary movement of public health. The uncritical prevalent belief of the 1950s that it had a droplet-nasal path of infection, even though the Swedish researcher Kling had shown as early as 1912 that the virus entered through the digestive tract, had disastrous consequences for the handling of the epidemic (Smith, 1989).

Antibiotics

Mackenbach and Looman, (1988) investigated the extent to which the introduction of antibiotics around 1947 affected mortality trends for 21 infectious diseases, analysing Dutch data from 1921–78. Regression models were used to test whether there was: (a) a sharp reduction in 1947; and (b) a more rapid decline subsequently. Although effects of mortality from the Second World War created measurement difficulties, changes of type (a) were present for 18 diseases and type (b) for 16, and some of these effects were quite large. For example, for puerperal fever, scarlet fever, rheumatic fever, erysipelas, otitis media, tuberculosis and bacillary dysentery, mortality fell by 10 per cent per annum or more. These effects were not apparent in 'all other' (mostly non-infectious) diseases. The findings suggest that antibiotics played a major role in the post-war decline in infectious disease mortality.

'Avoidable' deaths

One approach to measuring the outcome of medical intervention is to count adverse events, such as deaths, which, had appropriate treatment been given in time, were largely avoidable. The concept of 'avoidable' deaths as negative indices of the quality of health care derives from two papers by a working group on preventable and manageable diseases in the United States (Rutstein *et al.*, 1976, 1980). Charlton *et al.*, (1983) examined the geographical variation in mortality from conditions amenable to medical intervention in England and Wales. There were wide variations which persisted even after adjustment for socio-economic variables. Time-trend mortality comparisons were also made for five other developed countries that had experienced appreciable growth in health services during 1950–80 (Charlton and Velez, 1986). The disease groups and age-ranges were chosen so that mortality would reflect as much as possible the adequacy of medical treatment rather than, for example, primary preventive measures such as immunisation. However, changes in disease incidence, which may be related to preventive measures, are also important factors to take into account when interpreting the data. They found that in each country mortality from a heterogeneous group of 'avoidable' causes of death had declined faster than mortality from all other causes. Despite the difficulties inherent in making international comparisons where like is not always being compared with like, the consistency in mortality trends suggested that improvements in medical care were a feature in their rapid decline.

Studies have been undertaken to examine the extent to which health care resources are related to 'avoidable' mortality (Mackenbach *et al.*, 1990; Mackenbach, 1991). The 'avoidable' causes of death were selected on the basis of clinical trial evidence that medical treatment is effective, so these analyses do not tell us about effectiveness so much as whether differences in the availability of resources (as measured by the available data) make a difference to the outcome. The relationships found have been shown to be weak, and there are large international variations. It seems likely that the ways in which patients are treated are more important than the level of the resources available, and that there are wide variations in efficiency of health care delivery, which also depends on patient help-seeking behaviour and compliance. Mackenbach *et al.*, (1988) suggest that on the basis of analyses of 'avoidable' selected causes alone, medical care improvements have added 2.96 and 3.95 years of life expectancy at birth to Dutch males and females, between 1950 and 1984.

In this chapter we show trends for England and Wales from 1950 to 1994 for eight 'avoidable mortality' causes (see Table 14.1). The medical interventions specific to the diseases chosen are described elsewhere (EC Working Party, 1988). The data were drawn from ONS's historic deaths file using appropriate bridging across the different ICDs (Alderson, 1981). The mortality data have been age-standardised to the standard European population (Waterhouse *et al.*, 1976), using direct standardisation.

Figure 14.3 contrasts the trends in avoidable mortality at all ages with trends in mortality from all other (non-avoidable) causes of death for men and women separately (ages 1 and above). In both sexes the trends in avoidable deaths show a

Table 14.1

Comparison of mortality rates per million population in England and Wales in 1950 and 1994

Directly standardised to the European population*

Cause of death	1950	1994	% fall
All causes (all ages)	12,964	7,771	40
Eight 'avoidable' causes (all ages) *	513	102	80
All other	12,451	7,669	38
Tuberculosis (ages 5–64)	379	3	99
Hypertensive disease (ages 35–64)	282	20	93
Cerebrovascular disease (ages 35–64)	757	233	69
Chronic rheumatic heart disease (ages 5–64)	85	1	99
Appendicitis (ages 5–64)	22	1	96
Cholelithiasis and cholecystitis (ages 5–64)	12	1	92
Cervical cancer (ages 5–64)	46	20	56
Hodgkin's disease (ages 5–64)	15	4	73
Perinatal mortality**	37	8	79
Maternal mortality ***	87	8	91

*   *Tuberculosis, hypertensive disease, cerebrovascular disease, chronic rheumatic heart disease, appendicitis, cholelithiasis and cholecystitis, cervical cancer, Hodgkin's disease.*
** *Perinatal mortality expressed as deaths per 1000 births.*
*** *Maternal mortality expressed as deaths per 100,000 births.*

Figure 14.3

Mortality from all causes (ages 1+) between 1950 and 1994

Standardised to European population

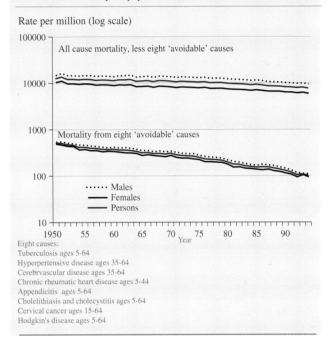

Eight causes:
Tuberculosis ages 5-64
Hyperpertensive disease ages 35-64
Cerebrvascular disease ages 35-64
Chronic rheumatic heart disease ages 5-44
Appendicitis ages 5-64
Cholelithiasis and cholecystitis ages 5-64
Cervical cancer ages 15-64
Hodgkin's disease ages 5-64

Figure 14.4

Hypertension and stroke mortality

Ages 35–64, standardised to European population

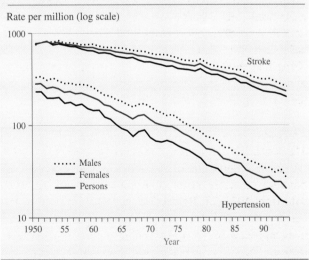

more rapid decline than deaths not so classified. Death rates from non-avoidable causes fell by about one third between 1950 and 1991, whereas avoidable mortality was reduced by 77 per cent. The selected 'avoidable' causes only account for a small proportion of total mortality, so in absolute terms the fall in 'other causes' is greater. Table 14.1 shows the percentage changes in mortality between 1950 and 1994.

Hypertensive and cerebrovascular disease (ages 35–64)

The main risk factor for stroke that is amenable to intervention is raised blood pressure, which can be reduced by changes in lifestyle (e.g. cessation of smoking, weight reduction, better nutrition) and by early detection and treatment (see Chapter 18). Clinical trials have shown that mortality from stroke may be reduced by half with intensive antihypertensive treatment (Hypertension Detection and Follow-up Co-operative Group, 1979, 1982; Collins *et al.*, 1990). A locally-based confidential enquiry into deaths from cerebrovascular and hypertensive disease in a UK health district identified avoidable factors that may have contributed to death in 29 per cent of cases (Payne *et al.,* 1993). In the United States, Bunker *et al.*, (1994) estimated that an increase in life expectancy of 5–6 months since 1950 can be attributed to the treatment of hypertension. However, mortality from hypertension and, to a lesser extent, that from stroke began falling before effective antihypertensive therapies were available (see Chapter 18). The standardised death rates for hypertension and stroke show falls of 93 and 69 per cent respectively between 1950 and 1994 (see Table 14.1).

Chronic rheumatic heart disease (ages 5–64)

Much of the observed fall in mortality from chronic rheumatic heart disease to near negligible levels has been due to the decline in incidence of rheumatic fever during the past 50 years. Factors in avoiding death include case detection of streptococci, antibiotics, prophylaxis and valve replacement surgery, which have been shown to be effective (Gordis, 1973; Feinstein *et al.*, 1966). Many patients who have developed rheumatic valvular disease have benefited from surgical intervention such as valvotomy or valve replacement under cardiopulmonary bypass with a prosthetic or heterograft valve.

Figure 14.5

Four 'avoidable' causes of mortality

Standardised to European population

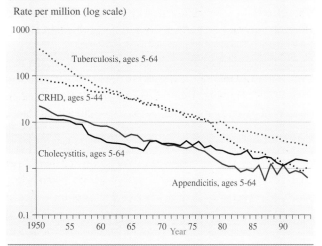

Appendicitis (ages 5–64)

Appendicectomy has been practised for over 100 years since the advent of general anaesthesia and antisepsis in the nineteenth century. Between 1901 and 1915 the mortality rate increased from about 40 to 70 per million population and this level was maintained until about 1935 (Donnan and Lambert, 1976). Since then death rates have fallen steeply to less than 1 per million of the population in 1994 (see Table 14.1). Undoubtedly, improvements in diagnosis and surgery and the introduction of antibiotics have played major roles in the decline in mortality, but changing incidence of the disease may also have played a role. Such incidence data as are available are based on hospital data, which are influenced by surgical rates that also may have been declining, making interpretation more difficult (Charlton and Velez, 1986).

Cholelithiasis and cholecystitis (ages 5–64)

Mortality from cholelithiasis and cholecystitis has fallen by 92 per cent since 1950 (see Table 14.1) and may fall still further as minimal access surgery (MAS) becomes more widely practised (Russell, 1993). With MAS a laparoscopic cholecystectomy or duct clearance enables gallstones to be removed with minimal morbidity and a short recovery period. Acute cholecystitis can be treated by percutaneous drainage followed by either a laparoscopic cholecystectomy or percutaneous cholecystolithotomy. MAS avoids the large open wounds and cut muscles of conventional surgery, and the large cholecystectomy scar with its subsequent incisional hernia has become a thing of the past.

Cervical cancer (ages 15–64)

Mass screening by cytology for the early detection of cancer of the cervix has been extremely successful in other countries, but the programme which has been in operation in Britain since 1964 has been less so (Editorial, 1976; Clark and Anderson, 1979; McGregor and Teper, 1978; Austoker, 1994; Sasieni *et al.*, 1996). In Scandinavia there is almost complete coverage of the target population (Hakama *et al.*, 1986). In

Britain there has been no reduction in the overall incidence of invasive disease and little evidence as yet that the screening programme has had any effect on the decline in mortality. Death rates from cervical cancer have fallen by 56 per cent since 1950 (see Table 14.1) but have not fallen as rapidly as in some other countries, possibly due to a combination of less vigorous screening and failure to reach older women from lower social classes who are most at risk.

Hodgkin's disease (ages 5–64)

Mortality from Hodgkin's disease has declined since the early 1970s from about 15 to 5 per million at ages 5–64 years (see Figure 14.6). The effectiveness of treatment has improved to the extent that there is practically 100 per cent 8-year survival, and 94 per cent disease-free survival at 8 years, based on a combination of multi-agent chemotherapy and radiotherapy (Coleman, 1991).

Figure 14.6

Mortality from cervical cancer and Hodgkin's disease

Standardised to European population

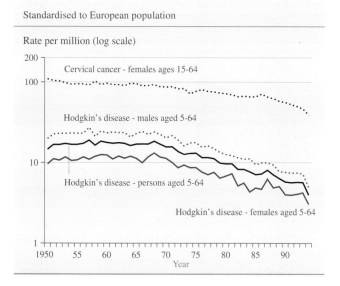

Perinatal and maternal mortality

Perinatal mortality rates are regarded as a good indicator for antenatal and obstetric care, as well as paediatric neonatal care, by hospitals and general practitioners (Alberman, 1982; Mersey RHA, 1982). Between 1950 and 1994 rates have fallen by 80 per cent, to 7.6 per thousand. Table 14.1 and Figure 14.1 show that maternal mortality, another indicator for antenatal and obstetric care, has also fallen dramatically, by 91 per cent since 1950. Women still die in childbirth, but for every 1 who dies today 50 died in the 1930s (Loudon, 1992). The most recent *Report on Confidential Enquiries into Maternal Deaths in the United Kingdom* covering the period 1991–93 showed a modest fall in the overall maternal mortality rate from 10.3 per 100,000 maternities in the 1988–90 triennium to 9.8 in the period covered by the report. In this most recent triennium, sub-standard care occurred in 40 per cent of deaths, with deficiencies in hospital care in 31 per cent, in general practitioner care in 7 per cent, and of mother/or family in 11 per cent (Department of Health *et al.*, 1996).

14.4 Iatrogenesis

Florence Nightingale was one of the first to suggest collecting statistics on the outcome of medical treatment, to establish whether 'treatment was doing more harm than good'. Although technological advances in medicine have made significant contributions to health, adverse effects of medical treatment and advice are increasingly a subject of concern to the general public, the medical profession, and other health professionals. Sudden infant deaths declined dramatically when doctors reversed the advice that they had previously given that babies should be made to lie in the prone position (Gilbert, 1994; Fleming, 1994; Golding and Colmer, 1994). An epidemic of asthma deaths occurred in the 1960s, coinciding closely with the rise and fall in sales of isoprenaline aerosol bronchodilators (Inman and Adelstein, 1969) (see Chapter 20 and Figure 20.9), Seidl *et al.,* (1966) found that 5 per cent of patients admitted to a medical ward at the Johns Hopkins Hospital were suffering from adverse drug reactions, and Hurwitz and Wade (1969) found that 10 per cent of all patients admitted to a general hospital in Belfast suffered from adverse reactions to drugs given to them while in hospital.

Drugs have always been potentially poisonous, but their unwanted side effects have increased with their power and widespread use. Many short-term unwanted effects of medical treatment are well known. Most occur within hours or weeks; they occur quite often, and in some cases, such as alopecia after chemotherapy, are sufficiently predictable for the patient to be warned, or for preventive measures to be adopted; and they are usually reversible (Coleman, 1991). Some, however, are serious, for example cyclosporin A, which has proved invaluable in renal transplantation, has been associated with serious nephrotoxicity (Johnson, 1992) and lymphoma (Tomatis *et al.*, 1990). Azathioprine has also been shown to induce cancers in organ-transplant recipients (Tomatis *et al.*, 1990). Rare side effects are unlikely to show up in clinical trials, because sample sizes tend to be too small, and they are carried out on selected homogeneous populations. The United Kingdom has formal licensing procedures for drugs, which were implemented following the epidemic of congenital deformities caused by thalidomide in the 1960s. Safety assessments of other technologies are not so systematic or comprehensive, and the safety of many medical procedures is crucially dependent on the vigilance of the professionals using them (Drummond, 1992). Spontaneous reporting schemes provide important early warning signals of potential hazards. Doctors in Britain are encouraged to use the yellow card system to report to the Committee on Safety of Medicines suspected adverse reactions to a wide range of products, including drugs, vaccines, blood products, X-ray contrast media, dental or surgical materials, intra-uterine contraceptive devices, absorbable sutures and contact lens fluids (ABPI, 1994). The yellow card system relies heavily on doctor co-operation, and the response rate is low. Recently the General Practice Research Database (GPRD), comprising 3.5 million current patients and data for over 20 million patient years, has been used to establish and quantify the risks of suspected treatments. Examples include the association between anti-

ulcer drugs and gynaecomastia (Rodriguez and Jick, 1994a), and estimates of the risks of upper gastrointestinal bleeding and perforation associated with individual non-steroidal anti-inflammatory drugs (Rodriguez and Jick, 1994b).

The effects of over-medication (e.g. from diazepam and flurezepam) can be a particularly serious problem in elderly people, because they often have difficulties taking drugs as prescribed, or with their bodies breaking them down (Boston Collaborative Drug Surveillance Program, 1973; Greenblatt *et al.*, 1977; Hurwitz, 1969). Learoyd (1972) found that 16 per cent of psychogeriatric admissions were directly attributed to the ill-effects of psychotropic drugs, and that at least 20 per cent of admissions were precipitated by the adverse effects of psychotropic agents. Hurwitz (1969) estimated that 21 per cent of the 70–79 year age-group suffered from adverse drug reactions. Peach (1989) similarly found rates of incidence of short-term adverse drug reactions in hospital practice of between 10 and 20 per cent. There have been few surveys of adverse drug reactions in the community. One survey in a London borough suggested that 15 per cent of adults living at home led restricted lives because of illness caused by the side effects of drugs (Peach and Charlton, 1986). The drugs being taken most frequently were analgesics, diuretics, sedatives, hypnotics and tranquillizers. Some disabling symptoms were similar to the effects, mainly adverse, of these commonly prescribed drugs. While it was difficult, except in a few cases, to exclude other explanations for the relation between symptoms and drugs, and temporal relationships were often unclear, symptomatic respondents taking these drugs were more disabled than respondents reporting similar symptoms who were not taking them.

One of the principal strategies in the chemotherapy of cancer has been the development of drugs that kill cancer cells by interacting with their DNA. However, these agents are not specific to tumour cells, and their interaction with the DNA of normal cells may subsequently result in the development of a new malignancy, after the first cancer has been successfully treated (Tomatis *et al.*, 1990). Leukaemia is by far the most frequently reported malignancy following chemotherapy, and the most clearly established as causally associated (Kaldor and Lasset, 1991). While the leukaemia risk following chemotherapy for Hodgkin's disease is considerable, before the advent of multi-agent chemotherapy advanced disease was almost universally fatal. The goal of several recent Hodgkin's disease trials has been to find new combinations of drugs which are as effective against advanced disease as the established ones, but which may be expected to be less leukaemogenic. Solid tumours are also induced by commonly used cancer chemotherapeutic agents (Tomatis *et al.*, 1990).

The therapeutic use of sex hormones has also been associated with the development of solid tumours (Tomatis *et al.*, 1990). Diethyl-stilboestrol induced vaginal and cervical carcinomas in the daughters of women treated for threatened miscarriage, possibly increased the risk of testicular cancer in their sons, and increased the risk of breast cancer in the women themselves. Assisted conception by means of drugs can lead to: hyperstimulation syndrome leading to acute renal failure; multiple pregnancies endangering mother and children; ectopic pregnancies; and possibly ovarian cancer (Davies, 1990; Schenker and Yossef, 1994).

Skin reactions after exposure to X-rays were reported as early as 1896, and by 1902 it had been noticed that skin cancers sometimes developed in frequently or heavily irradiated areas (Darby, 1991). By the 1930s radiation was an established treatment for a wide range of conditions both benign and malignant. However, it was not until the mid-1950s that it was fully realised that exposure to ionising radiation at doses insufficient to result in gross tissue damage could cause leukaemia and other cancers. Radiotherapy and cytotoxic chemotherapy are used mainly to treat diseases which are themselves serious or potentially fatal, and the risk of subsequent malignancy may be considered justifiable. In other cases, however, such as indolent tumours or disabling but rarely fatal diseases such as rheumatoid arthritis, the balance of risk and benefit may be harder to assess (Coleman, 1991).

Another important type of iatrogenesis is suffering caused by unevaluated and probably ineffective treatments. It has been suggested that in a number of instances electroconvulsive treatment (ECT) for depression and other psychiatric problems is an example of this (Robertson, 1993).

14.5 Evaluation of medical care and evidence-based medicine

Up to the end of the 1960s' boom there was considerable optimism that the new developments in medical technology were the means to better health. The 1950 *BMJ* special issue on medical progress (*BMJ*, 1950) was uncritical by today's standards. When it was realised that resources were not unlimited and that different health services would have to compete for limited funds, medical treatments came under the microscope, particularly the expensive ones. The principal critics of the current regime were Cochrane (1972), Illich (1974) and McKeown (1976).

Cochrane was concerned that the majority of therapeutic interventions had been introduced into routine practice without formal evaluation of their efficacy (does it produce the desired effect under ideal controlled conditions, e.g. randomised controlled trials?), effectiveness (does it work in practice for the intended population?) and efficiency (is it worth it in relation to the cost?). He maintained that all treatments should be evaluated on the basis of controlled clinical trials, 'the key to a rational health service' (Cochrane, 1972). He believed that there was a marked imbalance between the 'care' and 'cure' sectors of the NHS, the latter getting the lion's share of resources without having to justify expenditure.

McKeown argued that based on historical evidence the reduction in mortality had depended not so much on knowledge of mechanisms of disease as on control of the origins of disease: 'In order of importance the determinants of health were nutritional, environmental, and behavioural in

the past, and will probably be behavioural, environmental and nutritional in the future, at least in developed countries' (McKeown, 1976). He suggested that the role of medicine was 'to assist us to come safely into the world and comfortably out of it, and during life, to protect the well and care for the sick and disabled'. McKeown's analyses have been criticised, mainly for his failure to recognise the importance of the role of public health (Szretzer, 1988). In fact the work of public health pioneers has been proposed as a model for today's public health (Ashton, 1991; Warren and Francis, 1987). Cochrane and McKeown were influential in refocusing attention on the effects that medical interventions have on population health rather than individual cases, and providing a rational basis for resource allocation. In spite of the considerable influence that Cochrane and McKeown have had (Alvarez-Dardet and Ruiz, 1993), the health sector is still very much oriented towards therapeutic interventions rather than prevention, and there remain many medical treatments which have not been properly evaluated. However, one study recently undertaken in a GP training practice found that most interventions there were based on evidence from clinical trials (Gill *et al.*, 1996).

The recent growth in the numbers of systematic reviews or meta-analyses of randomised controlled trials in various fields reflects a growing awareness of their importance for improving knowledge about the effects of health care (Chalmers and Haynes, 1994). An important development has been the setting up in 1992 of the Cochrane Collaboration. This international group is undertaking a comprehensive evaluation and dissemination of all the evidence from randomised controlled trials so that treatments can be chosen on the basis of complete and up-to-date information instead of out-of-date research, anecdotes and conjecture (Godlee, 1994).

Most surgical procedures requiring a general anaesthetic entail some risk of death or complication. In most cases the risk of perioperative death is small and the anticipated benefit relatively large. However, since 1988, the national confidential enquiries into perioperative deaths have sought to identify the putative factors in order to provide better and safer care for patients in the future (Campling *et al.*, 1993). Clinical audit at national or local level is increasingly being undertaken as part of maintaining and improving standards of medical care, but there have been few studies establishing the effectiveness of this new approach.

14.6 Discussion and conclusions

The control of communicable diseases over the past 150 years owes much to the public health reforms of the nineteenth and twentieth centuries, but immunisation and the development of effective drug treatments have clearly played their part. A large part of the increase in life expectancy during this century has been due to the decline in infant mortality and in deaths from infectious diseases at comparatively young ages. More recently, an accelerating decline in death rates from many diseases in middle and early old age is also apparent – in women since the end of the Second World War, and in men since about 1970. The contribution made by the improvements in medical care has been estimated by Bunker *et al.*, (1994). Using data from the United States, they concluded that the clinical preventive and curative services had contributed about 5 years to the increase in life expectancy this century when averaged over the whole population, and had the potential for adding a further 2 years if therapies already known to be efficacious were extended to more people. Such analyses are of necessity crude, however, as the available data are not ideal, and it is also difficult to take account of competing risks between different diseases over such a long period.

Increasingly, medical care is sought and delivered in the expectation that it will improve not life expectancy, but rather the quality of that life. Much of surgery, for example, is intended primarily to improve, rather than save, life. Joint replacement relieves pain and improves function; implanted intraocular lenses improve vision; and cochlear implants improve hearing. Trends in health expectancy over the past two decades suggest that while life expectancy has continued to rise, there has not been an equivalent improvement in the expected years of life free from health-related limitation (Bebbington, 1991). Health expectancy is similar to life expectancy, but refers to the number of further years of good health (usually meaning without disability) someone of a particular age can expect to live. Methods for calculating health expectancy are a fairly recent development (Barendregt *et al.*, 1994; Bone *et al.*, 1995). Combined with information about mortality, health expectancy measures give some indication as to whether improvements in medical care are postponing the onset of disabilities into an increasingly brief period before death (compression of morbidity), or are simply extending the final period of ill health. This topic is complex and discussed in some detail in Chapters 25 and 26.

It must not be forgotten that most medical procedures also carry risks, and although the extent of iatrogenic disease is hard to quantify, it must always be considered in adopting new procedures and reviewing old ones.

The resources which can be devoted to health care will always be finite in the face of infinite demand. A major theme is the prevention of ill health, the promotion of good health, and reduction of avoidable disease and premature death. Medical advances towards these ends will continue to be made, but advances will be greatest if resources are first put into those areas where they can be most effective. There is also a need for people to change their behaviour as many of the main causes of premature death and ill health are related to lifestyle. The need for detailed evaluation remains as important as it was when Cochrane first drew our attention to it.

Acknowledgements

The graphs relating to perinatal and maternal mortality were kindly supplied by Alison Macfarlane of the National Perinatal Epidemiology Unit.

Appendix A

Codes of the International Classification of Diseases (ICD) used to define the diseases examined in this report
(unless otherwise stated in specific chapter)

Notes

1   Codes for ICD 1-5 refer to *computer codes* held on the historic data files. These are as similar as possible to the ICD codes but are numeric, e.g. the computer code for 4th ICD code 156a is 1561.
2   Diseases have been grouped into ICD Chapters for 1911-1994 consistent with ICD9 chapters.
3   For mortality data the following ICD revisions have been in operation:
ICD2=1911-1920; ICD3=1921-1930; ICD4=1931-1939; ICD5=1940-1949;
ICD6=1950-1957; ICD7=1958-1967; ICD8=1968-1978; ICD9=1979-

CHAPTER 4 CODES

ICD chapters (grouped according to ICD 9 concepts)

I Infections & Parasitic diseases (001-139)
ICD2   0010-0093, 0110-252, 0281-350, 0370-383, 0611, 0612, 0620, 0670, 1041-1047, 1060-1070, 1120, 1640
ICD3   0011-0100, 0120-422, 0710, 0720, 0760, 1131-1166, 1210, 1750
ICD4   0010-0100, 0120-446, 0790, 0800, 0830, 1191-1193, 1770
ICD5   0010-322, 0340-441, 0443-4, 0810, 1191-2, 1770
ICD6   0010-1389, 5710-9, 6960-9, 6970-9, 7640-9
ICD7   0010-1389, 5710-9, 6960-9, 7640-9
ICD8   0000-1369
ICD9   0010-1399

II Neoplasms (140-239)
ICD2   0390-463, 0531-2, 0743, 1290
ICD3   0430-500, 0651-2, 0842-1390
ICD4   0450-552, 0721-2
ICD5   0442, 0451-575, 0741-2
ICD6   1400-2209, 2220-39, 2940-9
ICD7   1400-2209, 2220-399, 2940-9
ICD8   1400-2089, 2100-399
ICD9   1400-2399

III Endocrine (240-279)
ICD2   0260-70, 0361-2, 0490-520, 0742, 0880
ICD3   0530-70, 0590-630
ICD4   0580-692
ICD5   0600-61, 0663-4, 0671-710
ICD6   2500-2899, 7720-9
ICD7   2500-899, 7720-9.
ICD8   2400-2799
ICD9   2400-799

Diabetes mellitus
ICD1 0750; ICD2 0500; ICD3 0570; ICD4 0590; ICD5 0610; ICD6 2600-9; ICD7 2600-9; ICD8 2500-9; ICD9 2500-9 (and multicoded data)

IV Diseases of blood & blood forming organs (280-289)
ICD2   0540-554, 1161-2
ICD3   0581-2, 0640, 0691-3,

ICD4   0701-13, 0731-40
ICD5   0721-34, 0751-64
ICD6   2900-2939, 2950-99
ICD7   2900-39, 2950-99
ICD8   2090-9, 2800-99
ICD9   2800-899

V Mental disorders (290-319)
ICD2   0560, 0590, 0680, 0741
ICD3   0660, 0680, 0770, 0841
ICD4   0750-60, 0841-2
ICD5   0770, 0792-3, 0841-4
ICD6   3000-3269
ICD7   3000-3269
ICD8   2900-3159
ICD9   2900-3199

Note: the following are not included in this chapter:
Suicide: ICD6 E9700-99, ICD7 E9700-99, ICD8 E9500-99, ICD9 E9500-99
Injury cause undetermined: ICD8 E9800-99, ICD9 E9800-99
Smoking related diseases — see Chapter 9.

VI Diseases of nervous system & sense organs (320-389)
ICD2   0600, 0612-3, -631-2, 0661-3, 0690, -731-2, 0744-62
ICD3   0701-2, 0730, 0751-2, 0780, 0820, 0843-62
ICD4   0781-2, 0811-4, 0826-7, 0850, 0872-92
ICD5   0801-2, 0821-4, 0833-4, 0850, 0872-92
ICD6   3400-3619, 3640-9, 3660-3989, 7810-9
ICD7   3400-3619, 3640-9, 3660-989, 7440-9, 7810-9
ICD8   3200-3519, 3540-3899, 7330-9, 7810-9
ICD9   3200-899

Dementia - ICD6 3040-69, 3090-9, 7940-9; ICD7 3040-69, 3090-9, 7940-9; ICD8 2900-9, 7940-9; ICD9 2900-9, 2970-9

VII Diseases of the circulatory system (390-459)
ICD2   0470, 0641-0650, 0720, 0770-853
ICD3   0510, 0741-4, 0810, 0830, 0870-960
ICD4   0560, 0821-5, 0871, 0900-0973, 0990-1030
ICD5   0581-4, 0831-2, 0871, 0901-0970, 0990-1030
ICD6   330-3349, 4000-549, 4560-689, 7820-9
ICD7   3300-349, 4000-549, 4560-689, 7820-9
ICD8   3900-4441, 4444-589, 7820-9
ICD9   3900-4599

VIII Diseases of the respiratory system (460-519)
ICD2   0100, 0860-73, 0891-0982, 1001
ICD3   0111-4, 0971-1073, 1091-2
ICD4   0111-4, 1041-1143, 1152
ICD5   0331-4, 1040-146, 1152-8
ICD6   2400-9, 2410-9, 4700-5279
ICD7   2400-9, 2410-9, 4700-5279
ICD8   4600-5199
ICD9   4600-5199

IX Disease of the digestive system (520-579)
ICD2   0991-4, 1002-32, 1080-110, 1131-50, 1170-82
ICD3   1081-3, 1100-22, 1170-200, 1221-70, ICD4 1151, 1154, 1160-82, 1210-90
ICD5   1151, 1160-82, 1211-90
ICD6   5300-709, 5720-879
ICD6   5300-709, 5720-879
ICD8   4442, 5200-5779
ICD9   5200-799

X Diseases of the genitourinary system (580-629)

ICD2   1190-282, 1301-30
ICD3   1280-382, 1400-20
ICD4   1300-1396
ICD5   1300-1396
ICD6   5900-6379, 7920-9
ICD7   5900-6379, 7920-9
ICD8   4443, 5800-6299, 7920-9
ICD9   5800-6299

XI Complications of pregnancy, childbirth and the puerperium (630-679)

ICD2   1341-410
ICD3   1431-500
ICD4   1400-503
ICD5   1401-503
ICD6   6400-899
ICD7   6400-689
ICD8   6300-679
ICD9   6300-679

XII Diseases of the skin and subcutaneous tissue (680-709)

ICD2   1430-1454
ICD3   1520-1544
ICD4   1510-30
ICD5   1510-30
ICD6   2210-9, 2430-2449, 6900-59, 6980-7169, 7660-9
ICD7   6900-59, 6980-7169, 2210-9, 2430-49, 7660-9
ICD8   6800-7099
ICD9   6800-7099

XII Diseases of the musculoskeletal system and connective tissue (710-739)

ICD2   0481-3, 1460-90
ICD3   0521-3, 1551-80
ICD4   0571-2, 1540-62
ICD5   0591-3, 1540-63
ICD6   3620-3639, 7200-439, 7450-99
ICD7   7200-439, 7450-99, 3620-39
ICD8   3520-39, 7100-329, 7340-89
ICD9   7100-7399

XIV Congenital anomalies (740-759)

ICD2   1501-4
ICD3   1591-3
ICD4   1571-9
ICD5   1571-85
ICD6   7500-99
ICD7   7500-99
ICD8   7400-599
ICD9   7400-599

XV Certain conditions originating in the perinatal period (760-779)

'Developmental and wasting diseases' (1848-1910) = 'congenital malformations' + 'early infancy' - 'birth injuries'.

ICD2   1511-24
ICD3   1601-12
ICD4   1580-615
ICD5   1589-615, 1617-8
ICD6   7600-39, 7650-9, 7670-719, 7730-69
ICD7   7600-39, 7650-9, 7670-719, 7730-69
ICD8   7600-799
ICD9   7600-799

XVI Symptoms, signs and ill-defined conditions (780-799)

ICD2   0701-12, 1421-4, 1541-2, 1870-96
ICD3   0790, 151-2, 1641-2, 2040-53
ICD4   0860-, 0981-2, 1621-2, 1990-2003
ICD5   0860, 0980, 1621-3, 1990-2004
ICD6   4550-9, 7800-19, 7830-919, 7930-59
ICD7   4550-9, 7800-9, 7830-919, 7930-59
ICD8   7800-9, 7830-919, 7930-69
ICD9   7800-799

XVII Injury and poisoning (800-999, E800-E999)

ICD2   0571-80, 1530, 1550-630, 1650-860
ICD3   0671-2, 1630, 1650-740, 1760-2030
ICD4   0771-2, 1630-760, 1780-980
ICD5   0662, 0781-2, 0794-5, 1631-1760, 1780-980
ICD6   2420-59, 3650-9, E8000-9999
ICD7   2420-9, 2450-9, 3650-9, E8000-9999
ICD8   E8000-E9999
ICD9   E8000-9999

Injury and poisoning: ICD6 E8000-9999; ICD7 E8000-9999; ICD8 E8000-9999; ICD9 E8000-9999
Accidental deaths: ICD6 E8000-9659; ICD7 E8000-9659; ICD8 E8000-9499; ICD9 E8000-9499
Road traffic accidents: ICD6 E8100-259; ICD7 E8100-259; ICD8 E8100-99
Suicide: ICD6 E9700-99; ICD7 E9700-99; ICD8 E9500-99; ICD9 E9500-99
Injury cause undetermined: ICD8 E9800-99; ICD9 E9800-99

CHAPTER 8 CODES

ICD9 (1979)

140-145	Oral cancer
146-149	Pharyngeal cancer
150	Cancer of oesophagus
155	Liver cancer
161	Laryngeal cancer
291	Alcoholic psychoses
303	Alcoholic dependence syndrome
305.0	Non-dependent abuse of alcohol
425.5	Alcoholic cardiomyopathy
571	Liver disease
571.0-571.3	Liver disease - alcohol mentioned
571.4-571.9	Liver disease - alcohol not mentioned
980	Toxic effect of alcohol
E860	Accidental poisoning by alcohol
E880	Falls on stairs

Appendix B

Chronology of major events

Although this report covers health from 1841 to 1994, the likelihood of a person succumbing to disease may depend on previous experiences. For example those dying in 1841 may have been affected by disability and unemployment caused by the Napoleonic Wars, previous periods of hardship, and other factors. Thus this chronology begins some time before 1841. It has been constructed in the main to place major events that may have influenced health or health statistics in time. A few other well known events have been added for interest.

1802	Act introduced to limit the employment of children to under 12 hours per day.
1806	Installation of first steam-operated loom.
1819	Peterloo Massacre. Factory Act forbade the employment of children under the age of 9 in cotton mills. Queen Victoria born.
1825	First public steam railway – Stockton to Darlington.
1830	Publication of William Cobbett's *Rural Rides* describing the plight of the rural poor.
1832	Cholera arrived in GB for first time (from India) and 22,000 died by June. Reform Act (abolition of rotten boroughs, franchisement of new industrial towns).
1833	Factory Act legislation banned any employment of children under nine, restricted working hours of older children, appointed factory inspectors. First government grant to education.
1834	Poor Law Amendment Act passed – benefits for the poor reduced and workhouses established. Tollpuddle Martyrs convicted.
1836	Births and Deaths Registration Act and Marriage Act established Office of Registrar General. Enabled first national statistics on numbers of births, deaths and marriages to be produced. Thomas Lister appointed the first Registrar General.
1837	Victoria's reign began. Registrar General introduced births, deaths and marriages registrations from 1 July.
1839	William Farr introduced the first classification of causes of death, published in the Registrar General's first report.

——————— BEGINNING OF PERIOD COVERED BY THIS VOLUME ———————

1841	First census of population to be conducted by Registrar General.
1842	Anaesthesia first used in an operation. Chadwick's *Report on the Condition of the Labouring Population of Great Britain. Coal Commission Report* published. *Children's Employment Commission Report* published.
1843	Royal Commission into state of large towns (reported 1844-45).
1844	Legislation extending protection of workers into mines and other industries.
1846	Corn Laws repealed. The office of Medical Officer of Health instituted in local authorities - responsible for producing an annual report (posts abolished 1974).
1848	Further major cholera outbreak (50-70,000 deaths, 14,000 in London). Public Health Act which created a central Board of Health, and empowered individual towns to set up local Medical Officers of Health. "The Communist Manifesto" was published.
1851	Lodging Houses Act – checked the worst abuses. The Great Exhibition. The 1851 census of population was the first to ask marital status and relationship to head of household.
1853-56	Crimean War.
1853	Smallpox vaccination of children within 4 months of birth made compulsory.
1854	Dickens published "Hard Times". 10,675 cholera deaths in London.
1855	General Register Office (Scotland) established. London's "great stink".
1856	First synthetic dye produced. Bessemer converter invented for cheap steel production.
1860	Florence Nightingale published her *Notes on nursing,* set up training school for nurses.
1861	Semmelweis published research results linking dirt with infection (discovered 1848).
1862	Pasteur demonstrated link between bacteria and disease, invented pasteurization.
1865	Mid-year population estimates first produced for large towns.
1866	Public Health Act. Local Authorities to improve sanitation and appoint sanitary inspectors. London cholera epidemic – 5,000 died within 3 weeks.
1867	Passing of second Parliamentary Reform Act. Lister introduced antiseptic surgery, using carbolic acid. Marx published *Das Kapital.*
1868	Trades Union Congress founded.
1869	Lister introduced antisepsis into surgery – surgical mortality fell by two thirds.
1870	Foster's Education Act, providing virtually free elementary education for anyone wanting it. Schools financed in part from the rates. Major smallpox outbreak, 40,000 died, 10,000 in London.
1872	Public Health Act.

1874	Factory act introduced a ten hour day, and raised age of employment of children to ten. Trade Unions acquired legal right to strike. Births and Deaths Registration Act transferred the obligation to register births and deaths from the registrar to the person directly concerned; certification of cause of death by a doctor now required.
1875	Public Health Act - set standards for sanitation in new houses. Compelled notification of all cases of cholera. Artisan's Dwelling Act - gave local authorities the power to clear slums.
1876	Robert Koch identified bacteria that cause tuberculosis, anthrax and cholera. Bell invented the telephone.
1880	Education up to age ten years of age was made compulsory.
1881-85	Cell division described by Walther Fleming. Pasteur used attenuated bacteria to confer immunity against rabies and anthrax. Motor cars invented by Karl Benz.
1881	Census of population. Mid-year population estimates produced for <u>all</u> registration counties and large towns.
1882	Koch discovered tuberculosis bacillus.
1883	Klebs and Loffler discovered diphtheria bacillus, leading to development of antitoxin.
1889	Notification of certain infectious diseases made compulsory in London. Sterilisation of surgical instruments by dry heat introduced.
1892	Diphtheria antitoxin isolated by Paul Ehrlich.
1893	Government established special education for blind and deaf children.
1894	Passing of third Parliamentary Reform Act.
1895-96	Roentgen discovered X-rays. Diesel invented the diesel engine. Becquerel discovered radioactivity.
1897-98	Ronald Ross discovered that malaria was transmitted by the mosquito. Beijerinck discovered viruses. Aspirin first marketed.
1899	Boer War. Notification of infectious diseases made compulsory in <u>every</u> urban, rural and port sanitary district in England and Wales. Local authorities given powers to provide special schools for the "educable mentally subnormal".
1900	Seebohm Rowntree investigated poverty in York.
1901	Queen Victoria died. Age of employment for children raised to 12. ABO blood grouping discovered.
1903-06	First sustained flight (Wright brothers). Einstein's special theory of relativity. Vitamins recognised as essential to health. Charles Booth - "Life and Labour of the People in London(1891-1903)".
1908	Old Age Pensions Act
1909	Chromosomes established as carriers of heredity.
1911	National Health Insurance Act. Census of population - first to ask fertility questions. Registrar General's "social classes" introduced as means of analysing population statistics according to the general standing in the community of occupation/ employment groups. Second revision of the International list of causes of deaths adopted by the Registrar General.
1914-1918	First World War
1917	Bolshevik Revolution in Russia.
1918	Representation of People Act. Gave the vote for all males over 21, and females over 30 with property qualifications.
1919-38	Great Depression. 2.8 million unemployed in 1932.
1919	Ministry of Health established.
1920	Age of employment of children raised to 14.
1922	Insulin isolated, and used for the first time to treat diabetics.
1926	General Strike. First Adoption of Children Act. Legitimacy Act. Births and Deaths Registration Act – made it unlawful to dispose of a body before the registrar's certificate or coroner's order had been issued. Also required the registration of stillbirths.
1927	Stillbirths first registered.
1928	Universal adult suffrage. Anti-bacterial activity of penicillium mould was discovered by Alexander Fleming (but not made stable enough for medical use until 1939).
1929	Act of Marriage Act – increased the minimum age from 12 for girls and 14 for boys to 16 years for both.
1931	Census of population – "usual address" question introduced.
1932	Sulphonamide antibiotic discovered, shown to be effective against streptococcal septicaemia. Modern drip methods perfected, enabling advanced surgery.
1934	First radioisotopes produced by the Curies.
1939-1945	Second World War. First nuclear reactor. Penicillin used for first time. Kidney machine invented. DDT invented. Synthetic fertilisers produced. First nuclear bombs used in war.
1939	National Registration Act – provided for establishment of a national register of the entire population maintained by GRO. Identity cards were issued. Penicillin manufactured in quantity.
1940s	Mass immunisation against diphtheria in Britain.
1941	Wartime Social Survey formed. National Insurance Act – compensated for "industrial diseases and injuries".
1944	Disabled Persons Act. Streptomycin discovered – active against tuberculosis.
1948	National Health Service Act. World Health Organisation established. Cancer registration scheme introduced. National Assistance Act – gave local authorities responsibility for providing accommodation and welfare services for people in their area who required it on account of age, infirmity, and other circumstances.
1950s	BCG vaccination against tuberculosis introduced in Britain. Betablockers developed for treating hypertension. Ultrasound developed.
1951	Census of population – questions about household amenities (e.g. WCs) introduced.
1952-55	Food rationing ended. Polio vaccine developed. Oral contraception introduced. Link between smoking and lung cancer proposed.
1952	National Health Service Central Register set up from National Registration records.
1953	Hospital In-patient Enquiry first carried out.
1956	Clean Air Act, after 4,000 died in 1952 London smog.

1957	Family Expenditure Survey started on behalf of Department of Employment.
1960s	Kidney machine developed. Benzodiazepines developed. First renal transplants undertaken. Cytotoxic chemotherapy became standard for a number of cancers including leukaemia and Wilms' tumour.
1961	Census of Population – some small area statistics published for first time.
1962	Royal College of Physicians report on *Smoking and Health* recommended restrictions on tobacco advertising, increasing taxation on cigarettes, etc. Doll and Hill published their findings linking cigarettes to lung cancer in the mid 1960s.
1964	Congenital malformations reported for first time on national basis.
1966	First heart transplant. Sample census – questions on car availability and means of transport to work introduced.
1967	Penicillin nucleus isolated, leading to new antibiotics.
1968	Legal abortions statistics collected for first time. Regional population projections started.
1969	Family Law Reform Act reduced age of majority from 21 to 18.
1970	General Register Office and Government Social Survey combined to form the Office of Population Censuses and Surveys – OPCS. The General Household Survey began. Chronically Sick and Disabled Persons Act – to help families cope with appreciably or severely handicapped members at home (unemployable and employable treated the same for first time).
1973	Britain joined European Community (EC). OPCS Longitudinal Study set up.
1975	Live birth weight information collected by OPCS.
1977	British scientist discovered complete genetic structure of a virus.
1978	British first test tube baby born.
1979	"Thatcher Revolution" – powers of unions curbed, number of home owners increased, Monetarism, privatisation.
1981	Industrial Diseases (Notification) Act – certification of deaths and recording of information relating to industrial diseases. Brixton and Liverpool riots. Over 3 million unemployed. First reported AIDS cases in UK. First heart-lung transplant. WHO published *Global Strategy for Health for All by the Year 2000*.
1982	Falklands War.
1983	Seat belts made compulsory. Labour Force Survey expanded to become annual and continuous.
1984	Coalminers' strike. Famine in Ethiopia.
1986	Chernobyl nuclear reactor meltdown. Greater London Council abolished.
1987	Regan and Gorbachev agreed to begin nuclear disarmament. Gorbachev began reforms of Soviet Union..
1989	Berlin Wall demolished. Fall of communist governments in Poland, East Germany, Hungary, Czechoslavakia, Bulgaria and Rumania.
1991	Germany reunited. Gulf War. Census of population – introduced new questions on ethnicity and limiting longstanding illness. Communism collapsed in the USSR. Treaty of Maastricht signed. Green Paper – *Health of the Nation* – published.

Appendix C Referees

Dr John Ashley
Dr John Ashton
Roger Black
Nick Bosenquet
Bev Botting
Carol Brayne
Peter Burney
Janet Cade
Mike Catchpole
Susan Cole
Michèl Coleman
Derek Cook
Cyrus Cooper
Mike D'Souza
Tim Devis
Stuart Donnon
Karen Dunnell
Grimley Evans
Douglas Fleming
Spence Galbraith
Adrian Gallop
Eileen Goddard
Jan Gregory
Andy Hall
Walter Holland
Jen Hollowell

Derek Jewell
Heather Joshi
Ken Judge
Sue Kelly
David Kerr
Tim Key
Johan Mackenbach
Netar Mallick
Hugh Markowe
Mark McCarthy
Anna McCormick
Alison Macfarlane
Mike Murphy
Clive Osmond
Stephen Palmer
Mike Quinn
Roberto Rona
Anthony Seaton
Gerry Shaper
Sally Sheard
Steve Smallwood
Jillian Smith
David Strachen
Robert Waller
Charles Warlow
Jean Weddle

References

Chapter 2 Monitoring health – data sources and methods

Acheson ED (1967), *Medical Record Linkage*, Oxford: Oxford University Press.

Alberman ED, Botting B, Blatchley N, Twidell A (1994), A new hierarchical classification of causes of infant deaths in England and Wales, *Archives Disease in Childhood*, 70: 403–409.

Alderson MR (1965), *The accuracy of certification of death, and the classification of the underlying cause of death from the death certification*, M.D. Thesis, London University.

Alderson MR (1974), Morbidity statistics, In *Reviews of United Kingdom statistical sources*, vol.II (ed. WF Maunder), pp.32–52. London: Heinemann.

Alderson MR (1981), *International Mortality Statistics*, London: MacMillan.

Allied Dunbar, Sports Council and Health Education Authority (1992), *Allied Dunbar National Fitness Survey*, London: The Sports Council.

Armitage RI (1986), Population projections for English local authority areas, *Population Trends*, 43: 31.

Armitage P (1971), *Statistical Methods in Medical Research*, New York: Blackwell.

Ashley JSA, Cole SK, Kilbane MPJ (1991), Health information resources: United Kingdom – health and social factors. In *Oxford Textbook of Public Health* vol.II, pp.29–53, Oxford: Oxford University Press.

Ashley J and Devis T (1992), Death certification from the point of view of the epidemiologist, *Population Trends*, 67: 22–28.

Bennett N, Dodd T, Flatley J, Freeth S, Bolling K (1995), *Health Survey for England 1993*, London: OPCS, HMSO.

Birch D (1993), Automatic coding of causes of death, *Population Trends*, 73: 36–38.

Black R, Sharp L and Kendrick SW (1993), *Trends in Cancer Survival in Scotland 1968–90*, Edinburgh: Information and Statistics Division, Directorate of Information Services, National Health Service in Scotland.

Blaxter M (1990), *Health and Lifestyles*, London and New York: Routledge.

Bolling K (1994), *Smoking among Secondary School children in 1993*, London: HMSO.

Bone MR, Bebbington AC, Jagger C, Morgan K, Nicolaas G (1995), *Health Expectancy and its Uses*, London: HMSO.

Botting B (1991), Trends in abortion, *Population Trends*, 64: 19–29.

Botting B (1995), Congenital anomalies, In: *The Health of our Children, Decennial Supplement*, OPCS Series DS no 11, London: HMSO.

Breeze E, Trevor G, Wilmot A (1991), *General Household Survey 1989*, London: HMSO.

Bridgwood A and Malbon G (OPCS, 1995), *Survey of the Physical Health of Prisoners 1994*, OPCS Series SS1376, London: HMSO.

Bridgwood A, Malbon G, Lader D, Matheson J (1996), *Health in England 1995*, London: HMSO.

Campbell H (1965), *Changes in Mortality Trends: England and Wales 1931–1961*, National Center for Health Statistics, Series 3 no.3, US DHEW, Washington DC: Public Health Service.

Carnegie (1951), In *The Urban Working-Class Diet 1940 to 1949: First report of the National Food Survey Committee*, Ministry of Food p.13, London: HMSO.

Carstairs V (1991), Dying away from home: the influence on mortality statistics, *Population Trends*, 66: 22–25.

Case RAM and Pearson JT (1954), Tumours of the urinary bladder in workmen engaged in the manufacture and use of certain dyestuff intermediates in the British Chemical Industry, *Br J Ind Med*, 11: 213–232.

Charlton JRH (1986), Use of mortality data in health planning, In *New Developments in the Analysis of Mortality and Causes of Death*, Hansluwka H, Lopez AD, Porapakkham Y, Prasartkul P (eds), Bangkok: World Health Organisation, Mahidol University,

Charlton J and Heady P (1995), Estimating local needs for GP services – a practical test of synthesised estimates. In *Proceedings of Data Needs in an era of Health Services Reform*, Washington DC: USDHHS.

Clarkson JA and Fine PFM (1985), The efficiency of measles and pertussis morbidity reporting in England and Wales, *International Journal of Epidemiology*, 14: 153.

Clayton DG and Schifflers E (1987), Models for temporal variation in cancer rates I: age-period and age-cohort models, *Statist Med*, 6: 449–467.

Colhoum H and Prescott-Clark P (eds) (1996), *Health Survey for England 1994*, Series HS no 4, London: HMSO.

CRC (1982), *Trends in Cancer Survival in Great Britain: cases registered between 1960 and 1974*, London: Cancer Research Campaign.

Daykin C (1986), Projecting the population of the United Kingdom, *Population Trends*, 44: 28.

Department of Health (1995), Executive letter EL(92)95.

Devis T (1990), The expectation of life in England and Wales, *Population Trends*, 60: 23–24.

DHSS (1963–94), *Social Security Statistics* (various years), London: HMSO.

Diamond A and Goddard E (OPCS, 1995), *Smoking among Secondary School Children in 1994*, London: HMSO.

Dight SE (OPCS, 1976), *Scottish Drinking Habits and Attitudes towards Alcohol*, London: HMSO.

Dobbs J and Marsh A (OPCS, 1983), *Smoking among Secondary School Children*, London: HMSO.

Dobbs J and Marsh A (OPCS, 1985), *Smoking among Secondary School Children in 1984*, London: HMSO.

Fenton Lewis A (1979), Morbidity data: what do we have? What do we need?, What are we likely to get? *Health Trends*, 11: 49–52.

Fleming DM, Crombie DL, Ross AM (1996), *Weekly Returns Service Report for 1995*, Birmingham: Birmingham Research Unit of the Royal College of General Practitioners.

Fox AJ and Goldblatt PO (1982), *Socio-demographic Differentials in Mortality*, Longitudinal Study series, LS no.1, London: HMSO.

Gillis RC (1971), *9th annual report of the Regional Cancer Committee for 1968*, Glasgow: Western Regional Hospital Cancer Registration Bureau.

Goddard E and Ikin C (OPCS, 1987), *Smoking among Secondary School Children in 1986*, London: HMSO.

Goddard E (OPCS, 1989), *Smoking among Secondary School Children in 1988*, London: HMSO.

Goddard E (1991), *Drinking in England and Wales in the late 1980s*, London: HMSO.

Goddard E and Savage D (OPCS, 1994), *People aged 65 and over*, Series GHS no 22, supplement A, London: HMSO.

Goldacre MJ and Miller DL (1976), Completeness of statutory notification of acute bacterial meningitis, *British Medical Journal*, ii: 501.

Gregory J, Foster K, Tyler H, Wiseman M (1990), *The Dietary and Nutritional Survey of British Adults*, London: HMSO.

Gregory J, Collins D, Davies P, Hughes J, Clarke P (1995), *National Diet and Nutrition Survey: children aged 1 1/2 to 4 1/2 years*, vol.1, London: HMSO.

Haward RA (1973), Scale of under-notification of infectious diseases by general practitioners, *Lancet*, I: 873.

Heasman MA and Lipworth L (1966), *Accuracy of Certification of Cause of Death*, OPCS Studies in medical and population subjects no. 20, London: HMSO.

Hey K, O'Donnell M, Murphy M, Jones N, Botting B (1994), Use of local neural tube defect registers to interpret national trends, *Arch Dis Child*, 71: f198–f202.

Hinds K and Gregory JR (1995), *National Diet and Nutrition Survey: children aged 1 1/2 to 4 1/2 years*, vol. 2: *Report of the Dental Survey*, London: HMSO.

Jette AM (1980), Health status indicators: their utility in chronic disease evaluation research, *J Chronic Dis*, 33: 567–579.

Kemp IW, Boyle P, Smans M, Muir CS (1985), *Atlas of Cancer in Scotland 1975–80, Incidence and Epidemiological Perspective*, IARC Scientific Publications no.72, Lyon: IARC

Kendrick S and Clarke J (1993), The Scottish record linkage system, *Health Bulletin*, 51(2): 72–79.

Knight I (1984), *The Heights and Weights of Adults in Great Britain*, London: HMSO

Lader D and Matheson J (OPCS, 1991), *Smoking amongst Secondary School Children in 1990*, London: HMSO.

Last JM (1963), The Iceberg, *Lancet*, 2: 28–31.

Last JM (1995), *A Dictionary of Epidemiology*, 3rd edn, Oxford: Oxford University Press.

Lee WC and Lin RS (1995), Analysis of cancer rates using excess risk age-period-cohort models, *Int Jnl of Epidemiology*, 24 no 4: 671–677.

Logan WPD (1950), Mortality in England and Wales from 1848–1947, *Population Studies*, 4: 132–78

Marsh A, Dobbs J, White A (1986), *Adolescent Drinking*, London: HMSO.

Martin J, Meltzer H, Elliot D (1988), *OPCS Surveys of Disability in Great Britain, Report 1: The Prevalence of Disability among Adults*, London: HMSO.

Meltzer H, Gill B, Petticrew M, Hinds K (1995a), *OPCS Surveys of Psychiatric Morbidity in Great Britain, Report 1: The Prevalence of Psychiatric Morbidity among Adults living in Private Households*, London: HMSO.

Meltzer H, Gill B, Petticrew M, Hinds K (1995b), *OPCS Surveys of Psychiatric Morbidity in Great Britain, Report 2: Physical Complaints, Service use and Treatment of Adults with Psychiatric Disorders*, London: HMSO.

McCormick A, Tillett H, Bannister B, Emslie J (1987), Surveillance of AIDS in the United Kingdom, *British Medical Journal*, 295: 1466.

McCormick A (1993), The notification of infectious diseases in England and Wales, *CDR Review*, 3: R19–25.

Ministry of Food (1951), *The Urban Working-Class Diet 1940 to 1949: First report of the National Food Survey Committee*, London: HMSO.

Ministry of Agriculture Fisheries and Food (1994), *Household Food Consumption and Expenditure 1993, Annual reports of the National Food Survey Committee*, London: HMSO.

Noble B and Charlton J (1994), Homicides in England and Wales, *Population Trends*, 75: 26–29.

O'Brien M (1994), *Children's Dental Health in the United Kingdom 1993*, Social Survey Report SS1350, London: HMSO.

ONS (1996), *Mortality Statistics: Cause 1993 (revised) and 1994, England and Wales*, Series DH2 no. 21, London: HMSO.

OPCS (1970), *Report of the Advisory Committee on Cancer Registration*, London: OPCS.

OPCS (1981,) *Report of the Advisory Committee on Cancer Registration*, Series MB1 no. 6, London: HMSO.

OPCS (1982), *A Comparison of the Registrar General's Annual Population Estimates for England and Wales compared with the results of the 1981 Census*, Occasional Paper no.29, London: OPCS.

OPCS (1982), *Cancer Statistics: Survival 1971–1975*, Series MB1 no.9, London: HMSO.

OPCS (1983), *Cancer Registration Surveillance 1968–78, England and Wales*, London: HMSO.

OPCS (1983), *Mortality Statistics, Comparison of 8th and 9th Revisions of the International Classification of Diseases, (1978 sample) England and Wales*, Series DH1 no. 10, London: HMSO.

OPCS (1985), *Mortality Statistics, Cause 1984, England and Wales*, Series DH2 no. 11, London: HMSO.

OPCS (1988), *Mortality Statistics: Cause, 1986*, DH2 no. 13, London: HMSO.

OPCS (1990a), *Review of the National Cancer Registration System, England and Wales*, Series MB1 no.17, London: HMSO.

OPCS (1990b), *Report of the Advisory Committee on Cancer Registration*, London: OPCS.

OPCS (1992), *Labour Force Survey 1990 and 1991*, London: HMSO.

OPCS (1993a), How complete was the 1991 Census?, *Population Trends*, 71: 22–25.

OPCS (1993b), Rebasing the annual population estimates, *Population Trends* 73: 27–31.

OPCS (1993c), *Uses of OPCS records for Medical Research*, OPCS Occasional Paper no. 41, London: OPCS.

OPCS (1994), *Cancer Statistics: Registrations 1989*, Series MB1 no. 22, London: HMSO.

OPCS (1995a), *Mortality Statistics, Cause, England and Wales*, Series DH2 no. 20, London: HMSO.

OPCS (1995b), *Monitoring Scheme for Congenital Malformations*, OPCS Occasional Paper no.43, London: OPCS.

OPCS (1995c), *Living in Britain. Preliminary results from the 1994 General Household Survey*, London: HMSO.

Orr JB (1936), *Food, Health and Income*, London: MacMillan.

Ransome A (1893), Vital statistics, In *A Treatise on Hygiene and Public Health II* (eds T Stevenson and SF Murphy), pp.465–509, London: Churchill.

Report of Committee on Medical Aspects of Abortion (1936), *Br Med J*, Supplement, 1: 230–238.

Royal College of General Practitioners (1968), Returns from general practice, *British Medical Journal*, iv: 63.

Sharp L, Black RJ, Harkness EF, Finlayson AR, Muir CS (1993), *Cancer Registration Statistics Scotland 1981–1990*, Edinburgh: Scottish Cancer Intelligence Unit, Information and Statistics Division, Directorate of Information Services, The National Health Service in Scotland.

Stiller CA, O'Connor CM, Vincent TJ and Draper GJ (1991), The National Registry of Childhood Tumours and the leukaemia/lymphoma data for 1966–83. In *The Geographical Epidemiology of Childhood Leukaemia and non-Hodgkin Lymphomas in Great Britain, 1966–83* (ed. G Draper), pp.7–16, Studies on Medical and Population Subjects no. 53, London: HMSO.

Stiller CA (1993), Cancer registration: its uses in research, and confidentiality in the EC, *Journal of Epidemiology and Community Health*, 47: 342–44.

Swerdlow AJ, Douglas AJ, Vaughan Hudson G, Vaughan Hudson B (1993), Completeness of cancer registration in England and Wales: an assessment based on 2145 patients with Hodgkin's disease independently registered by the British National Lymphoma Investigation, *British Journal of Cancer*, 67: 326–329.

Thomas M, Holroyd S, Goddard E (OPCS, 1993), *Smoking among Secondary School Children in 1992*, London: HMSO.

Tillett E and Spencer IL (1982), Influenza surveillance in England and Wales using routine statistics, *Journal of Hygiene*, 88: 33.

Todd JE and Whitworth A (1974), *Adult Dental Health in Scotland, 1972*, Social Survey Report SS1009, London: HMSO.

Todd JE (1975), *Children's Dental Health in England and Wales, 1973*, Social Survey Report SS1011, London: HMSO.

Todd JE and Walker AM (1980), *Adult Dental Health, vol. 1: England and Wales 1968–78*, Social Survey Report SS1112, London: HMSO.

Todd JE, Walker AM, Dodd T (1982), *Adult Dental Health, vol. 2: United Kingdom 1978*, Social Survey Report SS1112, London: HMSO.

Todd JE and Dodd T (1985), *Children's Dental Health in the United Kingdom 1983*, Social Survey Report SS1189, London: HMSO.

Todd JE (1988), *Scottish Children's Dental Health 1983–1986*, Social Survey Report SS1211, London: HMSO.

Todd JE and Lader D (1991), *Adult Dental Health 1988: United Kingdom*, Social Survey Report SS1260, London: HMSO.

Todd J, Lader D and Dodd T (OPCS, 1994), *Dental Crowns: report of a follow-up to the 1988 Adult Dental Health Survey*, London: HMSO.

Waldron HA and Vickerstaff L (1977), *Intimations of Quality: ante mortem and post mortem diagnosis*, London: Nuffield Provincial Hospitals Trust.

Weatherall JAC (1978), Congenital malformations: surveillance and reporting, *Population Trends* 11: 27.

West RR (1976), Accuracy of cancer registration, *British Journal of Preventive and Social Medicine* 30: 187–92.

Whitehead F (1985), Population statistics in the United Kingdom, *Population Trends* 41: 26.

Wilson P (1980) *Drinking in England and Wales*, London: HMSO.

World Health Organisation (1977), *Manual of the International Statistical Classification of Diseases, Injuries and Causes of Death*, I & II, Geneva: WHO.

World Health Organisation (1979), *Measurement of Levels of Health*, European series no. 7, Copenhagen: WHO.

World Health Organisation (1991), World Health Annual Statistics – based on *Cancer Incidence in Five Continents* (eds J Waterhouse *et al*), p.456, Lyon: IARC, 1976, Geneva: WHO.

Wrigley EA and Schofield RS (1989), *The Population History of England 1541–1871*, 2nd edn, Cambridge: Cambridge University Press.

Chapter 3 Trends in all-cause mortality: 1841–1994

Charlton JRH (1996), Which areas are healthiest? *Population Trends*, 83: 17-24.

GAD (forthcoming), *Cohort and Period Life Tables 1841-1991*.

Registrar General (1843), *Fifth Annual Report of the Registrar General of Births, Deaths and Marriages in England*, London: HMSO.

Shaw C (1995), Accuracy and uncertainty of the national population projections for the United Kingdom, *Population Trends* 77: 24–32.

Wilmoth JR and Lundstrom H (1996), Extreme longevity in five countries, *European Journal of Population* 12: 63–93.

Wrigley EA and Schofield RS (1989), *The Population History of England 1541–1871*, 2nd edn, Cambridge: Cambridge University Press.

Chapter 4 Trends in causes of mortality: 1841-1994 – an overview

Davenport F (1984), Influenza viruses. In *Viral Infections in Humans: Epidemiology and Control* (ed. AS Evans), New York: Plenum Press, pp. 373–396.

Dublin LI, Lotka AJ and Spiegelman M (1949), *Length of Life*, New York: The Roland Press Company.

d'Espaignet ET, van Ommeren M, Taylor F, Briscoe N and Petony P (1991), *Trends in Australian mortality 1921–1988*, Australian Institute of Health: Mortality Series no.1, Canberra: AGPS.

Gage TB (1993), The decline of mortality in England and Wales 1861 to 1964: decomposition by cause of death and component of mortality, *Population Studies*, 47: 47–66.

Goldacre MJ (1993), Cause specific mortality: understanding uncertain tips of the disease iceberg, *Journal of Epidemiology and Community Health*, 47: 491–496.

Kunitz SJ (1983), Speculations on the European mortality decline, *Economic History Review*, 36: 349–364.

Leitch DGM, Heller RF and O'Connor SJ (1987), Variation in death certification of ischaemic heart disease in Australia and New Zealand, *Australian and New Zealand Journal of Medicine*, 17: 309–315.

Logan WPD (1950), Mortality in England and Wales from 1848 to 1947, *Population Studies*, 4: 132–178.

Machenbach JP (1994), The epidemiologic transition theory, *J Epidemiol Community Health*, 48: 329–332.

Omran AR (1971), The epidemiologic transition: a theory of the epidemiology of population change, *Millbank Mem Fund Quart*, 49: 509–538.

OPCS (1983), *Mortality Statistics*, Series DH1 no. 14, Introduction, London: HMSO.

OPCS (1984), *Mortality Statistics: cause*, DH2 no. 11, Introduction: rule 3. London: HMSO.

OPCS (1984), *Mortality Statistics*, DH1 no. 16, Introduction: injury and poisoning rules, London: HMSO.

OPCS (1988), *Mortality statistics: cause, 1986*, Series DH2 no. 13, London: HMSO.

Trowell HC and Burkitt DP (1981), *Western Diseases: Their Emergence and Prevention*, London: Edward Arnold.

Chapter 5 Morbidity statistics from health service utilisation

Acheson ED (1967), *Medical Record Linkage*, Oxford: Oxford University Press.

de Alarcon J, Seagroatt V, Sellar C and Goldacre MJ (1993), Population-based trends in treatment rates in psychiatry in Oxfordshire, 1975–1986, *Journal of Public Health Medicine*, 15: 93–102.

Ashley JSA (1972), Present state of statistics from hospital in–patient data and their uses, *British Journal of Preventive and Social Medicine*, 26: 135–47.

Ashley JSA, Cole SK, and Kilbane MPJ (1991), Health information resources: United Kingdom – health and social factors, In *Oxford Textbook of Public Health* (ed. WW Holland), pp.29–53, Oxford: Oxford University Press.

Bennett N, Dodd T, Flatley J, Freeth S, Bolling K (1995), *Health Survey for England 1993*, OPCS, London: HMSO.

Charlton JRH, Heady P, Nicolaas G (1995), Demand for General Practitioner Services – A practical test of synthesised estimation In: *Data Needs in an Era of Health Reform, Proceedings of the 25th Public Health Conference on Records and Statistics 1995*, Washington DC: U.S. Department of Health and Human Services.

Coleman MP (1991), *Cancer Risk after Medical Treatment*, Oxford: Oxford University Press.

Curwen M, Dunnell K, Ashley J (1990), Hidden influenza deaths, *British Medical Journal*, 300: 896.

Department of Health (1994), *Hospital Episode Statistics*, vol.1: *Finished consultant episodes by diagnosis, operation and specialty, England: Financial year 1991–92*, Government Statistical Service.

Department of Health (1995a), *Hospital Episode Statistics*, vol.1 *Finished consultant episodes by diagnosis, operation and specialty 1988–89 to 1993–94*, Government Statistical Service.

Department of Health (1995b), *Asthma. An Epidemiological Overview*, Central Health Monitoring Unit Epidemiological Overview Series in collaboration with the Department of Health Statistics Division.

DHSS (1977), *In-patient Statistics from the Mental Health Enquiry for England*, Statistical and Research Report Series no. 17, London: HMSO.

DHSS (1986), Mental health statistics for England 1986, Booklet 1: *Mental Illness Hospitals and Units in England: Trends in Admissions, Discharges and Residents*, Government Statistical Service.

DHSS and OPCS (1972), *Report on Hospital In-patient Enquiry for the years 1949, 1957–1967: Historical Tables*, London: HMSO,

DHSS and OPCS (1978), *Hospital In-patient Enquiry: Main Tables 1975, England and Wales*, Series MB4 no. 5, London: HMSO.

DHSS and OPCS (1979), *Hospital In-patient Enquiry: Patterns of Morbidity 1962–1967, England and Wales*, Series MB4 no.3, London: HMSO.

DHSS and OPCS (1989), *Hospital In-patient Enquiry: In-patient and Day case Trends 1979–1985, England*, Series MB4 no. 29, London: HMSO.

DHSS, OPCS and Welsh Office (1981), *Trends in Morbidity 1968–1978: Applying Surveillance Techniques to the Hospital In-patient Enquiry*, Fareham: OPCS.

Dunnigan MG, Hartland WA and Fyfe T (1970), Seasonal incidence and mortality of ischaemic heart disease, *Lancet*, ii: 793–6.

Fedson DS, Hannoun C, Lees J, Sprenger MJW, Hampson AW, Bro-Jrgensen, Ahlbom A-M, Nokleby H, Valle M, Olafsson O, Garcia FS, Gugelman R, Andrade R, de Snacken R, Ambrosch F, Donatelli I (1995), Influenza vaccination in 18 developed countries, 1980–1992, *Vaccine*, 13: 623–627

Fleming DM (1991), Measurement of morbidity in general practice, *J.Epidemiol and Comm. Hlth*, 45: 180–183.

Fleming DM, Chakraverty P, Sadler C, Litton P (1995), *Combined Clinical and Virological Surveillance of Influenza in Winters of 1992 and 1993/94*.

Fleming DM and Crombie DL (1987), Prevalence of asthma and hay fever in England and Wales, *British Medical Journal*, 294: 279–283.

Fleming DM, Norbury CA, Crombie DL (1991), *Annual and Seasonal Variation in the Incidence of Common Diseases*, Occasional Paper 53, Royal College of General Practitioners.

Forster DF and Mahadevan S (1981), Information sources for planning and evaluating adult psychiatric services, *Community Medicine*, 3: 160–8.

Fraser P, Robinson N and Ashley JSA (1983), The pattern of disease in hospital, 1968–1978, *Health Trends*, 15: 1–6.

Goldacre M, Simmons H, Henderson J and Gill LE (1988), Trends in episode based and person based rates of admission to hospital in the Oxford record linkage study area, *British Medical Journal*, 296: 583–5.

Goldacre MJ, Ferguson JA, Kettlewell MGW (1993), Profiles of workload in general surgery from linked hospital statistics, *British Journal of Surgery*, 80: 1073–1077.

Goldacre MJ, Ferguson J, Bulstrode C (1994), Workload in trauma and orthopaedic surgery: use of linked statistics to profile a specialty, *Health Services Management Research*, 8: 55–63.

GRO (1958), *Morbidity statistics from general practice, 1955–6 (vols I–III)*, Studies on Medical and Population Subjects 14, London: HMSO,

Hedley AJ, Scott AM, Deans Weir R, Crooks J (1970), Computer-assisted follow-up register for the North-east of Scotland, *British Medical Journal*, 1: 556–8.

Hollowell J (1994), *General Practice Research Database (GPRD) – Scope and quality of data*, OPCS report (unpublished).

Howitt AJ and Cheales NA (1993), Diabetes registers: a grassroots approach, *British Medical Journal*, 307: 1046–8.

Hyndman SJ, Williams DRR, Merrill SL, Lipscombe JM and Palmer CR (1994), Rates of admission to hospital for asthma, *British Medical Journal*, 308: 1596–600.

Kiseley, Gater and Goldberg (1995), *Mental illness in general health care*, In Ustun TB, Sartorius N, Geneva: WHO.

LAIA (1993), *Seasonal Variations in Asthma*, Factsheet 93/4, Lung and Asthma Information Agency, Department of Public Health Sciences, St Georges Hospital Medical School, Cranmer Terrace, London SW1.

McCormick A, Fleming D, Charlton J (1995), *Morbidity Statistics from General Practice: fourth national study, 1992–92*, Series MB5 no. 3, London: HMSO.

McPherson K, Coleman D (1988), Chapter 11, Health, pp.398–461: In *British Social Trends since 1900* (ed AH Halsey), London: McMillan Press,

Meltzer H, Gill B, Petticrew M, Hinds K (1995), *OPCS Surveys of Psychiatric Morbidity in Great Britain, Report 1: The prevalence of psychiatric morbidity among adults living in private households*, London: HMSO.

Murray JE and Barnes BA (1971), Organ transplant registry, *Journal of the American Medical Association*, 217: 1546.

Newton J and Goldacre M (1993), Multiple hospital admissions to a calendar year, *Journal of Public Health Medicine*, 15: 249–254.

Nightingale F (1863), *Notes on Hospitals*, 3rd edn, London: Longman Green, Longman, Roberts and Green.

OHE Compendium of Health Statistics (1992), 8th edn, Office of Health Economics, 12 Whitehall London SW1A 2DY.

OPCS (1995), *Health Survey for England 1993* London: HMSO.

Paterson JG (1988), Surveillance systems from hospital data, In *Surveillance in Health and Disease* (eds. WJ Eylenbosch, ND Noah), pp.49–61, Oxford: Oxford University Press.

RCGP, OPCS and DH (1974), *Morbidity Statistics from General Practice: Second National Study, 1970–71*, Studies on Medical and Population Subjects 26, London: HMSO.

RCGP, OPCS and DH (1979), *Morbidity Statistics from General Practice, 1971–72: Second National Study*, Studies on Medical and Population Subjects 36, London: HMSO.

RCGP, OPCS and DH (1982), *Morbidity Statistics from General Practice, 1970–71: Socio-economic Analysis*, Studies on Medical and Population Subjects 46, London: HMSO.

RCGP, OPCS and DH (1986), *Morbidity Statistics from General Practice: Third National Study, 1981–82*, Series MB5 no. 1, London: HMSO.

RCGP, OPCS and DH (1990), *Morbidity Statistics from General Practice: Third National Study: Socioeconomic Analysis 1981–82*, Series MB5 no. 2, London: HMSO.

Ross AM, Fleming DM (1994), Incidence of allergic rhinitis in general practice, 1981–-2, *British Medical Journal*, 308: 897–900.

Sowden AJ, Sheldon TA and Alberti, G (1995), Shared care in diabetes, *British Medical Journal*, 310: 142–3.

Spear BE and Gould CA (1937), Mechanical tabulation of hospital records, *Proceedings of the Royal Society of Medicine*, XXX(1): 633–44.

Statistical Society (1842), Report of the committee on hospital statistics, *Journal of the Statistical Society*, 5: 168–76.

Statistical Society (1844), Second report of the committee on hospital statistics, *Journal of the Statistical Society*, 7: 214–31.

Statistical Society (1862), Statistics of the general hospitals of London, 1861, *Journal of the Statistical Society*, 25: 384–8.

Statistical Society (1866), Statistics of metropolitan and provincial general hospitals for 1865, *Journal of the Statistical Society*, 29: 596–605.

Steering Group on Health Services Information (1982a), *Converting Data into Information*, London: King's Fund.

Steering Group on Health Services Information (1982b), *First Report to the Secretary of State* (Chairman E Korner), London: HMSO.

Stiller CA (1994), Population based survival rates for childhood cancer in Britain, 1980–91, *British Medical Journal*, 309: 1612–16.

Strachan DP and Anderson HR (1992), Trends in hospital admission rates for asthma in children, *British Medical Journal*, 304: 819–20.

Waterhouse J, Muir C, Correa P and Powell J (1976), *Cancer Incidence in Five Continents* vol.III, p.456, IARC Scientific Publications no. 15, Lyon: International Agency for Research on Cancer.

Weddell JM (1973), Registers and registries: a review, *International Journal of Epidemiology*, 2: 221–8.

Wood J (1990), A review of diabetes care initiatives in primary care settings, *Health Trends*, 22: 39–43.

Chapter 6 Socio-economic and demographic trends

Atkinson AB and Harrison AJ (1978), *Distribution of Personal Wealth in Britain*, Cambridge: Cambridge University Press.

Beveridge WH (1924), *Insurance for All the Everything*, London: Daily News.

Beveridge WH (1943), *The Pillars of Security*, London: Allen & Unwin.

Bowley AL (1900), *Wages in the United Kingdom in the Nineteenth Century*, Cambridge: Cambridge University Press.

Boyd Orr J (1936), *Food Health and Income*, London: Methuen.

Burnett J (1989), *Plenty and Want: A Social History of Diet in England from 1815 to the Present Day*.

Calder A (1969), *The People's War: Britain 1939–1945*, London: Panther.

Carr-Saunders AM, Caradog Jones D and Moser CA (1958), *A Survey of Social Conditions in England and Wales*, Oxford: Clarendon.

Central Statistical Office (1990), *Social Trends*: no. 20, London: HMSO.

Chadwick (1842), *Report on the Sanitary Condition of the Labouring Population of Great Britain*, Edinburgh: Edinburgh University Press (Reprinted 1965).

Clarke JS (1943), *Beveridge on Beveridge: Recent speeches of Sir William Beveridge KCB*, London: Social Security League.

Coates K and Silburn R (1970), *Poverty: the Forgotten Englishman*, London: Penguin.

Cobbett W (1830), *Rural Rides*.

Coleman D and Salt J (1992), *The British Population: Patterns Trends and Processes*, Oxford: Oxford University Press.

Central Statistical Office (1995), *Households Below Averge Income: a Statistical Analysis*, London: HMSO.

Crowther MA (1981), *The Workhouse System*, London: Methuen.

Davey Smith G (1996), Income inequality and mortality: why are they related?, *British Medical Journal*, 312: 987–988.

Dingle AE (1972), Drink and working class living standards in Britain 1870–1914, *Economic History Review*, 25: 608–622.

Filakti H and Fox AJ (1995), Differences in mortality by housing tenure and by car access from the OPCS Longitudinal Study, *Population Trends*, 81: 27–30.

Flinn MW (ed.) (1965), *Report on the Sanitary Condition of the Labouring Population of Great Britain*, edited and with an introduction by MW Flinn, Edinburgh: Edinburgh University Press.

Frazer WM (1950), *A History of English Public Health*, London: Balliere Tindall and Cox.

Gilbert BB (1970), *British Social Policy 1914–1939*, London: Batsford.

Goldthorpe JH, Lockwood D, Bechhofer F and Platt J (1969), *The Affluent Worker in the Class Structure*, Cambridge: Cambridge University Press.

Goodman A and Webb S (1995), *The Distribution of UK Household Expenditure 1979-1992*, London: Institute for Fiscal Studies.

Gwatkin DR (1980), Indications of change in developing country mortality: the end of an era?, *Population and Development Review*, 6(4): 615–644.

Hall PH, Land R, Parker A and Webb (1975), *Change Choice and Conflict in Social Policy*. London: Heinemann.

Hansluwka H (1975), Health, population, and socioeconomic development. In *Population Growth and Development in the Third World* (ed. L.Tabah), vol. 1, pp.191–250, Belgium: Ordina Edition, Dolhain.

Harris B (1993), The demographic impact of the first world war: an anthropometric perspective, *Social History of Medicine*, 6: 343–366.

Hewetson J (1946), *Ill-health, Poverty and the State*, London: Freedom Press.

Hutton W (1995), *The State We're In*, London: Jonathan Cape.

Judge K (1995), Income distribution and life expectancy: a critical appraisal, *British Medical Journal*, 311: 1282–4.

Kearns G (1988), The urban penalty and the population history of England. In *Society, Health and Population during the Demographic Transition* (eds A Brandstrom and L-G Tedebran), Stockholm: Almqvist and Wiksell.

Kearns (1989), Zivilis or Hygeia: Urban public health and the epidemiological transition. In *The Rise and Fall of Great Cities* (ed. R. Lawton), London: Bellhaven.

Kennedy BP, Kawachi I, Prothrow-Stith D (1996), Income distribution and mortality: cross sectional ecological study using the Robin Hood index in the United States, *British Medical Journal*, 312: 1004–7.

Le Gros Clerk F and Titmuss RM (1939), *Our Food Problem*, London: Penguin.

Leete R and Fox J (1977), Registrar General's social classes: origins and uses, *Population Trends*, no.8.

Lesthaeghe R (1983), A century of demographic and cultural change in Western Europe: an explanation of underlying dimensions, *Population and Development Review*, 9(3): 411–35.

Logan WPD (1949), Fog and mortality, *Lancet*, p.73.

Logan WPD (1953), Mortality in the London fog incident, *Lancet*, p.336.

McCarron PG, Davey Smith G and Womersley J (1994), Deprivation and mortality in Glasgow, changes from 1980 to 1992, *British Medical Journal*, 309: 1481–2.

McKeown T (1976), *The Modern Rise of Population*, London: Edward Arnold.

McKeown T and Lowe CR (1966), *An Introduction to Social Medicine*, Oxford: Blackwell.

McKeown T (1979), *The Role of Medicine*, Oxford: Blackwell.

McLoone P and Boddy A (1994), Deprivation and mortality in Scotland, 1981 and 1991, *British Medical Journal*, 309: 1465–70.

Millward R and Sheard S (1995), The urban fiscal problem, 1870–1914: government expenditure and finance in England and Wales, *Economic History Review*, XLVII: 501–535.

Mitchell BR and Deane P (1962), *Abstract of British Historical Statistics*, Cambridge: Cambridge University Press.

Nickell S and Bell B (1995), The collapse in demand for the unskilled and unemployment across the OECD, *Oxford Review of Economic Policy*, 11: 40-62.

Notestein F (1953), *Economics of population change*, Eighth International Conference of Agricultural Economists, 1952, London: Oxford University Press.

Oddy DJ (1970), Working class diets in nineteenth century Britain, *Economic History Review*, 23: 314–322.

Phelps-Brown EH and Browne MH (1968), *A Century of Pay*, London: St Martin's.

Phillimore P and Beattie A (1994), *Health and Inequality: The Northern Region 1981–1991*, Department of Social Policy, University of Newcastle upon Tyne.

Phillimore P, Townsend P, Beattie A (1994), Widening inequality of health in northern England 1981–1991, *British Medical Journal*, 308: 1125–8.

Porter R (1987), *Disease, Medicine and Society in England 1550–1860*, London: Macmillan.

Rodgers GB (1979), Income and inequality as determinants of mortality: an international cross-section analysis, *Population Studies*, 33: 343–352.

Rose G and Marmot MG (1981), Social class and coronary heart disease, *Br Heart J*, 45: 13–19.

Rowntree BS (1901), *Poverty*, London.

Rowntree BS and Lavers GR (1951), *English Life and Leisure*, London: Longmans.

Ruzica LT and Hansluwka H (1982), Mortality transition in South and East Asia: technology confronts poverty, *Population and Development Review*, 8(3): 567–588.

Sheridan D (1990), *Wartime Women*, London: Heinemann.

Smith FB (1979), *The People's Health*, London: Croom Helm.

Stevenson J (1984), *British Society 1914-45*, London: Penguin.

Szreter S (1988), The importance of social intervention in Britain's mortality decline 1850–1914: a re-interpretation of the role of public health, *Social History of Medicine Journal*, 1: 1–37.

Taylor AJP (1945), *English History 1914–1945*, Oxford: Oxford University Press.

Townsend P (1979), *Poverty in the United Kingdom*, London: Penguin.

Variations Sub-Group of the Chief Medical Officer's Health of the Nation Working Group (1995), *Variations in Health. What can the Department of Health and the NHS do?* London: Department of Health.

Vernon HM (1936), *Preventive Methods for Improving National Health*, British Association for Labour Legislation.

Watt CM (1996), All together now: why social deprivation matters to everyone, *British Medical Journal*, 312: 1026–29.

Webb S and Webb B (1920), *The History of Trade Unionism*, 2nd edn, London: Longmans.

Webb S and Webb B (1929), English Local Government, vols 8–9 *English Poor Law History Part II The Last Hundred Years*, London: Cass.

Webster C (1985), Health, welfare and unemployment during the depression, *Past and Present*, 109: 204–30.

Wilkinson RG (1992), Income distribution and life expectancy, *British Medical Journal*, 304: 165–8.

Wilkinson RG (1994), The epidemiological transition: from material scarcity to social disadvantage?, *Daedalus*, 123: 61–77.

ibid (1995), Commentary: a reply to Ken Judge: mistaken criticisms ignore overwhelming evidence, *British Medical Journal*, 311: 1285–7.

Wilson E (1977), *Women and the Welfare State*, London: Tavistock.

Winter J (1976), Some aspects of the demographic consequences of the first world war in Britain, *Population Studies*, 30: 539–52.

Wood GH (1909), Real wages and the standard of comfort since 1850, *Journal of Royal Statistical Society*, 72: 91–103.

Woods RI (1987), Approaches to the fertility transition in Victorian England: models and patterns, *Population Studies*, 18: 27–54

Woodward M, Shewry M, Smith WC and Tunstall Pedoe H (1990), Coronary heart disease and socioeconomic factors in Edinburgh and North Glasgow, *The Statistician*, 39: 319–29.

Wrigley EA and Schofield RS (1981), *The Population History of England 1541–1871*, London: Edward Arnold.

Zweig F (1949), *Labour, Life and Poverty*, London: Gollancz.

Chapter 7 Trends in diet 1841-1994

Accum F (1920), *A Treatise on Adulterations of Food, and Culinary Poisons*.

Acheson KJ, Campbell IT, Edholm OG, Miller DS, Stock M (1990), Measurement of food and energy intake in man – an evaluation of some techniques, *American Journal of Clinical Nutrition*, 33: 1147.

Austoker Joan (1994), Diet and Cancer, *BMJ*, 308:1610–4.

Barker DJP (1994), *Mothers, Babies and Disease in Later Life*, London: BMJ Publishing Group.

Bennett N, Dodd T, Flatley J, Freeth S, Bolling K, (1995), *The Health Survey for England 1993*) London: HMSO.

Booth C (1889), *Life and Labour of the People in London*, First series: poverty.

Booth C (1902), *Life and Labour of the People in London*, Third series.

Bosanquet SR (1841), *The Rights of the Poor and Christian Almsgiving vindicated*.

Bowley AL (1985), Changes in average wages (nominal and real) in the UK between 1860 and 1891, *Journal of the Royal Statistical Society*, LVIII.

Bray GA (1985), Obesity: definitions, diagnosis and disadvantages, *Medical Journal of Australia*, 142: S2.

British Association for the Advancement of Science (1881), *Report of the Committee on the Present Appropriation of Wages etc*, 276 et seq.

British Medical Association's Committee on Nutrition (1950), in Ministry of Food (1952) *Domestic Food Consumption and Expenditure, 1950* p.111. London: HMSO.

Burkitt DP and Trowell HC (eds) (1975), *Refined Carbohydrate Foods and Disease: some Implications of Dietary Fibre*, New York: Academic Press.

Burnett J (1989), *Plenty and Want – a Social History of Diet in England from 1815 to the Present Day*, 3rd edn, London: Routledge.

Buss David H (1988), Is the British diet improving? *Proceedings of the Nutrition Society*, 47: 295–306.

Buss David H (1993), The British diet since the end of food rationing. In *Food, Diet and Economic Change Past and Present* (eds Geissler C and Oddy DJ), Leicester University Press.

Caird, J (1880), *The Landed Interest and the Supply of Food*.

Carnegie (1951), in *The Urban Working – Class Diet 1940 to 1949: First report of the National Food Survey Committee*, Ministry of Food, p.13, London: HMSO.

Chandra RK (1983), Nutrition, Immunity and Infection: Present Knowledge and Future Directions, *Lancet* (i) 688.

Chadwick E (1842), *Report on the Sanitary Condition of the Labouring Population by the Poor Law Commissioners*.

Cobbett W (1830), *Rural Rides*.

Crawford W and Broadley H (1938), *The People's Food*.

Cuckfield Rural District Council: *Annual Report of the Medical Officer of Health for the year 1936 by William Stott*, 5 and 10–12.

Davies D (1795), *The Case of Labourers in Husbandary*.

Department of Health and Social Security (1975), *A Nutrition Survey of Pre-School Children in 1967–68* Report on Health and Social Subjects no. 10, London: HMSO .

Department of Health and Social Security (1979), *Recommended Daily Amounts of Food Energy and Nutrients for Groups of People in the United Kingdom*, Report on Health and Social Subjects no. 15, London: HMSO.

Department of Health and Social Security (1984), *Diet and Cardiovascular Disease*, Report on Health and Social Subjects no. 28, London: HMSO.

Department of Health (1989), *Dietary Sugars and Human Disease*, Report on Health and Social Subjects no. 37, London: HMSO.

Department of Health (1991), *The Fortification of Yellow Fats with Vitamins A and D*, Report on Health and Social Subjects no. 40, London: HMSO.

Department of Health (1991a), *Dietary Reference Values for Food Energy and Nutrients for the United Kingdom*, Report on Health and Social Subjects no.41, London: HMSO.

Department of Health (1992), *The Health of the Nation: a Strategy for Health in England*, London: HMSO.

Department of Health (1994), *Weaning and the Weaning Diet*, Report on Health and Social Subjects no. 45, London: HMSO.

Department of Health (1994a), *Nutritional Aspects of Cardiovascular Disease, Report of the Cardiovascular Review Group Committee on Medical Aspects of Food Policy*. Report on Health and Social Subjects no. 46, London: HMSO.

Department of Health (1995), *Fit for the Future, Second progress report on the Health of the Nation*, Department of Health.

Dobson B, Beardsworth A, Keil T, Walker R (1994), *Diet, Choice and Poverty*, London: Family Policy Studies Centre.

Dowler Elizabeth (1995), *Factors affecting Nutrient Intake and Dietary Adequacy in Lone Parent Households*, London School of Tropical Hygiene.

Drummond JC and Wilbraham A (1957), *The Englishman's Food. A history of five centuries of English diet*.

Eveleth PB and Tanner JM (1990), *Worldwide Variation in Human Growth*, Cambridge: Cambridge University Press.

Falkner F and Tanner JM (1986), *Human Growth*, 3 vols., 2nd edn, New York: Plenum.

Fall CHD, Osmond C, Barker DJP, Clark PMS, Hales CN, Stirling Y, Meade TW (1995), Fetal and infant growth and cardiovascular risk factors in women, *BMJ*, 310: 428–32.

Floud R, Wachter K and Gregory A (1990), *Height, Health and History: Nutritional Status in the United Kingdom, 1750–1980*, Cambridge studies in population, economy and society in past time, no.9, Cambridge University Press.

Floud R (1991), Medicine and the decline of mortality: indicators of nutritional status. In *Decline in Mortality in Europe* (eds Schofield R, Raher D, Bedeau U) pp.146–157, Oxford: Clarenden Press.

Fogel RW (1986), Nutrition and the decline in mortality since 1700: some preliminary findings in Engerman SL and Gallman RE (eds.)

Foster K, Jackson B, Thomas M, Hunter P, Bennett N (1995), *General Household Survey 1993*, London: HMSO.

Foster JM, Chinn S and Rona RJ (1983), The relation of the height of primary school children to population density, *International Journal of Epidemiology*, vol. 12, no. 2: 199–204, Oxford University Press.

Flux A (1930), *Journal of the Royal Statistical Society*, 93: 538.

Friedman CI, Kim MH (1985), Obesity and its effect on reproductive function, *Clinical Obstetrics and Gynaecology*, 28: 645.

Gale CR, Martyn CN, Winter PD, Cooper C (1995), Vitamin C and risk of death from stroke and coronary heart disease in cohort of elderly people, *BMJ*, 310: 1563–6.

Garfinkel L (1985), Overweight and cancer, *Annals of Internal Medicine*, 103: 1034.

Garrow JS and Webster J (1985), Quetlet's Index (W/H2) as a measure of fatness, *International Journal of Obesity*, 9: 147.

Garrow JS (1991), Nutrition. In *Oxford Textbook of Public Health*, Oxford: OUP.

Gregory J, Foster K, Tyler H, Wiseman M (1990), *The Dietary and Nutritional Survey of British Adults*, London: HMSO.

Gregory J, Collins D, Davies P, Hughes J, Clarke P (1995), *National Diet and Nutrition Survey: children aged 1 1/2 to 4 1/2 years*, vol.1, London: HMSO.

Halsey AH (1987), Social trends since World War II, *Social Trends* vol. 17, p.11, London: HMSO, Central Statistical Office.

Hassall AH (1855), *Food and its Adulterations: comprising the reports of the Analytical Sanitary Commission of 'The Lancet' for the years 1851 to 1854 inclusive*, 278 et seq.

Herbert SM (1939), *Britain's Health*, prepared on the basis of the Report on the British Health Services by PEP, 171.

HMSO (1946), *How Britain was fed in Wartime, Food Control, 1939–1945*.

HMSO (1946), *The State of the Public Health during Six Years of War*.

Hobsbawm EJ (1975), The British standard of living 1790–1850. In *The Standard of Living in Britain in the Industrial Revolution* (ed Arthur J Tylor), pp.69–71.

Hubert HB (1984), The nature of the relationship between obesity and cardiovascular disease, *International Journal of Cardiology* , 6: 268.

Jones GS (1976), *Outcast London*, 127.

Keys A, Fidanza F, Karvonen MJ, Kimura N, Taylor HL (1972), Indices of relative weight and obesity, *Journal Chronic Dis*, 25: 329–43.

Khaw KT and Woodhouse P (1995), Interrelation of vitamin C, infection, haemostatic factors and cardiovascular disease, *BMJ*, 310: 1559–63.

Knight I (1984), *The Heights and Weights of Adults in Great Britain*, London: HMSO.

Kuskowska-Wolk A, Bergström (1993), Trends in body mass index and prevalence of obesity in Swedish men 1980–89, *Journal of Epidemiology and Community Health*, 47: 103–8

Levi L (1885), *Wages and Earnings of the Working Classes*, a report to Sir Arthur Bass, MP, 12.

Lopez (1986), Anthropometric nutritional evaluation of the hospitalised patient, *Bol. Med, Infant Mex* 43 (4): 233–6.

Lunn PG (1991), Nutrition, Immunity and Infection. In *The Decline of Mortality in Europe* (eds Schofield R, Reher D, Bideau), New York: Oxford University Press.

Marmot MG, Shipley MJ and Rose G (1984), Inequalities in death-specific explanations of a general pattern?, *Lancet*, 8384: 1003–6.

McGonigle GCM and Kirby J (1936), *Poverty and Public Health*.

McKenzie JC (1962), The composition and nutritional value of diets in Manchester and Dukinfield in 1841, Transactions of Lancashire and Cheshire Antiquarian Society, 72, 123–40. In J. Burnett (1989) *Plenty and Want: a social history of food diet in England from 1815 to the present day*, London: Routledge.

McKeown T (1976), *The role of Medicine – Dream, Mirage or Nemesis*, London: Nuffield Provincial Hospitals Trust.

McKeown T (1976), *The Modern Rise of Population*.

Ministry of Food (1951), *The Urban Working – Class Diet 1940 to 1949: First report of the National Food Survey Committee*, London: HMSO.

Ministry of Agriculture Fisheries and Food (1990), *Household Food Consumption and Expenditure 1989*, Annual reports of the National Food Survey Committee, London: HMSO.

Ministry of Agriculture Fisheries and Food (1991), *Household Food Consumption and Expenditure 1990*. Annual reports of the National Food Survey Committee, London: HMSO.

Ministry of Agriculture Fisheries and Food (1994), *Household Food Consumption and Expenditure 1993*. Annual reports of the National Food Survey Committee, London: HMSO.

Ministry of Agriculture Fisheries and Food (1992), *Fifty Years of the National Food Survey 1940–1990*, London: HMSO.

Money LC (1911), *Riches and Poverty*.

National Dairy Council Information Service (1939), Information Booklet no 2.

National Institutes of Health Consensus Development Panel (1985), Health Implications of Obesity, *Annals of Internal Medicine,* 103: 1073.

National Advisory Committee on Nutrition Education (1983), *A Discussion Paper on Proposals for Nutrition Guidelines for Health Education in Britain*, London: Health Education Council.

Nield W (1841), Comparative statement of the income and expenditure of certain families of the working classes in Manchester and Dukinfield in the years 1836 and 1841, *Journal of the Statistical Society of London* IV.

Oddy DJ (1970), Working-class diets in nineteenth-century Britain. In *Economic History Review* (2nd series) XXIII (1,2,3): 319.

Oddy DJ (1977), Discussion of `changing patterns of food consumption in the United Kingdom' by TC Barker. In *Diet of Man: Needs and wants* (ed. John Yudkin), p.181.

Oddy DJ (1981), Diet in Britain during industrialisation, paper at Leyden Colloquim The standard of living in Western Europe (September), p.15.

Oddy DJ (1982), The health of the people. In *Population and Society in Britain, 1850–1980* (eds Barker T and Drake M), p.127.

Orr JB (1936), *Food, Health and Income*. London: Macmillan.

Paneth N and Susser M (1995), Early origin of coronary heart disease (the "Barker hypothesis"), *BMJ*, 310: 411–2.

Powander MC (1977), Changes in body balance of nitrogen and other key nutrients: description and underlying mechanisms, *American Journal of Clinical Nutrition*, 30:1254.

Prentice AM, Black AE, Coward WA, et al (1986), High levels of energy expenditure in obese women, *British Medical Journal*, 292: 983.

Prentice Andrew M and Jebb Susan A (1995), Obesity in Britain: Gluttony or Sloth, *British Medical Journal*, 311: 437–9.

Rea JN (1971), Social and economic influences on the growth of pre-school children in Lagos, *Human Biology*, 43: 46–63.

Report (1899) on the Aged Deserving Poor, 1899.

Report of the Commissioners on Children's, young person's and women's employment in agriculture, 1867–70.

Report (1904) on Physical Deterioration, 1904.

Reports (1905–9) of the Royal Commission on the Poor Law 1905–9.

Report of the Sumner Committee on the Working Classes' Cost of Living (1918), Cd 8980, para 51.

Rona RJ (in press), Monitoring nutritional status in England and Scotland, In Essays on Auxology presented to James Mourilyon Tanner.

Rosenbaum S (1988), 100 years of heights and weights, *Journal of the Royal Statistical Society*, in Floud *et al* (1990), *Height, health and history: nutritional status in the United Kingdom, 1750–1980* (Cambridge studies in population, economy and society in past time; 9) Cambridge University Press.

Rowntree J and Sherwell A (1900), *The Temperance Problem and Social Reform.*

Rowntree BS (1901), *Poverty: A Study of Town Life*, London: MacMillan.

Rowntree BS and Kendall (1913), *How the Labourer Lives. A Study of the Rural Labour Problem.*

Rowntree BS (1937), *The Human Needs of Labour.*

Rowntree BS (1941), *Poverty and Progress.* Longmans, Green and Co. Ltd

Saarinen UM and Kajosaari M (1995), Breastfeeding as prophylax against atopic disease: prospective follow-up until 17 years old, *Lancet*, 346: 1065–69.

Salaman RN (1949), *The history and social influence of the potato*, Cambridge.

Scrimshaw NS (1977), Effect of Infection on Nutrient Requirements, *American Journal of Clinical Nutrition*, 30: 15362.

Scrimshaw NS (1981), Significance of the interations of nutrition and infection in children. In *Textbook of Paediatric Nutrition* (ed. Suskind RM), p.229. New York.

Smith E (1864), *Practical Dietary for Families, Schools and Labouring Classes*, 202–3.

Smith C (1940), *Britain's Food Supplies in Peace and War: a survey prepared for the Fabian Society by Charles Smith.*

Somerville A (1843), *A Letter to the Farmers of England on the Relationship of Manufactures and Agriculture by One who has Whistled at the Plough.*

Statistical Society (1904), Production and consumption of meat and milk, Second report from the committee appointed to inquire into the statistics available as a basis of estimating the production and consumption of meat and milk in the United Kingdom, *Journal of the Statistical Society* LXVIII: 368 et seq.

Stein Z, Susser M, Saenger G, Marolla F (1975), *Famine and Human Development: the Dutch Winter Hunger of 1944–1945*, New York: Oxford University Press.

Stephen AM and Sieber GM (1994), Trends in individual fat consumption in the UK, 1900–1985, *British Journal of Nutrition*, 71, 775–88.

Strachan DP, Cox BD, Erzinclioglu SW, Walters DE, Whichelow MJ (1991), Ventilatory function and winter fresh fruit consumption in a random sample of British adults, *Thorax*, 46: 624–9.

Thompson EP (1980), *The Making of the English Working Class*, Harmondsworth: Pelican, p.336.

Trichopoulou A, Kouris-Blazos A, Wahlqvist ML, Gnardellis C, Lagiou P, Polychronopoulos E, Vassilakou T, Lipworth L (1995), Diet and overall survival in elderly people, *BMJ*, 311: 1457–60.

Truswell AS (1983), Recommended dietary intakes around the world *Nutrition Abstracts and Reviews*, 53: 939 and 1075.

Waaler HTH (1984), *Height, Weight and Mortality: The Norwegian Experience'* Oslo: Gruppe for Helsetjenesteforskning.

Wenlock RW (1992), Trace element requirements and DRVs' *Food Chemistry*, 43: 225–231 Analytical Methods Section.

White A, Nicolaas G, Foster K, Browne F, Carey S (1993), *Health Survey for England 1991*, London: HMSO.

Williams EF (1976), The development of the meat industry. In *The Making of the Modern British Diet* (eds Derek J Oddy and Derek S Miller) p.50.

Winter JM (1977), The impact of the First World War on civilian health in Britain, *Economic History Review*, (2nd Series) XXX (3), 499.

Wrigley EA and Schofield RS (1989), *The Population History of England 1541–1871*, 2nd edn, Cambridge pp.228–48.

Chapter 8 Trends in alcohol and illicit drug-related diseases

Anderson K, Plant MA, Baillie R, Nevison C, Plant ML, Ritson B (1995), *Alcohol, tobacco, illicit drug use and sex education amongst teenagers*, Edinburgh: Alcohol Research Group (Report to the Western Isles Health Board).

Anderson K and Plant MA (1996), Abstaining and carousing: substance use among adolescents in the Western Isles of Scotland, *Drug Alc Dep*, 41: 181-96.

Bagnall G (1991), *Educating young drinkers*, London: Tavistock.

Berridge V(1979), Opiate use and legislative control: A nineteenth century case study, *Soc Sci Med*, 13A: 351-63.

Berridge V (ed.) (1990), *Drugs research and policy in Britain*, Aldershot: Avebury.

Berridge V and Edwards G (1979), *Opium and the people*, London: Allen Lane .

Binnie HL and Murdock G (1969), *The attitudes to drugs and drug takers of students of the university and colleges of further education in an English Midland city.* University of Leicester, Vaughan Papers, no. 14, pp.1-29.

Breeze E (1989), *Women and drinking*, London: HMSO.

Brewers' Society (1995), *Statistical handbook.* London: Brewers' Society.

Chambers G and Tombs J (eds) (1984), *The British crime survey, Scotland: A Scottish research study*, Edinburgh: HMSO.

Carpenter WB (1850), *On the use and abuse of alcoholic liquors in health and disease*, Philadelphia: Lea and Blanchard.

Christie M (1993), Drunken drivers and pedestrians. Paper presented at Addictions Forum conference: Alcohol: Problems and Solutions, Glasgow, October 13.

Coggans N, Shewan D, Henderson M, Davies JB, O'Hagen F, (1989) *National evaluation of drug education in Scotland,* Centre for Occupational and Health Psychology, University of Strathclyde.

Collins JJ Jr (ed.) (1982), *Drinking and crime*, London: Tavistock.

Crawford A and Plant MA (1986), Regional variations in alcohol dependence rates: A conundrum. *Q J Soc Affairs*, 2: 139-49.

Department of Transport (1990a), *Blood alcohol levels in fatalities in Great Britain 1988*, Transport and Road Research Laboratory.

Department of Transport (1990b), *Accident fact sheet 3/90*. London, Department of Transport).

Doll R, Peto R, Hall E, Wheatley K, Gray R (1994), Mortality in relation to consumption of alcohol: 13 years' observations on male British doctors, *British Medical Journal*, 309: 911-18.

Duffy JC and Plant MA (1986), Scotland's liquor licensing changes: an assessment. *British Medical Journal*, 292: 36-39.

Duffy JC and Sharples LD (1992), Alcohol and cancer risk. In *Alcohol and illness* (ed. Duffy JC), Edinburgh: University of Edinburgh Press, pp.64-127.

Edwards G (1971), *Unreason in an age of reason*, Edwin Stevens Lectures for the Laity, London: Royal Society of Medicine.

Edwards G, Anderson P, Babor TF, Casswell S, Ferrence R, Giesbrecht N, Godfrey C, Holder H, Lemmens P, Makela K, Midanik L, Norstrom T, Osterberg E, Romelsjo A, Room R, Simpura J, Skog O-J (1994), *Alcohol policy and the public good*, Oxford: Oxford University Press.

Edwards G and Busch C (eds) (1981), *Drug problems in Britain: A Review of Ten Years*, London: Academic Press.

Faculty of Public Health Medicine, Royal College of Physicians (1991), *Alcohol and the public health*, London: Macmillan.

Fossey E (1994), *Growing Up With Alcohol*, London: Tavistock.

Foster K, Wilmot A, Dobbs J(1990), *General Household Survey 1988*, London: HMSO.

Ghodse H (1994), Use of public health indicators of the extent and nature of drug problems during the 1970s and 1980s. In (*eds Strang J, Gossop M*), Oxford: Oxford Medical Publications, pp.66-78.

Giesbrecht N, Gonsalez R, Grant M, Osterberg E, Room R, Rootman I, Towle L (eds) (1989), *Drinking and Casualties: Accidents, Poisonings and Violence in an International Perspective*, London: Tavistock/Routledge.

Gronbaek M, Deis A, Sorensen TI, Becker U, Borsch-Johsen K, Muller C, Schnohr P, Jensen G (1994), Influence of sex, age, body mass index and smoking on alcohol intake and mortality, *British Medical Journal*, 308: 302-6.

Gronbaek M, Deis A, Sorensen TIA, Becker U, Schnohr P, Jensen G (1995), Mortality associated with moderate intakes of wine, beer, or spirits, *British Medical Journal*, 310: 1165-9.

Harrison B (1971), *Drink and the Victorians*. London: Faber & Faber.

Home Office (1979-96), *Statistics of drug addicts notified to the Home Office*, United Kingdom (annual reports), London: Home Office.

Home Office (1985), *Statistics of the misuse of drugs in the United Kingdom, supplementary tables 1984*, London: Home Office.

Home Office (1992), *Statistics of drug seizures and offenders dealt with, United Kingdom, 1991, area tables*, London: Home Office.

Home Office (1995), *Statistics of drug seizure and offenders dealt with, United Kingdom, 1994*, London: HMSO.

International Agency for Research on Cancer (1988), *Alcohol drinking*, Lyon: IARC.

Loretto W (1994), Youthful drinking in Northern Ireland and Scotland: Preliminary results from a comparative study, *Drugs: Education, Prevention and Policy*, 1: 143-51.

McKay AJ, Hawthorne VM, McCartney HN (1973), Drug-taking amongst medical students at Glasgow University, *British Medical Journal*, 1: 540-3.

Marsh A, Dobbs J, White A (1986), *Adolescent Drinking*, London: HMSO.

May C (1992), *Register of United Kingdom Alcohol Research 1991-1992*. London: Portman Group.

Miller P and Plant MA (1996), Drinking, smoking and illicit drug use among 15- and 16-year-olds in the UK, *British Medical Journal*, 313: 394-7.

Mott J (1989), Self-reported cannabis use in Great Britain in 1981. *Br J Addict*, 80: 30-43.

Mott J and Mirrlees-Black C (1995), *Self-reported drug misuse in England and Wales: Findings from the 1992 British Crime Survey*. Home Office, London: HMSO.

Noble B (1994), Deaths associated with the use of alcohol, drugs and volatile solvents, *Population Trends*, 76: 1-11.

NOP Market Research Ltd (1982), Survey conducted for the Daily Mail.

Parker H, Bakx K, Newcombe R (1988), *Living with heroin*, Milton Keynes: Open University Press.

Phillipson RV (ed.) (1970), *Drug addiction in Britain*, London: Robert Hale.

Pinot de Moira AC and Duffy JC (1994), Changes in licensing law in England and Wales and alcohol-related mortality. *Addict Res*, (in press).

Plant MA (1975), *Drug takers in an English town*, London: Tavistock.

Plant MA and Foster J (1991), Teenagers and alcohol: Results of a Scottish national survey, *Drug and Alcohol Dependence*, 28: 203-10.

Plant MA, Peck DF, Samuel E (1986), *Alcohol, drugs and school-leavers*, London: Tavistock.

Plant MA and Plant ML (1992), *Risk takers: alcohol, drugs, sex and youth*, London: Tavistock.

Plant M (1992), Alcohol and breast cancer: A review, *Int J Addict*, 27: 107-28.

Plant ML (1985), *Women, drinking and pregnancy*, London: Tavistock.

Plant ML (1996), *Women and alcohol*, London: Free Association Books.

Plant ML, Sullivan FM, Guerri C, Abel EL (1993), Alcohol and preg;nancy, In *Health issues related to alcohol consumption* (ed. Verschuren PM), Brussels: ILSI Press, pp.245-62.

Warner J (1992), 'North, south, male, female. Levels of alcohol consumption in late medieval Europe', Personal communication.

Pritchard C, Fielding M, Choudry N, Cox M, Diamond I (1986), Incidence of drug and solvent abuse in normal fourth and fifth year comprehensive school children - some socio-behavioural characteristics, *Br J Soc Work*, 16: 341-51.

Raab GM (1992), Alcohol and non-malignant disease, In *Alcohol and illness* (Duffy JC (ed.), Edinburgh: University of Edinburgh Press, pp.136-44.

Robertson JR (1987), *Heroin, AIDS and society*, London: Hodder & Stoughton.

Royal College of Psychiatrists (1986), *Alcohol: our favourite drug*, London: Tavistock.

Royal College of Physicians (1987), *A great and growing evil: the medical consequences of alcohol abuse*. London: Tavistock.

Sales J, Duffy J, Plant MA, Peck DF (1989), Alcohol consumption, cigarette sales and mortality in the United Kingdom: An analysis of the period 1970-1985, *Drug and Alcohol Dependence*, 24: 155-60.

Spring JA and Buss DH (1979), Three cultures of alcohol in Britain, In *Alcohol problems: reviews, research and commentaries* (ed. D Robinson), pp.22-30.

Strang J and Gossop M (eds) (1994), *Heroin Addiction and Drug Policy: The British System*, Oxford: Oxford University Press.

Strang J and Stimson GV (eds) (1990), *AIDS and Drug Misuse*, London: Tavistock/Routledge.

Taylor JC, Norman CL, Bland JM, Anderson HR, Ramsey JD (1995), *Trends in Deaths Associated with Abuse of Volatile Substances 1971-1991*, London: St George's Hospital Medical School, Report Number 6.

Trotter T (1813), *An essay, medical, philosophical and chemical on drunkenness, and its effects on the human body,* Boston, MA: Bradford and Read.

Verschuren PM (ed.) (1993), *Health issues related to alcohol consumption*, Brussels: ILSI Press.

Williams B, Chang K, Van Truong M, Saad F (1994), *International profile 1994: alcohol and drugs*, Toronto: WHO/Addiction Research Foundation.

Williams M (1986), The Thatcher generation, *New Society*, 21 February, 312-15.

Wilson G (1940), *Alcohol and the nation*, London: Nicholson and Watson.

Young J (1971), *The drug takers*. London: Paladin.

Chapter 9 Trends in mortality from smoking related diseases

Acheson ED and Gardner MJ (1979), *The Ill Effects of Asbestos on Health, Asbestos: Final Report of the Advisory Committee,* vol. 2, London: HMSO.

Barker DJP and Osmond C (1986), Childhood respiratory infection and adult chronic bronchitis in England and Wales, *British Medical Journal*, 293: 1271-75.

Bonser GM and Thomas GM (1959), Investigation of the validity of death certification of cancer of the lung in Leeds, *British Journal of Cancer*, 13: 1-12.

Breslow NE and Day N (1980), The analysis of case-control studies, *Statistical Methods in Cancer Research*, vol. 1, 227–33, IARC Scientific Publications, no.32, Lyon, France: IARC.

Brewers and Licensed Retailers Association (1994), *Statistical Handbook of Brewing Publications*, London: The Brewers and Licensed Retailers Association.

Cancer Research Campaign (1988), *Survival - England and Wales*, Factsheet 9.2, London: Cancer Research Campaign.

Case RAM, Hosker ME, McDonald DB and Pearson JT (1954), Tumours of the urinary bladder in workmen engaged in the manufacture and use of certain dyestuff intermediates in the District Chemical Industry, *British Journal of Industrial Medicine*, 11: 75-104.

Cederlöf R, Doll R, Fowler B, Friberg L, Nelson N and Vouk V (1978), Air pollution and cancer: risk assessment methodology and epidemiological evidence, *Environmental Health Perspectives*, 22: 1-12.

Davies JM, Somerville SM and Wallace DM (1976), Occupational bladder tumour cases identified during ten years' interviewing patients, *British Journal of Urology*, 48: 561-6.

Doll R and Peto R (1981), The causes of cancer: quantitative estimates of avoidable risks of cancer in the United States today, *Journal of the National Cancer Institute*, 66: 1191-308.

Doll R and Peto R (1976), Mortality in relation to smoking: 20 years' observations on male British doctors, *British Medical Journal*, 2: 1525-36.

Doll R, Forman D, La Vecchia C and Woutersen R (1993), Alcoholic beverages and cancers of the digestive tract and larynx. In *Health Issues related to Alcohol Consumption* (ed. PM Verschuren), pp.125–166, Washington: ILSI Press.

Doll R, Peto R, Wheatley K, Gray R and Sutherland I (1994), Mortality in relation to smoking: 40 years' observations on male British doctors, *British Medical Journal*, 309: 901–11.

Eriksson S (1964), Pulmonary emphysema and alpha-1-antitrypsin deficiency, *Acta Med Scand*, 175: 197-204.

Eriksson S (1965), Studies in alpha-1-antitrypsin efficiency, *Acta Med Scand*, 177, (suppl 432): 1-85.

Fletcher CM and Peto R (1977), The natural history of chronic airflow obstruction, *British Medical Journal*, 1: 1645-48.

Gunby JA, Darby SC, Miles JCH, Green BMR and Cox DR (1993), Factors affecting indoor radon concentrations in the United Kingdom, *Health Physics*, 64: 2-12.

Health Education Authority (1992), *The Smoking Epidemic: a Manifesto for Action in England*, London: Health Education Authority.

IARC (1974), *Some Aromatic Amines, Hydrazine and Related Substances, N-nitroso Compounds and Miscellaneous Alkylating Agents*, International Agency for Research on Cancer Monographs on the evaluation of the carcinogenic risk of chemicals to man, vol. 4, Lyon, France: IARC.

IARC (1982), *Some Industrial Chemicals and Dyestuffs*, International Agency for Research on Cancer Monographs on the evaluation of the carcinogenic risk of chemicals to humans, vol. 29, Lyon, France: IARC.

IARC (1986), *Tobacco Smoking*, International Agency for Research on Cancer Monographs on the evaluation of the carcinogenic risk of chemicals to humans, vol. 38, Lyon, France: IARC.

IARC (1987), *Overall Evaluations of Carcinogenicity: an Updating*, International Agency for Research on Cancer Monographs on the evaluation of carcinogenic risks to humans, vols. 1–42, Supplement 7, Lyon, France: IARC.

IARC (1990), Tomatis L (ed.), *Cancer: Causes, Occurrence and Control*, International Agency for Research on Cancer Scientific Publication no. 100, Lyon, France: IARC.

Parish S, Collins R, Peto R, Youngman L, Barton J, Jayne K, Clarke R, Appleby P, Lyon V, Cederholm-Williams S, Marshall J and Sleight P (1995), Cigarette tar yield and non-fatal myocardial infarction: 14,000 UK cases and 32,000 controls in the United Kingdom, The International Studies of Infarct Survival (ISIS) Collaborators, *British Medical Journal*, 311: 471–7.

Peto R, Lopez AD, Boreham J, Thun M and Heath C (1994), *Morbidity from Smoking in Developed Countries*, Oxford: Oxford University Press.

Sömmering ST (1795), *De morbis vasorum absorbentum corporis humani*, Frankfurt am Main: Vassentrapp and Wenner.

Sorsa M (1986), Experimental studies on the mutagenicity and related effects of low-tar are high-tar cigarettes in relation to smoker exposures. In *Tobacco* (eds Zaridze D and Peto R), International Agency for Research into Cancer Scientific Publications no. 74, pp.227–38, Lyon, France: IARC.

Stellman SD (1986), Influence of cigarette yield or risk of coronary heart disease and chronic obstructive lung disease. In *Tobacco* (eds Zaridze D and Peto R), International Agency for Research into Cancer Scientific Publications no. 74, pp.197–209, Lyon, France: IARC.

US Department of Health and Human Services (1979), *Smoking and health Report of the Surgeon General*, Washington DC: US Government Briefing Office.

US Department of Health and Human Services (1989), *Reducing the Health Consequences of Smoking: 25 years of Progress, Report of the Surgeon General*, Maryland: US Department of Health and Human Services, Office on Smoking and Health.

Wald N, Doll R and Copeland G (1981), Trends in tar, nicotine, and carbon monoxide yields of UK cigarettes manufactured since 1934, *British Medical Journal*, 282: 703-5.

Wald N and Nicolaides-Bouman A (eds.) (1991), *UK Smoking Statistics*, 2nd edn., Oxford: Oxford University Press.

Waller R (1991), Field investigations of air, in: Holland WW, Detels R and Knox G (eds.), *Oxford Textbook of Public Health*, vol. 2, Methods of public health, Oxford: Oxford University Press.

Waterhouse JAH (1974), *Cancer Handbook of Epidemiology and Prognosis*, Edinburgh: Churchill Livingstone.

Withey CA, Papacosta AO, Swan AV, Fitzsimons BA, Ellard GA, Burney PGJ, Colley TRT and Holland WW (1992), Respiratory effects of lowering tar and nicotine levels of cigarettes smoked by young male middle tar smokers, *Journal of Epidemiology and Community Health*, 46: 281-5.

World Health Organisation (1948), *Manual of the International Statistical Classification of Diseases, Injuries, and Causes of Death, Sixth Revision*, Geneva: World Health Organisation.

World Health Organisation (1957), *Manual of the International Statistical Classification of Diseases, Injuries, and Causes of Death, Seventh revision*, Geneva: World Health Organisation.

World Health Organisation (1967), *Manual of the International Statistical Classification of Diseases, Injuries, and Causes of Death. Eighth Revision*, Geneva: World Health Organisation.

World Health Organisation (1977), *Manual of the International Statistical Classification of Diseases, Injuries, and Causes of Death. Ninth Revision*, Geneva: World Health Organisation.

Wynder EL, Bross IJ and Day E (1956), A study of environment factors in cancer of the larynx, *Cancer*, 9: 86-110.

Wynder EL, Hultberg S, Jacobsen E and Bross IJ (1957), Environmental factors in cancer of upper alimentary tract, *Cancer*, 10: 470-87.

Chapter 10 Housing-related disorders

Acheson D (1991), Health and housing: Annual Lecture, *J R S Health*, 56: 236–43.

Akerblom H (1987), Coronary heart disease and risk factors in circumpolar areas, Seventh International Congress on Circumpolar Health, June 8–12, Umea, Sweden, *Abstr Arctic Med Res*, 45/87: 1.

Allander E, Rosenqvist U (1975), The diagnostic process in outpatient endocrine care with special reference to screening, *Scand J Soc Med*, 3: 117–21.

Audit Commission (1989), *Housing the Homeless: The Local Authority Role, A report*, London: HMSO.

BABIE (1989), *Survey on the Standards in B & B Accommodation used by Local Authorities in London,* London Research Centre & Bed and Breakfast Information Exchange.

Balarajan R, Yuen P, Machin D (1987), Inequalities in health: changes in RHAs in the past decade, *British Medical Journal*, 294: 1561–4.

Barker D, Osmond C (1986), Infant mortality, childhood nutrition and ischaemic heart disease, *Lancet*, i: 1077–81.

Barker D, Coggon D, Osmond C, Wickham C (1990), Poor housing in childhood and high rates of stomach cancer in England and Wales, *Br J Cancer*, 61: 575–8.

Bastenier H, Klosterkoetter W, Large J (1975), *Environment and the quality of life: damage and annoyance caused by noise*, EUR 5398e, Brussels: Commission of the European Communities.

Blackman T, Evason E, Melaughs M, Woods R (1989), Housing and health: a case study of two areas in West Belfast, *J Soc Policy*, 18: 1–26.

Boardman B (1991), *Fuel poverty*, London: Bellhaven Press.

Boyer J (1986), Homelessness from a health visitor's viewpoint, *Health Visitor*, 59: 340.

Bradford Hill A (1965), The environment and disease: association or causation? *Proc R Soc Med*, 58: 295–300.

Bradwell AR, Carmalt M, Whitehead T (1974), Explaining the unexpected abnormal results of biochemical profile investigations, *Lancet*, i: 10714.

Brennan M and Lancashire R (1978), Association of childhood mortality with housing status and unemployment, *J Epidemiol Commun Health*, 32: 28–33.

Brett GZ and Benjamin B (1957), Housing and TB in a mass radiography survey, *Br J Prevent Soc Med*, 11: 7–9.

British Medical Journal (1980), Blows from the winter wind, Editorial, *British Medical Journal*, i: 137–8.

British Medical Journal (1987), Deprivation and ill health, Editorial, *British Medical Journal*, 294:1305

Britten N, Davies J, Colley J (1987), Early respiratory experience and subsequent cough and peak expiratory flow rate in 36 year old men and women, *British Medical Journal*, 294: 1317–19.

Brotherston Sir J (1976), Inequality: is it inevitable? The Galton Lecture, 1975. In *Equalities and inequalities in health* (eds Carter CO and Peel J), Proceedings of the 12th Annual Symposium of the Eugenics Society, London: Academic Press, pp.73–104.

Brown G and Harris T (1978), *Social Origins of Depressions: A Study of Psychiatric Disorder in Women*, London: Tavistock.

Bryder L (1988), *Below the Magic Mountain*, Oxford: Oxford University Press.

Buckland FE and Tyrell DAJ (1962), Loss of infectivity on drying various viruses, *Nature*, 195: 1063–4.

Bull G and Morton J (1978), Environment, temperature and death rates, *Age Ageing*, 7: 210–24.

Burge H (1989), Indoor air and infectious diseases, *Occupational Medicine State of the Art Reviews*, 4: 713–22.

Burnett J (1978), *A Social History of Housing 1815–1970,* David and Charles, London: Newton Abbott.

Burr ML, Mullins J, Merrett T, Stott N (1988), Indoor moulds and asthma, *J R Soc Health,* 108: 99–102.

Byrne D, Harrison SP, Keithley J, McCarthy P, (1986), *Housing and Health: The Relationship between Housing Conditions and the Health of Council Tenants*, London: Gower.

Carswell F and Thompson SJ (1987), Percutaneous sensitisation to house dust mite may occur naturally in eczema, *Int Arch Allergy Appl Immunol*, 82, 453–5.

Chadwick E (1842), *Report to Her Majesty's Principle Secretary of State for the Home Department from the Poor Law Commissioners on an Inquiry into the Sanitary Condition of the Labouring Population of Great Britain*.

Chandler SE, Chapman A, Hollington S (1984), Fire incidence, housing and social conditions – the urban situation, *Fire Prevention*, 172: 15–20.

City of Glasgow (1989), *House Conditions Survey*, Glasgow District Council, Lomond House.

Collins KJ (1986), Low indoor temperatures and morbidity in the elderly, *Age Ageing*, 15: 212–20.

Connelly J, Kellehe C, Morton S, St George D, Roderick P (1991), *Housing or Homelessness: a public health perspective,* London: The Faculty of Public Health Medicine of the Royal College of Physicians.

Conway J (1988), *Prescription for Poor Health, The Crisis for Homeless Families,* LFC, Maternity alliance, London: SHAC & Shelter

Coull BM, Beamer N, De Garmo P, Sexton G, North F, Knox R, Nordt F, Seaman GVF (1991), Chronic blood hyperviscosity in subjects with acute stroke, transient ischaemic attack and risk factors for stroke, *Stroke*, 22: 162–8.

Dales RE, Zwanenburg H, Burnett R, Franklin CA (1991a), Respiratory health effects of home dampness and moulds among Canadian children, *Am J Epidemiol*, 134: 196–203.

Dales RE, Burnett R, Zwanenburg HO (1991b), Adverse health effects among adults exposed to home dampness and moulds, *Am J Epidemiol*, 134: 505–10.

Department of the Environment (1991), *English House Conditions Survey; preliminary report on unfit dwellings,* London: HMSO.

Department of Trade and Industry (1989), *Home and Leisure Accident Research: Eleventh annual report home accident surveillance system,* London: DTI.

Dorward A, Collof MJ, MacKay N, McSharry C, Thomson NC (1988), Effect of house dust mite avoidance measures on adult atopic asthma, *Thorax*, 43: 98–102.

Douglas A and Rawles J (1989), *Excess Winter Mortality: the Cardiovascular Component, Paper presented at Meeting of the Scottish Society of Experimental Medicine*, 3rd November, Aberdeen.

Dunleavy P (1981), *Mass Housing in Britain*, Oxford: Oxford University Press.

ECAO (1982), *Air Quality Criteria for Oxides of Nitrogen: Environmental Criteria and Assessment Office*, North Carolina: US Environment Protection Agency.

Engels F (1892), *The Condition of the Working Class in England*, Institute of Marxist-Leninism, Moscow, London: Panther.

Fanning D (1967), Families in flats, *British Medical Journal*, iv: 382–6.

Fergusson R, Milne L, Crompton G (1984), Penicillium allergic alveolitis: faulty installation of central heating, *Thorax*, 39: 294–8.

Filakti H and Fox J (1995), Differences in mortality by housing tenure and by car access from the OPCS Longitudinal Study, *Population Trends*, 81: 27–30.

Flinn MW (1965), *Report on the Sanitary Conditions of the Labouring Population of Great Britain* by Edwin Chadwick, 1842, Edinburgh: Edinburgh University Press.

Ford J (1988), *The Indebted Society*, London: Routledge .

Forrest R and Gordon D (1993), *People and Places: A 1991 Census Atlas of England*, University of Bristol, School for Advanced Urban Studies.

Fox J and Goldblatt P (1982), Household Mortality from the OPCS longitudinal study, *Population Trends*, London: HMSO.

Frazer WM (1947), *Duncan of Liverpool,* London: Bailliere, Tindall & Cox.

Garnier R (1895), *Annals of the British Peasantry*.

Gauldie E (1974), *Cruel Habitations*, London: Allen and Unwin.

Gavin H (1847), *The Unhealthiness of London and the Necessity of Remedial Measures,* London.

Gloag D (1980), Noise and health: public and private responsibility, *British Medical Journal*, 281: 1404–7.

Goldberg D (1972), *The Detection of Psychiatric Illness by Questionnaire,* Oxford: OUP,

Grasbeck R and Saris N (1969), Establishment and use of normal values, *Scand J Clin Lab Invest Suppl*, 110: 62–3.

Gyllerup S (1987), Cold and mortality in acute myocardial infarction. Seventh International Congress on Circumpolar Health, June 8–12, Umea, Sweden, *Abstr Arctic Med Res*, 45/87: 25.

Hall R, Horrocks J, Clamp S, Dedombal F (1976), Observer variation in assessment of results of surgery for peptic ulceration, *British Medical Journal*, i: 814–16.

Harrison J (1971), *The early Victorians 1832–1851*, London: Weidenfeld & Nicolson.

Hartup W (1978), Children and their friends, In *Man-environment Interactions: Evaluation and Applications,* (ed. Carson D), vol. 12, Childhood City, Milwaukee, Wisconsin: Environmental Design Research Association.

Hatch MT, Holmes MJ, Deig EF, *et al* (1976), Stability of airborne Rhinovirus Type 2 under atmospheric and physiological conditions, *Abstr Ann Meet Am Soc Microbiol*, 18: 193–8.

Haynes R (1991), Inequalities in health and health service use. Evidence from the General Household Survey, *Soc Science Med*, 33: 361–8.

Heasman M and Lipworth L (1966), *Accuracy of Certification and Cause of Death,* London: Studies on medical and population subjects no. 20, General Register Office.

Hopton J and Hunt SM (1990), *The Health Effects of Improved Heating in Domestic Dwellings: a Longitudinal Study,* Paper given at a conference on Unhealthy Housing University of Warwick .

Hopton J and Hunt SM (1996), Housing conditions and mental health in a disadvantaged area in Scotland, *Jnl of Epidemiology & Community Health*, 50: 56–61.

Hosen H (1978), Moulds in allergy, *J Asthma Res*, 15: 151–6.

Hunt D and Gidman MI (1982), A national field survey of house temperatures, *Building and Environment*, 17: 107–28.

Hunt SM (1990), Emotional distress and bad housing, *Health Hygiene*, 11: 72–9.

Hunt SM and Lewis C (1989), *Damp Housing, Mould Growth and Health Status Part II,* University of Edinburgh: Report to the funding bodies.

Hunt SM, Martin CJ, Platt SP (1986), *Health and housing in a deprived area of Edinburgh,* Paper given at a conference on Unhealthy Housing: a diagnosis, University of Warwick, 14–16 December.

Hunt SM, Martin CJ, Platt SP (1988), *Damp Housing, Mould Growth and Health Status,* Part I Report to the funding bodies. Glasgow and Edinburgh District Councils.

Hunt SM, McEwen J, McKenna S (1985), Social inequalities and perceived health, *Effective Health Care*, 3: 47–56

Hunter CA, Grant C, Flannigan B, Bravery AF (1988), Mould in buildings: the air spora of domestic dwellings, *Int Biodeterioration*, 24: 81–101.

Hyndman SJ (1990), Housing dampness and health among British Bengalis in East London, *Soc Sci Med*, 30: 131–41.

Ineichen B and Hooper D (1974), Wives' mental health and children's behaviour problems in contrasting residential areas, *Soc Sci Med*, 8: 369–74.

Jaakola J, Heinonen O, Seppanen O (1990), The occurrence of common cold and the number of persons in the office room. In *Indoor Air '90 Proceedings of the 5th International Conference on Indoor Air Quality and Climate,* Toronto, 29th July–3rd August .

Johnston L (1991), *Odds against Health: Children and Temporary Accommodation,* Edinburgh: Shelter..

Kannel W, Wolf P, Castelli WP, D'Angostino R (1987), Fibrinogen and risk of cardiovascular disease: the Framingham study, *JAMA*, 258: 1183–6.

Keatinge W, Coleshaw S, Cotter F, Mattock M, Murphy M, Chelliah R (1984), Increases in platelet and red cell counts, blood viscosity and arterial pressure during mild surface cooling: factors in mortality from coronary and cerebral thrombosis in winter, *British Medical Journal*, 289: 1405–8.

Keithley J, Byrne D, Harrisson S, McCarthy P (1984), Health and housing conditions in public sector housing estates, *Public Health*, 98: 344–53.

Kerribijn KF (1970), Endogenous factors in childhood CNSLD: methodological aspects in population studies. In *Bronchitis III* (eds Orie NGM, van der Lende R), Assen, Royal van Gorem, pp.38–48.

Kingdom KH (1960), Relative humidity and airborne infections, *Am Rev Respir Dis,* 81: 504–12.

Korsgaard J (1979), The effect of the indoor environment on the house dust mite. In *Indoor climate: Effects on Human Comfort, Performance and Health* (eds Fanger PO, Valbjorn O), Copenhagen: Danish Building Research Institute.

Kozak P, Gallup J, Cummins LH, Gillman SA (1980), Currently available methods for home mould surveys II: Examples of problem homes studied, *Ann Allergy,* 45: 167–75.

Kuh H, Wadsworth M (1989), Parental height: childhood environment and subsequent adult height in a national birth cohort, *Int J Epidemiol,* 18, 663–7.

Lancet (1983), Twenty-four hour blood pressure control, does it matter? Editorial, *Lancet,* i: 222–3.

Lovell B (1986), Health visiting homeless families, *Health Visitor,* 59: 340.

MacFarlane A (1977), Daily mortality and environment in English conurbations: air pollution, low temperature and influenza in Greater London, *Br J Prevent Soc Med,* 31: 54–61

Mant D and Muir Gray (1986) *J Health and Building Regulations - A report to the Building Research Establishment,* University of Oxford, Department of Community Medicine.

Marcus C (1974), Children's play behaviour in a low rise inner city housing development. In *Man-environment Interactions: Evaluation and Applications* (ed. Carson D), vol. 12, Childhood City, Milwaukee, Wisconsin: Environmental Design Research Association.

Marshall M (1989), Collected and neglected: Are Oxford hostels for the homeless filling up with disabled psychiatric patients?, *British Medical Journal,* 299: 706–7.

Martin AE (1967), Environment, housing and health, *Urban Studies,* 4: 1–21.

Martin CJ, Platt SP, Hunt SM (1987), Housing conditions and ill health, *British Medical Journal,* 294: 1125–7.

Maunsell K (1954), Sensitization risk from inhalation of fungal spores, *J Laryngol Otol,* 68: 765–75.

Maunsell K, Hughes A, Wraith DG (1970), Mite asthma: cause and management, *Practitioner,* 205: 779–83.

Mayon-White R (1992), *Buildings and health, Part 8. Sources of infection*, Building Research Establishment, Note N178/92,.

McCormick A, Fleming D, Charlton J (1995), *Morbidity Statistics from General Practice, Fourth National Morbidity Study 1991–1992,* London: HMSO.

McFarlane N (1989), *Hospitals, Housing and Tuberculosis in Glasgow,* The Society for the Social History of Medicine, pp.59-85.

McKeown T (1979), *The Role of Medicine: Dream, Mirage or Nemesis*? Oxford: Basil Blackwell.

McKinlay PL (1947), Tuberculosis mortality and overcrowding in Scotland, *Health Bull*, 37–39.

McMillan JS (1957), Examination of the association between housing conditions and pulmonary tuberculosis in Glasgow, *Br J Prevent Soc Med,* 11: 142–151.

Meade TW, Mellows S, Brozovic M, Miller G, Chakrabati T, North WR, Haines AP, Stirling Y, Imeson JD, Thompson SG (1986), Haemostatic function and ischaemic heart disease: principal results of the Northwick Park heart study, *Lancet*, ii: 533–7.

Melia R, Florey C, du V Chin S (1979), The relationship between respiratory illness in primary school children and the use of gas for cooking, I results from a national survey, *Int J Epidemiol,* 8: 383–7.

Meltzer H, Gill B, Petticrew M, Hinds K (1995), *The Prevalence of Psychiatric Morbidity among Adults living in Private Households. OPCS Surveys of Psychiatric Morbidity in Great Britain, Report 1*, London: HMSO.

Mitchell BR and Deane P (1962), *Population and Vital Statistics 2. United Kingdom population and intercensal increases 1801-1951*, London: HMSO.

M'Raihi L, Charpin D, Thibaudon M, Vervloet D (1990), Bronchial challenge to house dust can induce immediate bronchoconstriction in allergic asthmatic patients, *Ann Allergy*, 65: 485–8.

Murie A (1983), *Housing, Inequality and Deprivation*, London: Heinemann.

Murray R (1974), The influence of crowding on children's behaviour. In *Psychology and the Built Environment* (eds Canter D, Lee T), London: Architectural Press.

Neligman G, Prudham D, Steiner H (1974), *The Formative Years*, London: Oxford University Press and the Nuffield Trust.

Northup S and Kilburn K (1978), The role of mycotoxins in human pulmonary disease. In: *Mycotoxic Fungi and Mycotoxicosis, vol. 3: Mycotoxicosis of Man and Plants*, London: Academic Press.

OPCS (1988), *Mortality Statistics, 1985*, London: HMSO.

OPCS (1993), *1991 Census Topic Monitor: Housing and Availability of Cars*, London: OPCS.

Ostergaard PA, Ebbesen F, Nolte H, Skov PS (1990), Basophil histamine release in the diagnosis of house dust mite and dander allergy of asthmatic children. Comparison between prick test, RAST, basophil histamine release and bronchialprovocation, *Allergy*, 45: 231–5.

Page M (1986), *Child Safety and Housing*, London: Child Accident Prevention Trust.

Pedersen B and Gravesen S (1983), Allergic alveolitis precipitated by micro-organisms in the home environment, *Ugeskr Laeger*, 145: 580–1.

Platt SP, Martin CJ, Hunt SM (1989), Damp housing, mould growth and symptomatic health state, *British Medical Journal*, 298: 1673–8.

Platt-Mills T and Chapman M (1987), Dust mite: immunology, allergic disease and environmental control, *J Allergy Clin Immunol*, 80: 755–75.

Public Health (1895), *VII*, 8 July, 426: 1895.

Pyorala K, Punsar S, Siltanen P, Savolainen E, Sarna S (1977), The coronary heart disease mortality of Helsinki policemen born in west and east Finland, *Nord Coun Arct Med Res Report*, 19: 70–7.

Qizilbash N, Jones L, Warlow C, Mann J (1991), Fibrinogen and lipid concentration as risk factors for transient ischaemic attacks and minor ischaemic strokes, *British Medical Journal*, 303: 605–9.

Rasmussen F, Borchsenius L, Winslow J, Ostergaard E (1991), Associations between housing conditions, smoking habits and ventilatory lung function in men with clean jobs, *Scand J Respir Dis*, 59: 264–76.

Reed C (1981), Allergenic agents, *Bull NY Acad Med*, 57: 897–906.

Richman N (1974), The effects of housing on pre-school children and their mothers, *Develop Med Child Neurol*, 16: 53–8.

Richman N, Roderick P, Victor C, Lissauer T (1991), Use of acute hospital services by children, *Public Health*, 105: 297–302.

Riley R (1974), Airborne infections, *Am J Med*, 57: 466–75.

Rose G and Marmot M (1981), Social class and coronary heart disease, *Br Heart J*, 45: 13–19.

Rutter M (1974), Attainment and adjustment in two geographical areas. III Some factors accounting for area differences, *Br J Psychiatry*, 125: 520–33.

Sainsbury P (1983), Hypothermia in the elderly, *NZ Med J*, 16: 16–18.

Salonen JK, Puska P, Kottke TE, Tuomilento J, Nissinen A (1983), Decline in mortality from coronary heart disease in Finland from 1969–1979, *British Medical Journal*, 286: 1857–60.

Samet J, Marbury M, Spengler J (1987), Health effects and sources if indoor air pollution, Part I, *Am Rev Respir Dis*, 136: 1486–508.

Samet J, Marbury M, Spengler J (1988), Health effects and sources of indoor air pollution, Part II, *Am Rev Respir Dis*, 137: 221–42.

Satsangi M and McLennan I (1991), *Glasgow House Conditions Survey: People and Dwellings*, Centre for Housing Research, University of Glasgow.

Scottish Development Department (1978), *Statistical Bulletin; Condensation in Housing*, Edinburgh: HMSO.

Scottish Development Department Building Directorate (1984), *Condensation in Housing. A Report on Local Authority Returns, Survey Results and Remedial Measures*, Edinburgh: Scottish Office.

Sewell E and Scholes W (1984), *Sound Insulation Performance between Dwellings built in the early 1970s*, Garston: Building Research Establishment.

Shanks N (1988), Medical morbidity of the homeless, *J Epidemiol Commun Health*, 42: 183–8.

Shanks N and Carroll K (1982), Improving the identification rate of pulmonary tuberculosis among inmates of common lodging houses, *J Epidemiol Commun Health*, 36: 130–5.

Shanks N and Carroll N (1984), Persistent tubercular disease among inmates of common lodging houses, *J Epidemiol Commun Health*, 38: 66–9.

Shibasaki M, Hori T, Shimizu T, Isoyama S, Takeda K, Takita H (1988), Relationship between asthma and seasonal allergic rhinitis in schoolchildren, *Ann Allergy*, 65: 489–95

Skrimshire A (1978), *Area Disadvantage. Social Class and the Health Service*, Social Evaluation Unit, University of Glasgow.

Smith CA, Smith CJ, Kearns RA, Abbott MW (1993), Housing stressors, social support and psychological distress, *Soc Sci Med*, 37: 603–12.

Smith E (1875, 1876), *The Peasant's Home 1760--865*, Howard Prize Essay.

Smith FB (1988), *The Retreat of Tuberculosis – 1850–1950*, London: Macmillan.

Smith JE and Moss MO (1985), *Mycotoxins: Formation, Analysis and Significance*, Chichester: John Wiley and Sons Ltd.

Smith S (1990), Health status and the housing system, *Soc Sci Med*, 31: 753–62.

Solomon WR (1974), Fungus aerosols arising from cold mist vaporizers, *J Allergy*, 54: 222–8.

Spengler J and Sexton K (1983), Indoor air pollution: a public health perspective, *Science*, 221: 9–17.

Sporik R, Holgate S, Platt-Mills T, Cogswell J (1990), Exposure to house dust mite allergen (Der pI) and the development of asthma in childhood, *N Engl J Med*, 323: 502–7

Stein L (1952), Tuberculosis and the Social Complex, *Br J Soc Med*, 6: 1–48.

Stewart W (1970), *Children in Flats: a Family Study*, London: NSPCC.

Stone MC and Thorp JM (1985), Plasma fibrinogen a major cardiovascular risk factor, *J R Coll Gen Practit*, 35: 565–9.

Stout RW and Crawford V (1991), Seasonal variations in fibrinogen concentrations among elderly people, *Lancet*, 338: 9–13.

Strachan D and Elton P (1986), Relationship between respiratory morbidity in children and the home environment, *Fam Pract*, 3: 137–42.

Strachan D and Sanders C (1989), Damp housing and childhood asthma: respiratory effects of indoor air temperature and relative humidity, *J Epidemiol Commun Health*: 43: 7–14.

Thomas A and Niner P (1989), *Survey of Temporary Accommodation: Homeless People placed in Temporary Accommodation*, London: HMSO.

Tobin R, Baranowski E, Gilman A, *et al* (1987), Significance of fungi in indoor air: report of a working party, *Can J Public Health*, 78 (suppl), 1–14.

Toon P, Thomas K, Doherty M (1987), Audit of work at a medical centre for the homeless over one year, *J R Coll Gen Practit*, 37: 120–4.

Torok M, De Weck A, Scherner M (1981), allergische alveolitis infolge Verschimmelung der Schlafzimmerwand, *Schmeiz med Wochenschr*, 111: 924–9.

Tunstall-Pedoe H (1989), Heart disease mortality, *British Medical Journal*, i: 751–2.

Tuomilheto J, Geboers J, Salonen JT, Nissinen A, Kuulasmaa K, Puska P (1986), Decline in cardiovascular mortality in North Karelia and other parts of Finland, *British Medical Journal*, ii: 1068–76

Victor C, Connelly J, Roderick P, Cohen C (1989), Use of hospital services by homeless families in an inner London health district, *British Medical Journal*, 299: 725–7.

Voorhorst R, Spieksman F, Th M, Vareskamp, H (1969), *House Dust Atopy and the House Dust Mite*, Leiden: Staflein's Publishing Co.

Wardlaw A and Geddes D (1992), Allergic bronchopulmonary aspergillosis: a review, *J R Soc Med*, 85: 747–51.

Weaver L (1926), *Cottages*, London: Country Life.

West R, Lloyd S, Roberts C (1973), Mortality from ischaemic heart disease – association with the weather, *Br J Prevent Soc Med*, 27: 36–40.

Whitehead M (1987), *The Health Divide: Inequalities in Health in the 1980s*, London: Health Education Council.

Wicks M (1978), *Old and Cold*, London: Heinemenn.

Wilhelmsen L, Svardssudd K, Korsan-Bengsten K, Larsson B, Welin L, Tibblin G (1984), Fibrinogen as a cardiovascular risk factor for stroke and myocardial infarction, *N Engl J Med*, 311: 501–5.

Williams M (1991), *Housing Health and the Longitudinal Study*, Paper given at a conference on Unhealthy Housing: The Public Health Response, December, The Legal Research Institute, University of Warwick,

Wilner D, Walkley R, Pinkerton T, Tayback M (1969), *The Housing Environment and Family Life*, Baltimore: The Johns Hopkins Press.

Wohl AS (1983), *Endangered Lives – Public Health in Victorian Britain*, London: Dent.

Wolfe M and Golan M (1976), *Privacy and Institutionalisation*, Paper presented at a meeting of the Environmental Design Research Association Vancouver, BC.

Woodhouse P, Kay-tee Khaw, Plummer M (1993), Seasonal variations of blood pressure and its relationship to ambient temperature in an elderly population, *J Hypertens*, 11: 1267–74.

World Health Organisation (1982), *The Effects of Indoor Housing Climate on the Health of the Elderly*, Regional Office for Europe, Copenhagen. Report of a WHO working group Graz.

World Health Organisation (1987), *Health Impact of Low Indoor Temperatures*, Copenhagen: WHO.

Chapter 11 Family and household structure: the association of social support and living arrangements with health

Ader R, Cohen N, Felten D (1995), Psychoneuroimmunology: interactions between the nervous system and the immune system, *Lancet*, 345: 99–103.

Allnutt D and Gelardi A (1980), Inner cities in England, *Social Trends*, London: HMSO.

Anson O (1989), Marital status and women's health revisited: the importance of a proximate adult, *Journal of Marriage and the Family*, 51: 185–194.

Arber S (1991), Class, paid employment and family roles: making sense of structural disadvantage, gender and health status, *Social Science and Medicine*, 32: 425–436.

Beatson-Hind P, Yuen P, Balarajan R (1989), Single mothers: their health and health service use, *Journal of Epidemiology and Community Health*, 43: 385–390.

Ben-Shlomo Y, Davey-Smith G, Shipley M, Marmot MG (1993), Magnitude and causes of mortality differences between married and unmarried men, *Journal of Epidemiology and Community Health*, 47: 200–205.

Berkman LF and Syme L (1979), Social networks, host resistance and mortality: a nine year follow-up study of Alameda county residents, *American Journal of Epidemiology*, 109: 186–204.

Blaxter M (1990), *Health and Lifestyles*, London: Tavistock/Routledge.

Britton M (1990), *Mortality and Geography - a Review in the mid-1980s*. OPCS Series DS no.9, London: HMSO.

Butler JR and Morgan M (1977), Marital status and hospital use, *British Journal of Preventative and Social Medicine*, 31: 192–198.

Charlton J, Wallace M, White I (1994), Long-term illness: results from the 1991 Census, *Population Trends*, 75: 18–25.

Charlton JRH (1996), Which areas are healthiest? *Population Trends*, 83: 17–24.

Coombs RH (1991), Marital status and personal well-being: a literature review, *Family Relations*, 40: 97–102.

Craig J (1975), Population density and concentration in Great Britain 1931, 1951 and 1961, *OPCS Studies on Medical and Population Subjects* no. 30, London: HMSO.

Dalgard OS (1980), Mental health, neighbourhood and related social variables in Oslo, *Acta Psychiatrica Scandinavica*, 62, 298–304. In *Epidemiological research as a basis for the organisation of extramural psychiatry*, Supplement 285.

Drever F and Whitehead M (1995), Mortality in regions and local authority districts in the 1990's: exploring the relationship with deprivation, *Population Trends*, 82: 19–26.

Dorling D and Atkins D (1995), Population density, change and concentration in Great Britain 1971, 1981 and 1991, *OPCS Studies on Medical and Population Subjects no. 58*, London: HMSO.

Eames M, Ben-Shlomo Y, Marmot MG (1993), Social deprivation and premature mortality: a regional comparison across England, *British Medical Journal*, 307: 1097–1102.

Farr W (1858), The influence of marriage on the mortality of the French people, Transactions of the National Association for the Promotion of Social Science, 504–512. (Published in full in: *Influence of Marriage on the Mortality of the French people*, London: Savill and Edwards, 1859.).

Fox AJ and Goldblatt PO (1982), *Longitudinal study: Sociodemographic Mortality Differentials 1971–75*, OPCS Series LS. no.1, London: HMSO.

Glenn ND (1975), The contribution of marriage to the psychological well-being of males and females, *Journal of Marriage and the Family*, 37: 594–601.

Gove WR (1974), Sex, marital status and mortality, *American Journal of Sociology*, 79: 45–67.

Gove WR and Geerken MR (1977), The effect of children and employment on the mental health of married men and women, *Social Forces:* 56, 66–76.

Graham H (1991), The informal sector of welfare: a crisis in caring, *Social Science and Medicine*, 32: 507–515.

Griffiths M (1991), Nuns, virgins, and spinsters, Rigoni-Stern and cervical cancer revisited, *British Journal of Obstetrics and Gynaecology*, 98: 797–802.

Hajdu P, Mckee M, Bojan F (1995), Changes in premature mortality differentials by marital status in Hungary and in England and Wales, *European Journal of Public Health*, 5: 259–264.

Haskey J (1987), Trends in marriage and divorce in England and Wales, *Population Trends*, 48: 11–19.

Healing TD, Hoffman PN, Young SEJ (1995), The infection hazards of human cadavers, *Communicable Disease Review*, 5: R61–R68.

House JS, Landis KR, Umberson D (1988), Social relationships and health, *Science*, 241: 540–44.

Hu Y and Goldman N (1990), Mortality differentials by marital status: an international comparison, *Demography*, 27: 233–250.

Joung IMA, van de Mheen H, Stronks K, van Poppel FWA, Mackenbach JP (1994), Differences in self-reported morbidity by marital status and by living arrangement, *International Journal of Epidemiology*, 23: 91–97.

Joung IMA (1996), *Marital Status and Health, Descriptive and Explanatory Studies*, Doctoral Thesis, Erasmus Universiteit, Rotterdam, The Netherlands.

Joung IMA, van de Meer JWB, Mackenbach JP (1995a), Marital status and health care utilisation, *International Journal of Epidemiology*, 24: 569–575.

Joung IMA, Stronks K, van de Mheen H, Mackenbach JP (1995b), Health behaviours explain part of the differences in self reported health associated with partner/marital status in the Netherlands, *Journal of Epidemiology and Community Health*, 49: 482–488.

Joung IMA, Glerum JJ, van Poppel FWA, Kardaun JWPF, Mackenbach JP (1996), The contribution of specific causes of death to mortality differences by marital status in the Netherlands, *European Journal of Public Health*, 6: 142–149.

Judge K, Benzeval M (1993), Health inequalities: new concerns about the children of single mothers, *British Medical Journal*, 306: 677–680.

Kandel DB, Davies M, Raveisl VH (1985), The stressfulness of daily social roles for women: marital, occupational and household roles, *Journal of Health and Social Behaviour*, 26: 64–78.

Kawachi I, Colditz GA, Ascherio A, Rimm EB, Giovannucci E, Stampfer MJ, Willett WC (1996), A prospective study of social networks in relation to total mortality and cardiovascular disease in men in the USA, *Journal of Epidemiology and Community Health*, 50: 245–251.

Kiernan KE (1988), Who remains celibate, *Journal of Biosocial Science*, 20: 253–263.

Kiernan KE (1989), Who remains childless, *Journal of Biosocial Science*, 21: 387–398.

Kinlen LJ and John SM (1994), Wartime evacuation and mortality from childhood leukaemia in England and Wales in 1945–49, *British Medical Journal*, 309: 1197–1202.

Knodel J and Hermalin AI (1984), Effect of birth rank, maternal age, birth interval and sibship size on infant and child mortality: evidence from 18th and 19th century reproductive histories, *American Journal of Public Health*, 74: 1098–1106.

Kvikstad A, Vatten LJ, Tretli S (1995), Widowhood and divorce in relation to overall survival among middle-aged Norwegian women with cancer, *British Journal of Cancer*, 71: 1343–1347.

McAllister F (1995), *Marital Breakdown and the Health of the Nation*, 2nd edn, London: One Plus One.

Macintyre S (1992), The effects of family position and status on health, *Social Science and Medicine*, 35: 453–464.

Macintyre S, Maciver S, Soomans A (1993), Area, class, and health: should we be focusing on places or people?, *Journal of Social Policy*, 22: 213–234.

Macintyre S (1994), Understanding the social patterning of health: the role of the social sciences, *Journal of Public Health Medicine*, 16: 53–59.

Mackenbach J (1993), Inequalities in health in the Netherlands according to age, gender, marital status, level of education, degree of urbanisation and region, *European Journal of Public Health*, 3: 112–118.

McCormick A, Fleming D, Charlton J (1995), *Morbidity Statistics from General Practice: Fourth National Study, 1991–92*, OPCS Series MB5 no.3, London: HMSO.

Marsh C and Teague A (1992), Samples of anonymised records from the 1991 Census, *Population Trends*, 69: 17–26.

Martikainen P and Valkonen T (1996), Mortality after death of spouse in relation to duration of bereavement in Finland, *Journal of Epidemiology and Community Health*, 50: 264–268.

Meltzer H, Gill B, Petticrew M, Hinds K (1995), *The Prevalence of Psychiatric Morbidity among Adults living in Private Households*, OPCS Surveys of Psychiatric Morbidity in Great Britain, Report 1, London: HMSO.

Mercer A, Goldblatt P, Pugh H (1989), *Family and Demographic Circumstances and Mortality among Married Women of Working Ages*, OPCS LS working paper number 65, London: SSRU City University.

Mercer A (1990), *Disease, Mortality, and Population in Transition*, Leicester: Leicester University Press.

Mercer A (1991), *Support from a spouse and survival differentials among parents by family circumstances and employment*, Research Paper 91–2, Centre for Population Studies, London School of Hygiene and Tropical Medicine.

Morgan M (1980), Marital status, health, illness and service use, *Social Science and Medicine*, 14A: 633–643.

Murphy MFG (1996), Marital status and mortality: an epidemiological viewpoint, *Zeitschrift fur Bevolherungswissenschaft*, vol. 3. Neale AV, Tilley BC, Vernon SW (1986), Marital status, delay in seeking treatment and survival from breast cancer, *Social Science and Medicine*, 23: 305–312.

Olsen O (1993), Impact of social network on cardiovascular mortality in middle aged Danish men, *Journal of Epidemiology and Community Health*, 47: 176–180.

Popay J and Jones G (1990), Patterns of Health and Illness amongst lone parents. *Journal of Social Policy*, 4: 499–534.

RCGP, OPCS and DH (1974), *Morbidity Statistics from General Practice: Second National Study, 1970–71*, Studies on Medical and Population Subjects no. 26, London: HMSO.

RCGP, OPCS and DH (1979), *Morbidity Statistics from General Practice, 1971–72: Second National Study*, Studies on Medical and Population Subjects no. 36, London: HMSO.

RCGP, OPCS and DH (1982), *Morbidity Statistics from General Practice, 1970–71: Socio-economic Analysis*, Studies on Medical and Population Subjects no. 46, London: HMSO.

RCGP, OPCS and DH (1986), *Morbidity Statistics from General Practice: Third National Study, 1981–82*, OPCS Series MB5 no. 1, London: HMSO.

RCGP, OPCS and DH (1990), *Morbidity Statistics from General Practice, Third National Study: Socioeconomic Analysis 1981–82*, OPCS Series MB5 no. 2, London: HMSO.

Renne KS (1971), Health and marital experience in an urban population, *Journal of Marriage and the Family*, 34: 338–350.

Reves R (1985), Declining fertility in England and Wales as a major cause of the twentieth century decline in mortality, The role of changing family size and age structure in infectious disease mortality in infancy, *American Journal of Epidemiology*, 122: 112–126.

Riessman C and Gerstel N (1985), Marital dissolution and health, Do males or females have greater risk?, *Social Science and Medicine*, 20: 627–635.

Rigoni-Stern (1842), Statistical facts about cancers on which Doctor Rigoni-Stern based his contribution to the surgeon's subgroup of the IV congress of the Italian Scientists on 23 September 1842. Translated by Bianca de Stavola, *Statistics in Medicine* (1987) 6: 881–84.

Sawchuk LA (1993), Societal and ecological determinants of urban health: a case study of pre-reproductive mortality in 19th century Gibraltar, *Social Science and Medicine*, 36: 875–892.

Shouls S, Congdon P, Curtis S (1996), Modelling inequality in reported long-term illness in the UK: combining individual and area characteristics, *Journal of Epidemiology and Community Health*, 50, 366–376.

Sloggett A and Joshi H (1994), Higher mortality in deprived areas: community or personal disadvantage, *British Medical Journal*, 309: 1470–1474.

Smith S, Baker D, Buchan A, Bodiwala G (1992), Adult domestic violence, *Health Trends*, 24: 97–99.

Stone L (1990), *The Family, Sex and Marriage in England 1500–1800*, Harmondsworth: Penguin, abridged edn.

Susser M (1981), Widowhood: a situational life stress or a stressful life event, *American Journal of Public Health*, 71: 793–795.

Verbrugge LM and Madans JH (1985), Social roles and health trends of American Women, *Millbank Memorial Fund Quarterly/Health and Society*, 63: 691–735.

Verbrugge L (1979), Marital status and health, *Journal of Marriage and the Family*, 41: 267–285.

Wetherall R, Joshi H, Macran S (1994), Double burden or double blessing: employment, motherhood and mortality in the longitudinal study of England and Wales, *Social Science and Medicine,* 38: 285–97.

Woods RI, Watterson PA, Woodward JH (1988), The causes of rapid infant mortality decline in England and Wales 1861-1921, Part I, *Population Studies,* 42: 343–366 .

Woods RI, Watterson PA, Woodward JH (1989), The causes of rapid infant mortality decline in England and Wales, 1861–1921, Part II, *Population studies,* 43: 113–132.

Wyke S and Ford G (1992), Competing explanations for associations between marital status and health, *Social Science and Medicine,* 34: 523–532.

Chapter 12 Air pollution, climate and health: short-term effects and long-term prospects

Abercrombie GF (1953), December fog in London and the Emergency Bed Service, *Lancet,* i: 234–235.

Adams F (1849), *The Genuine Works of Hippocrates,* Translated from the Greek, with a preliminary discourse and annotations, vol. 1. London: Sydenham Society: 203.

Anderson HR, Limb ES, Bland JM, Ponce de Leon A, Strachan DP, Bower JS (1995a), *The Health Effects of an Air Pollution Episode in London, December 1991. Report to the Department of Health,* London: Department of Public Health Sciences, St George's Hospital Medical School.

Anderson HR, Limb ES, Bland JM, Ponce de Leon A, Strachan DP, Bower JS (1995b), The health effects of an air pollution episode in London, December 1991, *Thorax,* 50:1188-1193.

Anderson HR, Ponce de Leon A, Bland JM, Bower JS, Strachan DP (1996), Air pollution and daily mortality in London, *BMJ,* 312: 665–9.

Apling AJ, Sullivan EJ, Williams ML, Ball, DJ, Bernard RE, Derwent RG, Eggleton EJ, Hampton L, Waller RE (1977), Ozone concentrations in south east England during the summer of 1976, *Nature,* 269: 569–573.

Aris R, Christian D, Sheppard D, Barnes JR (1991), The effects of sequential exposure to acidic fog and ozone on pulmonary function in exercising subjects, *American Review of Respiratory Disease,* 43: 85–91.

Auliciems A and Burton I (1973), Trends in smoke concentrations before and after the Clean Air Act of 1956, *Atmospheric Environment,* 7: 1063–1070.

Bailey DLR and Clayton P (1982), The measurement of suspended particle and total carbon concentrations in the atmosphere using standard smokeshade methods *Atmospheric Environment,* 16: 2683–90.

Bellomo R, Gigliotti P, Treloar A, Holmes P, Suphioglu, Singh MB (1992), Two consecutive thunderstorm associated epidemics of asthma in the city of Melbourne. the possible role of rye grass pollen, *Medical Journal of Australia,* 156: 834–837.

Bernstein HT (1975), The mysterious disappearance of Edwardian London fog, *London Journal,* 1: 189–206.

Biersteker K and Evendijk JE (1976), Ozone, temperature, and mortality on Rotterdam in the summer of 1974 and 1975, *Environmental Research,* 12: 214–217.

Bower JS, Broughton GFJ, Stedman JR, Williams ML (1994), A winter NO_2 smog episode in the UK, *Atmos Environ,* 28: 461-475.

Bower JS, Broughton GFJ, Willis PG, Clark H (1995), *Air Pollution in the UK: 1993/94,* Harwell: AEA Technology.

Bower JS, Stevenson KJ, Broughton GFJ, Lampert JE, Sweeney BP, Wilken J et al (1990), *Ozone in the UK: a Review of 1989/90 Data from Monitoring Sites operated by Warren Spring Laboratory,* Report LR 793(AP)M Stevenage: Warren Spring Laboratory: 32-33.

Bradley HM, Logan WPD, Martin AE (1958), The London fog of December 2nd–5th 1957, *Monthly Bulletin of the Ministry of Health and Public Health Laboratory Service* 17: 156–166.

Brodie FJ (1891), On the prevalence of fog in London during the 20 years 1871–1890, *Quarterly Journal of the Royal Meteorological Society,* 18: 40–45.

Brodie FJ (1905), Decrease of fog in London during recent years, *Quarterly Journal of the Royal Meteorological Society,* 51: 15–28.

Brimblecombe P (1987), *The Big Smoke,* London: Methuen.

Burnett RT, Dales R, Krewski D, Vincent R, Dann T, Brook JR (1995), Associations between ambient particulate sulfate and admissions to Ontario hospitals for cardiac and respiratory diseases, *American Journal of Epidemiology* 142(1): 15–22.

Burnett RT, Dales RE, Raizenne ME, Krewski D, Summers PW, Roberts GR, Raad-Young M, Dann T, Brook J (1994), Effects of low ambient levels of ozone and sulfates on the frequency of respiratory admissions to Ontario hospitals, *Environmental Research,* 65(2): 172–194.

Campbell-Hewson G, Cope A, Egleston C, Sherriff HM, Robinson SM, Allitt U (1994), Epidemic of asthma possibly associated with electrical storms, *BMJ,* 309: 1086–87.

Cameron K, Maynard DR (1992), A new look at the health effects of air pollution, *Health Trends,* 24: 82–85.

Cellenza A, Fothergill J, Kupek E, Shaw RJ (1996), Thunderstorm associated asthma: a detailed analysis of environmental factors, *BMJ,* 312: 604–607.

Cody RP, Weisel CP, Birnbaum G, Lioy PJ (1992), The effect of ozone associated with summertime photochemical smog on the frequency of asthma visits to hospital emergency departments, *Environmental Research,* 58: 184–194.

Cook GC (1992), Effect of global warming on the distribution of parasitic and other infectious diseases: a review, *Journal of the Royal Society of Medicine,* 85: 688–691.

Craxford SR, Gooriah BD and Weatherley M-L PM (1970), *Air Pollution in Urban Areas in the United Kingdom: Present Position and Recent National and Regional Trends,* National Survey of Air Pollution, Warren Spring Laboratory, SGGB 74/6.

Curwen M (1990), Excess winter mortality: a British phenomenon? *Health Trends,* 22: 169–175.

Delfino RJ, Becklake MR, Hanley JA (1994), The relationship of urgent hospital admissions for respiratory illnesses to photochemical air pollution levels in Montreal, *Environmental Research,* 67(1): 1-19.

Department of Environment (1992), *The UK Environment* (ed. A Brown), London: HMSO

Department of Health Advisory Group on the Medical Aspects of Air Pollution Episodes (1991), *Ozone,* London: HMSO.

Department of Health Advisory Group on the Medical Effects of Air Pollution episodes (1992), *Sulphur Dioxide, Acid Aerosols and Particulates in the UK,* London: HMSO.

Department of Health Advisory Group on the Medical Aspects of Air Pollution Episodes (1993), *Oxides of Nitrogen,* London: HMSO.

Department of Health Advisory Group on the Medical Aspects of Air Pollution Episodes (1995a), *Health Effects of Exposures to Mixtures of Air Pollutants,* London: HMSO.

Department of Health Committee on the Medical Effects of Air Pollutants (1995a), *Asthma and Outdoor Air Pollutants,* London: HMSO.

Department of Health Committee on the Medical Effects of Air Pollutants (1995b), *Non-biological Particles and Health,* London: HMSO,

Dockery DW and Pope III CA, Xu X, Spengler JD, Ware JH, Fay ME, Ferris BG, Speizer FE (1993), An association between air pollution and mortality in six US cities, *New England Journal of Medicine,* 329: 1753-1759.

Dockery DW and Pope III CA (1994), Acute respiratory effects of particulate air pollution, *Ann Rev Public Health,* 15:107-132.

Ellis FP (1972), Mortality from heat illness and heat-aggravated illness in the United States, *Environmental Research,* 5: 1–58.

Evans BG (1985), The emergency bed service – the past illustrates the present, *Community Medicine,* 7: 265–271.

Evelyn J (1659), *A Character of England,* (cited in Brumblecombe (1987).

Evelyn J (1661), *Fumifugium or the inconvenience of the aer and smoak of London dissipated,* London: Gabriel Bedel and Thomas Collins.

Farr W (1840), *Letter to the Registrar General. Second report of the Registrar General 1838–1839*, London: HMSO, p.88.

Farr W (1841), *Letter to the Registrar General. Third report of the Registrar General 1839–1840*, London: HMSO, p.102.

Farr W (1843), *Causes of High Mortality in Town Districts. Fifth report of the Registrar General 1841*, London: HMSO, p.416.

Farr W (1867), *Twenty eighth report of the Registrar General 1865*, London: HMSO, pp.18–19. Quoted in Farr (1885).

Farr W (1885), *Vital Statistics: a Memorial Volume of Selections from the Reports and Writings of William Farr*, Edited by NA Humphreys. London: Sanitary Institute of Great Britain.

Fleming DM, Norbury CA, Crombie DL (1991), *Annual and Seasonal Variation in the Incidence of Common Diseases*, Occasional Paper 53, London: Royal College of General Practitioners.

Fry J (1953), Effects of a severe fog on a general practice, *Lancet*, i: 235–236.

General Register Office (1868), *Report on the Cholera Epidemic of 1866. Supplement to the 29th Report of the Registrar General*, London: HMSO.

Gore AT and Shaddick CW (1958), Atmospheric pollution and mortality in the County of London. *British Journal of Preventive and Social Medicine*, 12: 104–113.

Goubet S (1993), The potential effect of high concentrations of ozone on mortality, MSc dissertation, Birkbeck College, University of London.

Gover M (1938), Mortality during periods of excessive temperature, *Public Health Reports (US)*, 53: 1122 –1143.

Graunt J (1662), Natural and political observations ... Made upon the the Bills of Mortality.

Gray DP (1992), *Planning Primary Care*, Occasional Paper 57, London: Royal College of General Practitioners.

Greenwood M (1921), Galen as an epidemiologist, *Proceedings of the Royal Society of Medicine*, 14: 3–16.

Gribbin J (1978), *The Climate Threat, What's wrong with our Weather?*, Glasgow: Fontana/Collins 1978.

Guy WA (1843), An attempt to determine the influence of the seasons and weather on sickness and mortality, *Journal of the Statistical Society*, vi: 133–150.

Guy WA (1881), On temperature and its relation to mortality: an illustration of the application of the numerical method to the discovery of truth, *Journal of the Statistical Society*, xliv: 235–261.

Haines A, Epstein PR, McMichael AJ (1993), Global health watch: monitoring impacts of environmental change, *Lancet*, 342: 1464–69.

Haines A and Fuchs C (1991), Potential impacts on health of atmospheric change, *J Pub Health Med*, 13: 69–80.

Haines A and Parry M (1993), Potential effects on health of global warming, *World Resources Review*, 5: 430–448.

Hartley H (1962), The Macfarlane memorial lecture, *Journal of the Institute of Fuel*, 35: 196–209.

Haviland A (1855), *Climate, weather and disease, being a sketch of the opinions of the most celebrated antient and modern writers with regard to the influence of climate and weather in producing disease*, London: John Churchill.

Hazucha MJ, Bates BV, Bromberg PA (1989), Mechanism of action of ozone on human lung, *J Appl Physiol*, 67: 1535–1541.

Higgins BG, Francis HC, Yates CJ, Warburton CJ, Fletcher AM, Reid JA, Pickering CA, Woodcock AA (1995), Effects of air pollution on symptoms and peak expiratory flow measurements in subjects with obstructive lung disease, *Thorax*, 50: 149-155.

Holland WW, Bennett AE, Cameron IR, Florey CduV, Leeder SR, Schilling RSF, Swan AV, and Waller RE (1979), Health effects of particulate pollution reappraising the evidence, *American Journal of Epidemiology*, 110: 527–659.

Houghton JT, Jenkins GJ, Ephraums JJ (1990), *Climate Change: The IPCC Scientific Assessment*, Cambridge: Cambridge University Press.

Houghton JT, Meira Filho LG, Callender BA, Harris N, Kattenberg A, Maskell K, eds (1996), *Climate Change 1995: the Science of Climate Change*, contribution of working group I to the second assessment report of the Intergovernmental panel on climate change, Cambridge, New York: Cambridge University Press.

Kalkstein LS (1991a), A new approach to evaluate the impact of climate upon human mortality, *Environ Health Perspectives*, 96: 145–150.

Kalkstein LS (1991b), Potential impact of global warming: climate change and human mortality, In *Global Climate Change and Life on Earth* (ed. Wyman RL), London: Chapman and Hall, pp.216–223.

Kalkstein LS (1993), Health and climate change: direct impacts in cities, *Lancet*, 342: 1397–1399.

Kalkstein LS and Davis RE (1989), Weather and human mortality: an evaluation of demographic and interregional responses in the United States, *Annals of the Association of American Geographers*, 79(1): 44–64.

Katsouyanni K (1996), Foreword. The APHEA project. Short term effects of air pollution on health: a European approach using epidemiological time series data, *Journal of Epidemiology and Community Health*, 50 (Supplement 1): S2.

Katsouyanni K, Pantozopoulou A, Youloumi G, Tselepidali I, Moustris K, Asimakopoulos D, Poulopoulou G, Trichopoulos D (1993),

Evidence for interaction between air pollution and high temperature in the causation of excess mortality, *Archives of Environmental Health*, 48(4): 235–242.

Katsouyanni K, Schwartz J, Spix C, Touloumi G, Zmirou D, Zanobetti A, Wojtyniak B, Vonk JM, Tobias A, Ponka A, Medina S, Bacharova L, Anderson HR (1996), Short term effects of air pollution on health: a European approach using epidemiologic time series data: the APHEA protocol, *Journal of Epidemiology and Community Health (Supplement 1)*: S12–S18.

Kunst AE, Looman CWN, Mackenback JP (1993), Outdoor air temperature and mortality in the Netherlands: a time-series analysis, *American Journal of Epidemiology*, 137(3): 331–341.

Langford IH and Bentham G (1995), The potential effects of climate change on winter mortality in England and Wales, *International Journal of Biometeorology*, 38: 141–147.

Lawther PJ, Ellison JMcK, Waller RE (1968), Some aspects of aerosols research, *Proc Roy Soc A*, 307: 223–234.

Lawther PJ, Waller RE, Henderson M (1970), Air pollution and exacerbations of chronic bronchitis, *Thorax*, 25: 525–539.

Lee RE, Caldwell JS, Morgan GB (1972), The evaluation of methods for measuring suspended particulates in air, *Atmospheric Environment*, 6: 593–622.

Logan WPD (1949), Fog and mortality, *Lancet*, i: 78.

Logan WPD (1956), Mortality from fog in London, January 1956, *BMJ*, 1: 722–5.

MacDowall AB (1895), *Weather and Disease: a Curve History of their Variations in Recent Years*, London: The Graphotone Co.

Macfarlane AJ (1976), Daily Deaths in Greater London, *Population Trends*, 5: 20–25.

Macfarlane AJ (1977), Daily mortality and climate in English conurbations. 1. Air pollution, low temperature, and influenza in Greater London, *British Journal of Preventive and Social Medicine*, 31: 54–61.

Macfarlane AJ (1978), Daily mortality and environment in English conurbations II. Deaths during summer hot spells in Greater London, *Environmental Research*, 15: 332–341.

Macfarlane AJ (1984), A time to die?, *International Journal of Epidemiology*, 13: 38–44.

Macfarlane AJ and Waller R (1976), Short-term increases in mortality during heatwaves, *Nature*, 264: 434–436.

Martin AE (1961), Epidemiological studies of air pollution. A review of British methodology, *Monthly Bulletin of the Ministry of Health and the Public Health Laboratory Service*, 19: 56–72.

Martin AE (1964), Mortality and Morbidity Statistics and Air Pollution, *Proceedings of the Royal Society of Medicine*, 57: 969–975.

Martin AE and Bradley WH (1960), Mortality, fog and air pollution – an investigation during the winter of 1958-59, *Monthly bulletin of the Ministry of Health and the Public Health Laboratory Service*, 19: 56–72.

Mazumdar S, Schimmel H, Higgins ITT (1982), Relation of daily mortality to air pollution: an analysis of 14 London winters, 1958/59–1971/72, *Arch Environ Health*, 37: 213–220.

McMichael AJ (1993), Global environmental change and human population health: a conceptual and scientific challenge for epidemiology, *International Journal of Epidemiology*, 22: 1–8.

McMichael AJ, Haines A, Slooff R, Kovars S eds. (1996), *Climate Change and Human Health*, Geneva: World Health Organisation.

Medical Research Council (1920), *The Science of Ventilation and Open Air Treatment*, Special Report series, no. 52.

Ministry of Health (1954), *Mortality and Morbidity during the London Fog of December 1952*, Reports on Public Health and Medical Subjects no.95.

Molfino NA, Wright SC, Katz I, Tarlo S, Silverman S, McClean PA, Szalai JP, Raizenne M, Slutsky AS, Zamet N (1991), Effects of low concentrations of ozone on inhaled allergen responses in asthmatic subjects, *Lancet*, 338: 199–203.

Mortality and Morbidity Weekly Report (1995), Heat-related mortality – Chicago, July 1995, *MMWR*, 44: 577–579.

Murray V, Venables K, Laing-Morton T, Partridge M, Thurston J, Williams D (1994), Episodes of asthma possibly related to thunderstorms, *BMJ*, 309: 131–132.

Ostro B (1984), A search for a threshold in the relationship of air pollution to mortality: a reanalysis of data on London winters, *Environmental Health Perspectives*, 58: 397–399.

Packe GE and Ayres JG (1985), Asthma outbreak during a thunderstorm, *Lancet*, ii: 199–204.

Parry ML and Rosenzweig C (1993), Health and climate change: food supply and risk of hunger, *Lancet*, 342; 1345–1347.

Photochemical Oxidants Review Group (1993), *Ozone in the United Kingdom*, London: Department of Environment.

Ponce de Leon A, Anderson HR, Bland JM, Strachan DP, Bower JS (1996), The effects of air pollution on daily hospital admissions for respiratory disease in London: 1987/88 to 1991/92, *J Epidemiol Community Health*, 50 (Supplement): S63–S70.

Pope III CA, Dockery DW, Spengler JD, Raizenne ME (1991), Respiratory health and PM$_{10}$ pollution: a daily time series analysis, *American Review of Respiratory Diseases 1991*, 144: 668–674.

Pope III CA, Schwartz J and Ransom MR (1992), Daily mortality and PM$_{10}$ pollution in Utah Valley, *Archives of Environmental Health*, 47(3): 211–216.

Quality of Urban Air Review Group (1993a), *Urban air quality in the United Kingdom*, Bradford: Department of the Environment.

Quality of Urban Air Review Group (1993b), *Diesel Vehicle Emissions and Urban Air Quality*, Institute of Public and Environmental Health, University of Birmingham.

Ramlow JM and Kuller LH (1990), Effects of the summer heat wave of 1988 on daily mortality in Allegheny County PA, *Public Health Reports* 105(3): 283–288.

Roener W, Hoeck G, Brunekreef B (1993), Effect of ambient winter air pollution on respiratory health of children with chronic respiratory symptoms, *American Review of Respiratory Disease*, 147: 118–124.

Rosenzweig C, Parry ML, Fischer G, Frohberg K (1993), *Climate Change and World Food Supply*, Research report no.3, Environmental Change Unit, University of Oxford.

Russell WT (1924), The influence of fog on mortality from respiratory diseases, *Lancet*, 2: 335–339.

Russell WT (1926), The relative influence of fog and low temperature on the mortality from respiratory disease, *Lancet*, 2: 1128–1130.

Scarlett JF, Abbott KJ, Peacock JL, Strachan DP, Anderson HR, Acute effects of summer pollution on respiratory function in primary school children in southen England, *Thorax*, (in press).

Schwartz J (1991a), Particulate air pollution and daily mortality: a synthesis. *Public Health Reviews*, 19:39-60.

Schwartz J (1991b), Particulate air pollution and daily mortality in Detroit, *Environmental Research*, 56: 204–213.

Schwartz J (1992), What are people dying of on high air pollution days?, *Environmental Research*, 64: 26–35.

Schwartz J (1994a), Air pollution and daily mortality: a review and meta analysis, *Environmental Research*, 64: 36-52.

Schwartz J (1994b), PM$_{10}$, ozone and hospital admissions for the elderly in Minneapolis St-Paul, Minnesota, *Archives of Environmental Health*, 49(5): 366–374.

Schwartz J (1994c), Air pollution and hospital admissions for the elderly in Detroit, Michigan, *Am J Respira Crti Care Med*, 150(3): 648–655.

Schwartz J (1994d), Total suspended particulate matter and daily mortality in Cincinnati, Ohio, *Environmental Health Perspectives*, 102(2): 186–189.

Schwartz J (1994e), Air pollution and hospital admissions for the elderly in Birmingham, Alabama, *American Journal of Epidemiology*, 139: 589–598.

Schwartz J (1996), Air pollution, respiratory disease and mortality. In *Health at the crossroads: transport policy and urban health* (eds Fletcher AC and McMichael AJ), London: London School of Hygiene and Tropical Medicine.

Schwartz J and Dockery DW (1992a), Increased mortality in Philadelphia associated with daily air pollution concentrations, *Am Rev Respir Dis*, 148: 600–604.

Schwartz J and Dockery DW (1992b), Particulate air pollution and daily mortality in Steubenville Ohio, *Am J Epidemiol*, 135: 12–20.

Schwartz J and Marcus A (1990), Mortality and air pollution in London: a time series analysis, *Am J Epidemiol*, 131: 185–194.

Schwartz J, Slater D, Larson T V, Pierson W E, Koenig J Q (1993), Particulate air pollution and hospital emergency room visits for asthma in Seattle, *American Review of Respiratory Diseases*, 147: 826–831.

Schwartz J, Spix C, Touloumi G, Bacharova L, Barumamdzadeh T, le Tertre A, Piekarski T, Ponce de Leon A, Ponka A, Rossi G, Saez M, Schouten JP (1996), Methodological issues in studies of airpollution and daily counts of deaths or hospital admissions, *Journal of Epidemiology and Community Health*, 50 (Supplement 1): S3–S11.

Shope R (1991), Global climate change and infectious diseases, *Environmental Health Perspectives*, 96: 171–174.

Streetly A and Markowe H (1995), Changing trends in the epidemiology of malignant melanoma: gender differences and their implications for public health, *International Journal of Epidemiology*, 24: 897–907.

Thurston GD, Ito K, Hayes CG, Bates DV, Lippmann M (1994), Respiratory hospital admissions and summertime haze air pollution in Toronto, Ontario: consideration of the role of acid aerosols, *Environmental Research*, 65(2): 271–290.

Thurston GD, Ito K, Lippmann M, Hayes C (1989), Reexamination of London, England, mortality in relation to exposure to acidic aerosols during 1963–1972 winters, *Environmental Health Perspectives*, 79: 73–82.

Wadsworth M (1995), *Changing influences on research into lower respiratory illness since 1915*, Paper given at 'Has epidemiology a history?', Conference organised by Society for Social Medicine. March 31 1995.

Waller RE (1984), *Assessing effects of suspended particualte matter on health*, European Community Workshop RIVM-Bilthoven. European Economic Community, 1984.

Waller RE, Lawther PJ, and Martin AE (1969), *Clean air and health in London*, Proceedings of the Clean Air Conference, Eastbourne, October 1969, Part 1. London: National Society for Clean Air.

Walters S, Griffiths RK, Ayres J (1994), Temporal association between hospital admissions for asthma in Birmingham and ambient levels of sulphur dioxide and smoke, *Thorax*, 49:133-140.

Walters S, Miles J, Ayres JG, Archer G (1993), Effect of an air pollution episode on respiratory function of patients with asthma (abstract), *Thorax*, 48:1063.

Watson RT, Zinyowera MC, Moss RH, eds (1996), Climate change 1995 Impacts, adaptations and mitigation of climate change: Scientific-Technical analyses. Contribution of Working Group II to the Second Assessment Report of the Intergovernmental Panel on Climate Change, Cambridge, New York: Cambridge University Press.

Woods HM (1927), The influence of external factors on mortality from pneumonia in childhood and later adult life, *Journal of Hygiene*, 26: 36–43.

Wright GP and Wright HP (1945), The influence of weather conditions on the mortality from bronchitis and pneumonia in children, *Journal of Hygiene*, 23: 151–175.

Young M (1924), The influence of weather conditions on the mortality from bronchitis and pneumonia in children, *Journal of Hygiene*, 23: 151–175.

Chapter 13 Excess winter mortality in England and Wales, with special reference to the effects of temperature and influenza

Alderson MR (1985), Season and Mortality, *Health Trends*, 17: 87-96.

Ashley J, Smith T, Dunnell K (1991), Deaths in Great Britain associated with the influenza epidemic of 1989/90, *Population Trends*, 61: 16-20.

Betts RF (1989), Amantadine and rimatadine for the prevention of Influenza A, *Seminars in Respiratory Infections*, 4: 304-10.

Bull GM and Morton J (1978), Environment, temperature and death rates, *Age and Ageing*, 7: 210-224.

Clifford RE, Smith JWG, Tillett HE, Wherry PJ (1977), Excess mortality associated with influenza in England and Wales, *International Journal of Epidemiology*, 6: 115–128.

Curwen M (1991), Excess winter mortality: a British phenomenon?, *Health Trends*, 22: 169–175.

Curwen M and Devis T (1988), Winter mortality, temperature and influenza: has the relationship changed in recent years? *Population Trends*, 54: 17-20.

Curwen M, Dunnell K, Ashley J,(1990), Hidden influenza deaths 1989/90, *Population Trends*, 61: 31-42.

Dab W, Quenel P, Cohen JM, Hannoun C,(1991), A new influenza surveillance system in France: the Ile-de-France "Gro~" (2) , *European Journal of Epidemiology*, 7: 579-587.

Diepersloot RJ, Bouter KP, Hoekstra JB (1990), Influenza infection and diabetes: case for annual vaccination, *Diabetes Care*, 13: 876-882.

Fleming DM and Crombie DL (1985), The incidence of common infectious diseases: the weekly returns service of the Royal College of General Practitioners, *Health Trends*, 17: 13-16.

Fleming DM and Cross KW (1993), Respiratory syncytial virus or influenza?, *Lancet*, 342: 1507-10.

Fleming DM, Norbury CA, Crombie DL (1991), *Annual and Seasonal Variation in the Incidence of Common Diseases*, London: Royal College of General Practitioners.

Fox AJ and Goldblatt PO (1882), *Longitudinal Study: Socio-demographic Mortality Differentials*, OPCS Series LS no. 1, London: HMSO.

General Register Office (1841), *Third Annual Report of Births, Deaths and Marriages in England*, London: HMSO, pp.102-9.

General Register Office (1874), *Weekly Return of Births and Deaths in London*, 51, London: HMSO, pp.427-8.

Keatinge WR, Coleshaw SRK, Holmes J (1989), Changes in seasonal mortalities with improvement in home heating in England and Wales from 1964 to 1984, *International Journal of Biometeorology*, 33: 71-76.

Keatinge W and Holmes J (1990), Changes in seasonal mortality in the 80-84 age group with increase in central heating, *Environmental Stress*, 307-316.

Kunst AE, Looman CWN, Mackenbach JP (1990), The decline in winter excess mortality in The Netherlands, *International Journal of Epidemiology*, 20: 971-7.

Langmuir AD (1976), William Farr: founder of modern concepts of surveillance, *International Journal of Epidemiology*, 5: 13–18.

Larsen U (1990), The effects of monthly temperature fluctuations on mortality in the United States from 1921 to 1985, *International Journal of Biometeorology*, 34: 136-145.

MacFarlane A (1976), Daily deaths in Greater London, *Population Trends*, 5: 20–25.

MacFarlane A (1977), Air pollution, low temperature and influenza in Greater London, *British Journal of Preventive and Social Medicine*, 31: 54–61.

MacFarlane A (1984), "A time to die?", *International Journal of Epidemiology*, 13: 38–44.

MacKee M (1991), (letter) *Health Trends*, 23: 2: 86.

McDowell M, (1981), Long term trends in seasonal mortality, *Population Trends*, 26: 16–19.

McKee CN (1989), Deaths in winter: can Britain learn from Europe?, *European Journal of Epidemiology*, 5: 178-182.

McKee CM (1990), Deaths in winter in Northern Ireland: the role of low temperature, *Ulster Medical Journal*, 59: 17-22.

Mackenbach JP, Kunst AE, Looman CWN, (1992), Seasonal variation of mortality in The Netherlands, *Journal of Epidemiology and Community Health*, 46: 261-265.

Mannino JA and Washburn RA (1989), Environmental temperature and mortality from acute myocardial infarction, *International Journal of Biometeorology*, 33: 32-35.

Ministry of Health (1954), Mortality and morbidity during the London fog of December 1952, *Reports on Public Health and Medical Subjects no. 95*, London: HMSO.

Nguyen VT and Nicholson KG (1992), Influenza deaths in Leicestershire during the 1989-90 epidemic: implications for prevention, *Epidemiology and Infection*, 108: 537-545.

OPCS (1987), *Trends in Respiratory Mortality, 1951-1975*, Series DH1 no.7, London: HMSO pp.13-22.

OPCS (1975), *General Household Survey 1972*, London: HMSO.

OPCS (1994), *General Household Survey 1992*, London: HMSO.

Royal College of Physicians of London (1966), *Report of Committee on Accidental Hypothermia*, London: Royal College of Physicians.

Ruggiero G and Utiliti R (1992), Usefulness and limitations of vaccination against influenza, *Recenti progressi in medicina*, 83: 337-40.

Sakamoto-Momiyama (1977), *Seasonality in Human Mortality*, Tokyo: University Press.

Sprenger MJ, Mulder PG, Beyer WE, Masurel N (1991), Influenza: relation of mortality to morbidity parameters - Netherlands, 1970-1989, *International Journal of Epidemiology*, 20: 1118-24.

Sprenger MJW, Mulder PGH, Beyer WEP, Van Strik R, Masurel NIC (1993), Impact of influenza in mortality in relation to age and underlying disease 1667–1989, *International Journal of Epidemiology*, 22: 334–340.

Stout RW and Crawford V (1991), Seasonal variations in fibrinogen concentrations among elderly people, *Lancet*, 338: 9-13.

Tillett HE, Nicholas S, Watson JM (1991), Unusual pattern of influenza mortality in 1989/90, *Lancet*, 338: 1590-91.

Tillett HE, Smith JW, Gooch CD (1983), Excess deaths attributable to influenza in England and Wales: age at death and certified cause, *International Journal of Epidemiology*, 12: 344-352.

Tillett HE and Spencer I (1982), Influenza surveillance in England and Wales using routine statistics, *Journal of Hygiene, Cambridge*, 88: 83-94.

United Nations (1985), *Demographic Yearbook*, New York: UN.

Vuori 1 (1987), The heart and the cold, *Annals of Clinical Research*, 19: 156-162.

Chapter 14 Medical advances and iatrogenesis

ABPI (1994), Code of Practice for the Pharmaceutical Industry (1994), in *ABPI Data Sheet Compendium 1994–95* pp.vii–xxvii. Datapharm Publications Limited.

Alberman E (1982), Perinatal audit (editorial), *Community Medicine*, 4: 95–6.

Alderson M (1981), Alignment of the Revisions of the International Classification of Diseases, in *International Mortality Statistics*, pp.91–109, London: Macmillan Press Ltd.

Alvarez-Dardet C and Ruiz MT (1993), Thomas McKeown and Archibald Cochran: a journey through the diffusion of ideas, *British Medical Journal*, 306: 1252–5.

Ashton J (1991), Sanitarian becomes ecologist: the new environmental health, *British Medical Journal*, 302: 189–90.

Austoker J (1994), Screening for cervical cancer, *British Medical Journal*, 309: 241–8.

Barkun SB, Barkun AN, Sampalis JS, Fried G, Taylor B, Wexler MJ, Wexler MJ, Goresky CA and Meakins JL (1992), Randomised controlled trial of laparoscopic versus mini cholecystectomy, *Lancet*, 340: 1116–9.

Barendregt JJ, Bonneux L and Van der Maas PJ (1994), for the Technology Assessment Methods Project Team, Healthy expectancy: an indicator for change?, *Journal of Epidemiology and Community Health*, 48: 482–7.

Bebbington AC (1991), The expectation of life without disability in England and Wales: 1976–88, *Population Trends*, 66: 26–9.

Begg N and Nicoll A (1994), Immunisation, *British Medical Journal*, 309: 1073–5.

Biraben JN (1991), Pasteur, pasturisation and medicine. In *The Decline of Mortality in Europe* (eds Schofield R, Reher D and Bideau A), Oxford: Clarendon Press.

Bishop PJ (1967), The Brompton Hospital and its First Medical Report, *Tubercle*, 48: 344.

BMJ (1950), Fifty Years of Medicine, *British Medical Journal*, 7 January 1950.

Bolton RG (1994), The Ethics of Gene Therapy, *Journal of the Royal Society of Medicine*, 87: 302–4.

Bone MR: Bebbington AC, Jagger C, Morgan K and Nicolaas G (1995), *Health Expectancy and its Uses*, London: HMSO.

Boston Collaborative Drug Surveillance Program (1973), Clinical depression of the central nervous system due to diazepam and chlordiazepoxide in relation to cigarette smoking and age, *New England Journal of Medicine*, 288: 277–80.

Brewster SF (1994), Gene theapy for cancer: what's it all about? *Hospital Update*, 20: 140–50.

Bunker JP, Frazier HS and Mosteller F (1994), Improving health: measuring effects of medical care, *The Millbank Quarterly*, 72: 225–58.

Burdon DW (1982), Advances in antibiotics, *The Practitioner*, 226: 1701–8.

Campling EA, Devlin HB, Hoile RW and Lunn JN (1993), *The Report of the National Confidential Enquiry into Perioperative Deaths 1991/1992*.

Chalmers I and Haynes B (1994), Reporting, updating, and correcting systematic reviews of the effects of health care, *British Medical Journal*, 309: 862–5.

Charlton JRH, Hartley RM, Silver R and Holland WW (1983), Geographical variation in mortality from conditions amenable to medical intervention in England and Wales, *Lancet*, i: 691–6.

Charlton JRH and Velez R (1986), Some international comparisons of mortality amenable to medical intervention, *British Medical Journal*, 292: 295–301.

Clark BA and Anderson TW (1979), Does screening by 'PAP' smears help prevent cancer? *Lancet*, ii: 1–4.

Cochrane AL (1972), *Effectiveness and Efficiency*, London: National Provincial Hospital Trust.

Collins R, Peto R, MacMahon S, Hebert P, Fiebach NH, Eberlain KA et al (1990), Blood pressure, stroke, and coronary heart disease, Part 2: Short–term reductions in blood pressure: overview of randomised drug trials in their epidemiological context, *Lancet*, 335: 827–38.

Coleman MP (1991), *Cancer Risk after Medical Treatment*, Oxford University Press.

Darby SC (1991), Irradiation for non–malignant conditions, in *Cancer Risk after Medical Treatment* (ed. MP Coleman), pp.29–49, Oxford University Press.

Davies OK (1990), Complications of assisted conception techniques, *Current Opinion in Obstetrics and Gynaecology*, 2: 721–5.

Department of Health, Welsh Office, Scottish Office Home and Health Department, Department of Health and Social Security Northern Ireland (1996), *Report on Confidential Enquiries into Maternal Deaths in the United Kingdom 1991–1993*, London: HMSO.

Department of Health (1992), *The Health of the Nation: A Strategy for Health in England*. London: HMSO.

Dhillon S (1993), A bitter pill to swallow, *Health Service Journal*, 103, No. 5343: 30–1.

Doll R and Peto R (1976), Mortality in relation to smoking: 20 years' observations on male British doctors, *British Medical Journal*, 2: 1525–36.

Doll R, Peto R, Wheatley K, Gray R and Sutherland I (1994), Mortality in relation to smoking: 40 years' observations on male British doctors, *British Medical Journal*, (in press).

Donnan SPB and Lambert PM (1976), Appendicitis: incidence and mortality, *Population Trends*, 5: 26–8.

Dwork D (1987), *What is Good for Babies and Other Young Children: A History of the Infant and Child Welfare Movement in England 1898–1918*, in Morel (1991) op cit.

EC Working Party on Health Services and Avoidable Mortality (1988), *European Community Atlas of Avoidable Deaths*, Appendix A, London: Oxford University Press.

Editorial (1976), (Editorial and whole issue on cancer of cervix), Screening for carcinoma of the cervix, *Canadian Medical Association Journal*, 114: 1013–26.

Emmerson AM, Enstone JE, Griffin M, Kelsey MC, Smyth ETM (1996), The Second National Prevalence Survey of Infection in Hospitals: overview of the results, *Journal of Hospital Infection*, 32: 175–190.

Feinstein AR, Stern EK and Spagnuola M (1966), The prognosis of acute rheumatic fever, *American Heart Journal*, 68: 817–34.

Fleming P (1994), The Avon infant mortality study: risk factors for SIDS before and after a risk reduction campaign, presented at *Infant Sleep Position and Risk for Sudden Infant Death Syndrome*, National Institutes of Health, Bethesda, MD, January 13, 1994.

Flinn MW (1965), *Introduction to Edwin Chadwick's The sanitary condition of the labouring population of Great Britain*, Edinburgh: Edinburgh University Press, pp.1–73.

General Register Office (1938), *The Registrar General's Decennial Supplement, England and Wales 1931 Part IIa: Occupational mortality*, London: HMSO.

Gilbert R (1994), The changing epidemiology of SIDS, *Archives of Disease in Childhood*, 70: 445–9.

Gill P, Dowell AC, Neal RD, Smith N, Heywood P and Wilson E (1996), Evidence based general practice: a retrospective study of interventions in one training practice, *British Medical Journal*, 312: 819–21.

Godlee F (1994), The Cochrane Collaboration, *British Medical Journal*, 309: 969–70.

Golding J and Colmer S (1994), Sleeping position, health and development: a preliminary report from the ALSPAC (Avon Longitudinal Study of Pregnancy and Childhood) Study. Presented at *Infant Sleep Position and Risk for Sudden Infant Death Syndrome*, Bethesda, MD: National Institutes of Health, January 13, 1994.

Gordis L (1973), Effectiveness of comprehensive programs in preventing rheumatic fever, *New England Journal of Medicine*, 289: 331–35.

Greenblatt DJ, Allen MD and Shader RI (1977), Toxicity of high dose fluezepam in the elderly, *Clinical Pharmacologic Therapy*, 21: 355.

Hakama M, Miller AB and Day NE (1986), *Screening for cancer of the uterine cervix*, IARC Scientific Publications No.76, Lyon: International Agency for Research on Cancer.

Harris R and Rhind J (1993), Uncorking the gene, *Health Service Journal*, 103, no. 5335: 24–5.

Hey K, O'Donnell M, Murphy M, Jones N and Botting B (1994), Use of local neural tube defect registers to interpret national trends, *Archives of Disease in Childhood*, 71: f198–f202.

Hull HF, Ward NA, Hull BP, Milstien JB and de Quadros C (1994), Paralytic poliomyelitis: seasoned strategies, disappearing disease, *Lancet*, 343: 1331–1337.

Hurwitz N (1969), Predisposing factors in adverse reactions to drugs, *British Medical Journal*, 1, 536–9.

Hurwitz N and Wade OL (1969), Intensive hospital monitoring of adverse reactions to drugs, *British Medical Journal*, 1: 531–9.

Hypertension Detection and Follow-up Program Co-operative Group (1979), Five-year findings of the hypertension detection and follow-up program, I. Reduction in mortality of persons with high blood pressure, including mild hypertension, *Journal of the American Medical Association*, 242: 2562–71.

Hypertension Detection and Follow-up Program Co-operative Group (1982), Five-year findings of the hypertension detection and follow-up program, II, Reduction in stroke incidence among persons with high blood pressure, *Journal of the American Medical Association*, 247: 633–8.

Illich I (1974), Medical nemesis, *Lancet*, i: 918–21.

Inman WHW and Adelstein AM (1969), Rise and fall of asthma mortality in England and Wales in relation to use of pressurised aerosols, *Lancet*, ii: 279-84.

ISIS-1 Collaborative Group (1986), Randomised trial of intravenous atenolol among 16,027 cases of suspected acute myocardial infarction, *Lancet*, ii: 57–66.

Johnson AP, Speller DCE, George C, Warner M, Domingue G, Efstratiou A (1996). Prevalence of antibiotic resistance and serotypes in pneumococci in England and Wales: results of observational surveys in 1990 and 1995, *British Medical Journal*, 312: 1454–1456.

Johnson R (1992), Part exchange, *Health Service Journal*, 102, No. 5331: 24–5.

Kaldor JM and Lasset C (1991), Cytotoxic chemotherapy for cancer, in *Cancer Risk after Medical Treatment*, (ed. MP Coleman), pp.50–70, Oxford University Press.

Learoyd BM (1972), Psychotropic drugs and the elderly patient, *Medical Journal of Australia*, 1: 1131–33.

Leitch I (1945), Diet and tuberculosis, *Proceedings of the Nutrition Society*, 3: 156–64.

Lewis J (1991), The origins and development of public health in the UK, in *Oxford Textbook of Public Health* (ed. Holland WW), Oxford.

Logan WPD (1950), Mortality in England and Wales from 1848 to 1947, *Population Studies*, 4: 132–178.

Loudon I (1986), Obstetric care, social class, and maternal mortality, *British Medical Journal*, 293: 606–8.

Loudon I (1992), *Death in Childbirth: an International Study of Maternal Care and Maternal Mortality 1800–1950*, Oxford: Clarendon Press.

McCloy R (1992), Through the keyhole, *Health Service Journal*, 102, No. 5328: pp.26–7.

McCormick A (1993), The notification of infectious diseases in England and Wales. *Communicable Disease Report Review*, 3(2): 19–25.

McGinn FP, Miles AJG, Uglow M, Ozmen M, Terzi C, Humby M (1995), Randomized trial of laparoscopic cholecystectomy and minicholecystectomy, *British Journal of Surgery*, 85: 1374–7.

McGregor JE and Teper S (1978), Mortality from carcinoma of the cervix uteri in Britain, *Lancet*, ii: 774–6.

McKeown T and Record RG (1962), Reasons for the decline of mortality in England and Wales in the 19th century, *Population Studies*, 16: 94–122.

McKeown T (1976), *The Role of Medicine: Dream, Mirage or Nemesis*, London: Nuffield Provincial Hospital Trust.

McMahon AJ, Russell IT, Baxter JN, Ross S, Anderson JR, Moran CJ, Sutherland G, Galloway D, Ramsay G and O'Dwyer PJ (1994), Laparoscopic versus minilaparotomy cholecystectomy: a randomised trial, *Lancet*, 343: 135–8.

Macfarlane A and Mugford M (1984), *Birth Counts. Statistics of Pregnancy and Childbirth*, National Perinatal Epidemiology Unit (in collaboration with OPCS), London: HMSO.

Mackenbach JP and Looman CWN (1988), Secular trends of infectious disease mortality in the Netherlands, 1911–1978: quantitave estimates of changes coinciding with the introduction of antibiotics, *International Journal of Epidemiology*, 17: 618–624.

Mackenbach JP, Looman CWN, Kunst AE, Habema DF, Van der Maas PJ (1988), Post-1950 mortality trends and medical care: gains in life expectancy due to declines in mortality from conditions amenable to medical intervention in the Netherlands, *Social Science & Medicine*, 27(9): 889–894.

Mackenbach JP, Bouvier-Colle MH, Jougla E (1990), 'Avoidable' mortality and health services: a review of aggregate data studies, *Journal of Epidemiology and Community Health*, 44: 106–111.

Mackenbach JP (1991), Health care expenditure and mortality from amenable conditions in the European Community, *Health Policy*, 19: 245-255.

Majeed AW, Troy G, Nicholl JP, Smythe A, Reed MWR, Stoddard CJ, Peacock J and Johnson AG (1996), *Lancet*, 347: 989–94.

Marche J and Grunelle H (1950), The relation of protein scarcity and modification of blood protein to tuberculosis among undernourished subjects, *Millbank Memorial Fund Quarterly*, 28.

Mersey RHA (1982), Report of working part, Confidential enquiry into perinatal deaths in Mersey Region, *Lancet*, i: 491–4.

Morel M-F (1991), The care of children: the influence of medical intervention and medical institutions on infant mortality 1750–1914. In *The Decline of Mortality in Europe,* (eds Schofield R, Reher D, Bideau A), Oxford: Clarendon Press.

Miller E (1994), The new measles campaign, *British Medical Journal*, 309: 1102–3.

MRC Vitamin Study Group (1991), Prevention of neural tube defects: Results of the Medical Research Council Vitamin Study, *Lancet*, 338: 131–37.

Obaro SK, Monteil MA, Henderson DC (1996), The pneumococcal problem, *British Medical Journal*, 312: 1521–1525.

OPCS (1992), *Mortality Statistics, Serial tables, 1841–1990, England and Wales*, Series DH1 no.25. London: HMSO.

Paul JR (1971), *A History of Poliomyelitis*, New Haven/London: Yale University Press.

Payne JN, Milner PC, Saul C, Bowns IR, Hannay DR and Ramsay LE (1993), Local confidential inquiry into avoidable factors in deaths from stroke and hypertensive disease, *British Medical Journal*, 307: 1027–30.

Peach H (1989), Disability and iatrogenesis. In *Disablement in the Community*, pp.101–13, Oxford University Press.

Peach H and Charlton J (1986), Illness, disability, and drugs among 25 to 75 year olds living at home, *Journal of Epidemiology and Community Health*, 40(1), 59–66.

Puranen B (1991), Tuberculosis and the decline of mortality in Sweden. In Schofield R, Reher D, Bideau A (eds), *The Decline of Mortality in Europe*, Oxford: Clarendon Press.

Quinn M and Allen E (1996), Changes in incidence of and mortality from breast cancer in England and wales since introduction of screening, *British Medical Journal*, 311: 1391–5.

Richmond S and Longson M (1982), Recent advances in antiviral agents, *The Practitioner*, 226: 711–8.

Robertson I (1993), To a man with a hammer, everything looks like a nail, *British Medical Journal*, 306: 937.

Rodriguez LA and Jick H (1994a), Risk of gynaecomsatia associated with cimetidine, omeprazole and other antiulcer drugs, *British Medical Journal*, 308: 503–6.

Rodriguez LA and Jick H (1994b), The risk of upper gastrointestinal bleeding and/or perforation associated with individual nonsteroidal anti-inflamatory drugs, *Lancet*, 343: 769–772.

Russell RCG (1993), General surgery: biliary surgery, *British Medical Journal*, 307: 1266–69.

Rutstein DD, Berenberg W, Chalmers TC, Child CG, Fishman AP, Perrin EB (1976), Measuring the quality of medical care, *New England Journal of Medicine*, 294: 582–8.

Rutstein DD, Berenberg W, Chalmers TC, Child CG, Fishman AP, Perrin EB (1980), Measuring the quality of medical care: second revision of tables of indices, *New England Journal of Medicine*, 302: 1146–50.

Sanchez-Guerrero J and Liang MH (1994), Silicone breast implants and connective tissue diseases, *British Medical Journal*, 309: 822–3.

Seidl LG, Thornton GF, Smith JW, Cluff LE (1966), *Bulletin of the Johns Hopkins Hospital*, 119: 299.

Sasieni PD, Cuzicj J, Lynch-Farmery E, National Coordinating Network for Cervical Screening Working Group (1996), Estimating the efficiency of screening by auditing smear histories of women with and without cervical cancer, *British Journal of Cancer*, 73: 1001–1005.

Schenker JG and Yosset E (1994), Complications of assisted conception techniques, *Fertility and Sterility*, 61 (3): 411–422.

Smith B (1989), The Victorian poliomyelitis epidemic In *What we know about health transition: The cultural, social and behavioural determinants of health: Procedings of an international workshop* (ed. Caldwell JC), Canberra: Australian National University.

Stoker N (1994), Tuberculosis in a changing world. *British Medical Journal*, 309: 1178–9.

Szretzeer S (1988), The importance of social intervention in Britain's mortality decline c 1850–1914: a re-examination of the role of public health, *Social History of Medicine*, 1: 1–37.

Tomatis L, Aitio A, Day NE, Heseltine E, Kaldor J, Miller AB, Parkin DM and Riboli E (1990), Drugs and exogenous sex hormones, In *Cancer: Causes, Occurrence and Control*, IARC Scientific Publications no.100, pp.148–154, Lyon: National Agency for Research on Cancer.

Walton J, Barondess JA, Lock S (1994), *The Oxford Medical Companion*, Oxford: Oxford University Press.

Warren M and Francis H (1987), *Recalling the Medical Officer of Health. Writings by Sidney Chave*, London: King Edward' Hospital Fund for London.

Waterhouse J, Muir C, Correa P and Powell J (1976), *Cancer Incidence in Five Continents*, vol.III, p.456. IARC Scientific Publications no.15, Lyon: International Agency for Research on Cancer.

Willinger M, Hoffman HJ, Hartford RB (1994), Infant sleep position and risk for Sudden Infant Death Syndrome: report of meeting held January 13 and 14, 1994, Bethesda, MD: National Institutes for Health, *Pediatrics*, 93: 814–20.

Index

Notes: (I) and (II) are volume numbers, *italic* page numbers refer to figures and graphs and **bold** numbers to tables.

266

mortality (I) 43, 51; (II) 142–3
musculoskeletal symptoms (II) **156**
nomenclature (II) 141–2
physical disability (II) 156–7
prevalence rates (I) **62**
soft tissue rheumatism (II) 154–5, *154*
mycoplasmae
chemotherapy (I) 222
pneumoniae (II) *9*, 10
mycotoxins (I) 164
myelomatosis (II) 115
myocardial degeneration (I) **130**, 151, **153**
myocardial infarction (II) 61, 64
death attributes (I) 151
morbidity comparison (I) **65**
winter deaths (I) 165

NADOR (Notification of Accidents and Dangerous Occurrences Regulations, 1980) *see* Reporting of Injuries, Diseases and Dangerous Occurrences Regulations
2-naphthylamine, bladder cancer (I) 146
narcotics (I) 101, **123**
National Ankylosing Spondylitis Society, United Kingdom (II) 146
National Assistance (I) 89–90
National Deterioration of Health and Physique, Committee of (I) 85
National Diet and Nutrition Survey (I) 109
National Food Surveys (NFS) (I) 107–9
National Health Service Central Register (NHSCR) (I) 8, 10–11
National Health Service (NHS) (I) 48, 74, 90
utilisation rates (I) 179–81, **181**
National Insurance Act (1911) (I) 88–9; (II) 191–2
National Milk Scheme (I) 104
National Morbidity Surveys in General Practice (I) 60–7, 181 2
abdominal symptoms (II) 136
accidents (II) 166–7, *167*, **167**
back pain (II) 152, **153**, 154
digestive system diseases (II) 132
gout (II) 147
GP consultations (II) 195–6
IP morbidity (II) 161
musculoskeletal diseases (II) 143
osteoarthritis (II) 150
patient consulting rates (II) **196–7**
renal diseases (II) 114–15, 117, 126
soft tissue rheumatism (II) 154–5
'national prosperity, barometer' (I) 172
National Renal Review (II) 122–3
National Study of Health and Growth (I) 112
National Survey of Sexual Attributes and Lifestyles (II) 28–9
neonatal death certificates (I) 5, 7
neoplasms
see also cancers
data sources (I) **59**
deaths by ICD chapter (I) **43**
episode-based rates (I) **69**, **71**
mortality (I) 34–6, 45–6, *46*
post-mortem examinations (I) 7
prevalence (I) **62**, 63–4
years of life lost (I) **57**
nephropathy (IgA) (II) 120
nephrotoxicity (I) 227

Netherlands (I) 95
death rates (I) 199
Excess Winter Mortality (I) 206, 215
family studies (I) 180, 182, 185
influenza mortality (I) 209
mortality data (I) 176–7
neurological system diseases (II) 82–92
cancer (II) 38–9, *38*, **44**, **54**
crude death rates (I) **32**
data sources (I) **59**
episode-based rates (I) **69**, **71**, 72
ICD chapter (I) **43**, 45, 48
mortality (I) 33, **34–6**, 49
prevalence rates (I) **62**
New Poor Law Act (1834) (I) 87
New York criteria, ankylosing spondylitis (II) 146
New Zealand (I) 167, 191
NFS *see* National Food Surveys
NHL see non-Hodgkin's lymphoma
NHSCR *see* National Health Service Central Register
NIDDM *see* non-insulin dependent diabetes mellitus
Nightingale, Florence (I) 67, 227
nitrogen dioxide (I) 168, 192, 195, *195*, 198
nitrogen oxides (I) 190
noise, mental health (I) 167
non-Hodgkin's lymphoma (NHL) (II) 39–40, *40*, **44**, **56**
non-insulin dependent diabetes mellitus (NIDDM), ethnicity (II) 121
non-resiratory tuberculosis (II) 9
non-specific genital infection (II) **23**
non-steroidal anti-inflammatory drugs (NSAIDs) (II) 134
non-ulcer dyspepsia (II) 129, 132
Norfolk Arthritis Register (II) 144
Northern Ireland, renal diseases (II) 119–20
nosology (I) 130
Notes on Hospitals (1863) (I) 67
notifiable diseases (I) 2, **9**
Notification of Accidents and Dangerous Occurrences Regulations 1980 (NADOR) *see* Reporting of Injuries, Diseases and Dangerous Occurrences Regulations
NSAIDs *see* non-steroidal anti-inflammatory drugs
NSHG *see* National Study of Health and Growth
nutrition (I) 84
diseases (I) 47, 95–6
health status (I) 94–8
improvement (II) 1
intake (I) **99**
sanitation (I) 94
social policy (I) 88
status (I) 96–7, **96**
tobacco (I) 141
Nutritional and Dietary Survey (I) 110

OA *see* osteoarthritis
obesity (II) 174
cardiovascular disease (I) 93
changes since 1980 (I) 112–13, *112*
health (I) 97–8
ischaemic heart disease (II) 61, 70
obstructive lung disease (I) 196, *197*
occupational mortality (I) 11
odds ratio, definition (I) 15
oesophagitis (II) 132–3

oesophagus
cancer (I) 46, **129**, 141–3; (II) *32*, 33, **44–5**
mortality rate (I) *142*, **142**
smoking-related diseases (I) **130**
disorders (I) 117
Office for National Statistics (ONS)
cancer mortality rates (II) 31
coding changes (I) 41, 47; (II) 31, 37, 41–2
Dental Health Surveys (I) 2, 12
Disability Surveys (I) 2, 12
ischaemic heart disease (II) 61
Labour Force Surveys (I) 2
Longitudinal Study (I) 2, 11
'medical enquiry' form (I) 7
National Food Surveys (I) 2, 12
Omnibus Surveys (I) 12
Psychiatric Morbidity Surveys (I) 2, 12
renal diseases (II) 116
respiratory diseases (II) 95
stroke (II) 76
underlying cause of death (I) 6
Office of Population Censuses and Surveys (OPCS) (I) 110
old age (I) 88, 95
older adults
see also elderly
activities of daily living (II) **202**
cohort survivorship (II) *201*
data sources (II) 186
definition (II) 183–4, *184*
disability (II) **202**
General Household Survey (II) 193
GP consultation (II) **196–7**
health (II) 182–203
1840-1920 (II) 187–92
1921-1994 (II) 192–8
dental (II) 195
trends (II) 198–203
hospital usage (II) 196–8
incapacity days (II) **194**
life expectancy 1841-1921 (II) **187**
life expectancy 1921-1991 (II) **192**
long-standing illness (II) 198–201, *199–200*
mobility restrictions (II) 194–5, **194**
morbidity (II) 187–8, *188*, 192–3
mortality (II) *184*, **185**, 187, 192, 203
residential status (II) *199*
sickness episodes (II) **193**
Survey of the Elderly at Home (1976) (II) 202
Survey of Sickness (1947-1951) (II) 193
one-roomed dwelling (I) **158**
ONS *see* Office for National Statistics
OPCS *see* Decennial Occupational Supplement; Office of Population Censuses and Surveys
OPD *see* out patient departments
open air living, related disorders (I) 159
Open Spaces Act (1906) (I) 85
opium (I) 119, 123
opthalmia neonatorum, notification (I) **9**
oral cavity cancers (I) 140–1, *140*, **141**
smoking-related diseases (I) **130**
oral contraceptives
ovarian cancer (II) 37
rheumatoid arthritis (II) 144
oral infections (II) 4
organs, transplantation (I) 223
ORLS see Oxford Record Linkage Study
orthostatic albuminuria (II) 117, **126**

*Printed in the United Kingdom
for* The Stationery Office
3/97